THE YEAR IN
HYPERTENSION
2002

THE YEAR IN HYPERTENSION

2002

GREGORY YH LIP, WAI KAENG LEE

University Department of Medicine, City Hospital, Birmingham, UK

CLINICAL PUBLISHING SERVICES

OXFORD

Clinical Publishing Services Ltd

Oxford Centre for Innovation
Mill Street, Oxford OX2 0JX, UK

Tel: +44 1865 811116
Fax: +44 1865 251550
Web: www.clinicalpublishing.co.uk

Distributed by:

Plymbridge Distributors Ltd
Estover Road
Plymouth PL6 7PY, UK

Tel: +44 1752 202300
Fax: +44 1752 202333
E mail: orders@plymbridge.com

A catalogue record for this book is available from the British Library

ISBN 1-904392-00-8

The publisher makes no representation, express or implied, that the dosages in this book are correct. Readers must therefore always check the product information and clinical procedures with the most up-to-date published product information and data sheets provided by the manufacturers and the most recent codes of conduct and safety regulations. The authors and the publisher do not accept any liability for any errors in the text or for the misuse or misapplication of material in this work

Commissioning editor: Jonathan Gregory
Project manager: Rosemary Osmond
Typeset by Footnote Graphics, Warminster, Wiltshire
Printed in Spain by T G Hostench SA, Barcelona

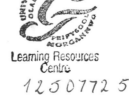

Contents

Authors

PROFESOR GREGORY YH LIP, MD, FRCP, FACC, FESC, Consultant Cardiologist and Professor of Cardiovascular Medicine, Director-Haemostasis Thrombosis and Vascular Biology Unit, University Department of Medicine, City Hospital, Birmingham, UK.

DR WAI KAENG LEE, MB, BCh, MRCP, Cardiology Research Fellow, University Department of Medicine, City Hospital, Birmingham, UK.

Part I

Basic science

1

Epidemiology

'High-normal' blood pressure

Introduction

The benefits and risks of lowering blood pressure (BP) are not uniform across the whole population, but vary greatly in individuals according to each person's total cardiovascular (CV) risk profile. This concept is now well recognized and indeed has been incorporated into major guidelines for the management of hypertension such as the Sixth Joint National Committee on Prevention, Detection, Evaluation and Treatment of High Blood Pressure (JNC VI) and the World Health Organization/International Society of Hypertension (WHO/ISH) Guidelines.

Periodic monitoring of BP in non-hypertensive adults to detect the onset of hypertension has been recommended by many guidelines for the management of hypertension. Nevertheless, the suggested frequency of monitoring varies widely. Data from the Framingham Study indicates that people with 'high-normal' BP – defined as a systolic BP of 130–139 mmHg, diastolic BP of 85–89 mmHg, or both – are at increased risk of developing hypertension in the short run, and should have their BP checked annually.

However, it is of note that the JNC VI guideline did not distinguish between stage 1 isolated systolic hypertension (ISH) and higher stages regarding treatment. Indeed, because of the large number of individuals in these stages, 'high-normal' BP and 'stage 1 hypertension' have the highest population-attributable risk for future cardiovascular disease (CVD). Furthermore, high-normal BP has been associated with altered cardiac morphologic features, an increased thickness of the carotid intima and media and diastolic ventricular dysfunction, all of which may be precursors of CV events.

Indeed, the recent Framingham group (below) have reinforced the clear gradations of risk within the 'normotensive' range, with definite stepwise increases in the risk of CV disease as the BP increases from 'optimal' to 'normal' to 'high-normal' using the WHO/ISH and JNC VI definitions.

However, outcomes studies are needed to look at whether drug treatment of hypertension in this range would prevent CV events, and whether such approach is cost-effective. The focus on treating older patients and those with coronary heart disease, cerebrovascular disease or diabetes may be justified because of the higher absolute risk of CV events, and thus making treatment more cost-effective.

Assessment of frequency of progression to hypertension in non-hypertensive participants in the Framingham Heart Study: a cohort study.
Vasan RS, Larson MG, Leip EP, *et al. Lancet* 2001; **358**: 1682–6.

BACKGROUND. Patients with optimum (< 120/80 mmHg), normal (120–129/80–84 mmHg), and high-normal (130–139/85–89 mmHg) BP may progress to hypertension (≥140/90 mmHg) over time.

INTERPRETATION. High-normal BP and normal BP frequently progress to hypertension over a period of 4 years, especially in older adults. These findings support recommendations for monitoring individuals with high-normal BP once a year, and monitoring those with normal BP every 2 years, and they emphasize the importance of weight control as a measure for primary prevention of hypertension.

Comment

The study aimed to establish the best frequency of BP screening by assessing the rates and determinants of progression to hypertension on follow-up among 9845 participants – predominantly white – who were non-hypertensive at baseline in the Framingham Heart Study. The rates of progression to hypertension for each of their six categories of individuals (those under 65 years of age with optimum BP, normal BP, and high-normal BP, and those over 65 within these three BP classes) was determined, and subsequently evidence-based suggestions for the optimum frequency of BP screening were made.

A stepwise increase in hypertension incidence occurred across the three non-hypertensive BP categories. Older individuals and persons with higher BP at baseline were found to be more likely to develop hypertension at 4 years. At greatest risk of hypertension were patients > 65 who had high-normal BP at baseline. Half of this cohort had developed hypertension by 4 years follow-up. About 23% of the cohort had developed stage II or greater hypertension (>160/100 mmHg). Assuming that the annual progression rate is constant over the 4 years, 11%–16%

Table 1.1 Rates of progression to hypertension over 4 years in individuals < 65 years

BP class	Number of patients	4-year rate of hypertension* (95% CI)
Optimum (<120/80 mmHg)	4067	5.3% (4.4–6.3)
Normal (120–129/80–84 mmHg)	2399	17.6% (15.2–20.3)
High-normal (130–139/85–89 mmHg)	1778	37.3% (33.3–41.5)

* Hypertension defined as ≥ 140/90 mmHg.

Source: Vasan *et al.* (2001).

Table 1.2 Rates of progression to hypertension over 4 years in individuals > 65 years

BP class	Number of patients	4-year rate of hypertension* (95% CI)
Optimum (<120/80 mmHg)	432	16.0% (12.0–20.9)
Normal (120–129/80–84 mmHg)	545	25.5% (20.4–31.4)
High-normal (130–139/85–89 mmHg)	624	49.5% (42.6–56.4)

* Hypertension defined as ≥ 140/90 mmHg.

Source: Vasan *et al.* (2001).

of participants with high-normal BP would have progressed to hypertension within the first year, suggesting that annual screening might be desirable for this group. Almost a third of individuals with normal BP developed hypertension within 2 years (in older individuals) or 3 years (in younger individuals), suggesting a strategy of screening every 2 years might be reasonable in this group. Factors influencing the rate of progression to hypertension, other than age and baseline BP class, were weight gain and increases in body mass index (BMI) over the 4 years ($P < 0.0001$). Rates of progression to hypertension did not vary with sex ($P = 0.31$).

However, it is of note that the current guidelines recommend follow-up of people with normal and high-normal BP at an interval of 5 years. Further research is now called for to determine the cost-effectiveness, the risk associated with new-onset hypertension, and the benefits of BP lowering.

Impact of high-normal blood pressure on the risk of cardiovascular disease.
Vasan RS, Larson MG, Leip EP, *et al. N Engl J Med* 2001; **345**(18): 1291–7.

BACKGROUND. Information is limited regarding the risk of CVD in persons with high-normal BP (systolic pressure of 130 to 139 mmHg, diastolic BP (DBP) of 85 to 89 mmHg, or both).

INTERPRETATION. High-normal BP is associated with an increased risk of CVD. The findings emphasize the need to determine whether lowering high-normal BP can reduce the risk of CVD.

Comment

This study investigated the association between BP category at base line and the incidence of CVD on an average follow-up of 11.1 years among 6859 participants in the Framingham Heart Study who were initially free of hypertension and CVD.

Table 1.3 Cumulative incidence of first CV event according to BP category at baseline

Subjects	Crude 10-year cumulative incidence of first CV event (95% CI)	Age-adjusted* 10-year cumulative incidence of first CV event (95% CI)
Men with optimal BP	4.9% (3.5–6.2%)	5.8% (4.2–7.4%)
Women with optimal EP	1.3% (0.8–1.8%)	1.9% (1.1–2.7%)
Men with normal BP	7.8% (6.1–9.4%)	7.6% (6.0–9.1%)
Women with normal BP	2.9% (1.9–3.9%)	2.8% (1.9–3.8%)
Men with high-normal BP	10.3% (8.3–12.3%)	10.1% (8.1–12.1%)
Women with high-normal BP	6.4% (4.8–8.0%)	4.4% (3.2–5.5%)

*Numbers adjusted by direct standardization to overall age distribution in sample in four age groups (< 50 years, 50–59 years, 60–69 years, and ≥70 years)

Source: NHLBI/NIH; Vasan et al. (2001).

When compared with optimal BP, high-normal BP was associated with an adjusted hazard ratio for CVD of 2.5 in women and 1.6 in men. The association between high-normal BP and increased risk of CVD was particularly strong in elderly patients aged over 65. A stepwise increase in CV event rates was noted across the three non-hypertensive BP categories: optimal, normal, and high-normal. Hence, the number of people at risk of hypertensive CV events is much higher than previously thought.

Such findings were not unexpected as high-normal BP has been associated with altered cardiac morphologic features, an increased thickness of the carotid intima and media and diastolic ventricular dysfunction, all of which may be precursors of CV events. Indeed, the accompanying editorial has postulated impaired endothelial function as another possible mechanism. However, further large clinical trials are needed to determine whether lowering BP (non-pharmacological measures or drugs) in this category would actually reduce the risk of CVD and whether such treatment would be cost-effective.

Relationship of blood pressure to 25-year mortality due to coronary heart disease, cardiovascular diseases, and all causes in young adult men. The Chicago Heart Association Detection Project in Industry.

Miura K, Daviglus ML, Dyer AR, et al. Arch Intern Med 2001; **161**: 1501–8.

BACKGROUND. Data are limited on BP in young adults and long-term mortality. Moreover, screening and hypertension treatment guidelines have been based mainly on findings for middle-aged and older populations. This study assesses relationships of BP measured in young adult men to long-term mortality due to coronary heart disease (CHD), CVD, and all causes.

INTERPRETATION. In young adult men, BP above normal was significantly related to increased long-term mortality due to CHD, CVD, and all causes. Population-wide primary prevention, early detection, and control of higher BP are indicated from young adulthood on.

Comment

In this analysis of 10 874 men aged 18–39 at baseline who were not receiving antihypertensive drugs and showed no CHD or diabetes from the Chicago Heart Association Detection Project in Industry, young men with even high-normal BP or stage 1 hypertension according to the Sixth Joint National Committee on Prevention, Detection, Evaluation and Treatment of High Blood Pressure (JNC VI) criteria have higher 25-year risks for death by CHD and CVD, and all-cause mortality rate than those with normal or optimal BP.

Table 1.4

Classification	$n = 10\ 874$	BP range (mmHg)
Optimal	930 (8.6%)	SBP < 120 and DBP < 80
Normal	2194 (20.2%)	SBP 120–129 and DBP < 85 OR SBP < 130 and DBP 80–84
High-normal	2773 (25.5%)	SBP 130-139 and DBP < 90 OR SBP < 140 and DBP 85–89
Stage 1 hypertension	3963 (36.4%)	SBP 140–159 and DBP < 100 OR SBP < 160 and DBP 90–99

Source: Miura *et al.* (2001).

Table 1.5 Baseline JNC VI classification and mortality

Classification	Adjusted relative risk for CHD mortality (95% CI)	Adjusted relative risk for CVD mortality (95% CI)	RR for all-cause mortality (95% CI)
Optimal	1.39 (0.67–2.86; P = NS)	1.28 (0.68–2.41; P = NS)	1.29 (0.94–1.77; P = NS)
Normal	1.00 (reference)	1.00 (reference)	1.00 (reference)
High-normal	1.37 (0.81–2.30; P = NS)	1.36 (0.87–2.13; P < 0.1)	1.15 (0.91–1.46; P = NS)
Stage 1 hypertension	1.62 (1.00–2.61; P < 0.05)	1.50 (0.99–2.27; P < 0.1)	1.31 (1.05–1.63; P < 0.05)

Source: Miura *et al.* (2001).

Stage I isolated systolic hypertension

One-year study of felodipine or placebo for stage 1 isolated systolic hypertension.

Black HR, Elliott WJ, Weber MA, *et al*. *Hypertension* 2001; **38**: 1118–23.

BACKGROUND. A substantial number of older hypertensive patients have stage 1 isolated systolic BP (SBP) between 140 and 159 mmHg and DBP < 90 mmHg, but there are currently no data showing that drug treatment is effective, safe and/or beneficial.

INTERPRETATION. There were no clinically significant differences between treatments in tolerability or adverse effects. Stage 1 isolated systolic hypertension (ISH) can be effectively and safely treated pharmacologically. Treatment reduced progression to the higher stages of hypertension, reduced the incidence of left ventricular hypertrophy and improved an overall measure of the quality of life. Larger and longer studies will be needed to document any long-term reduction in CV event rates associated with treating stage 1 systolic hypertension.

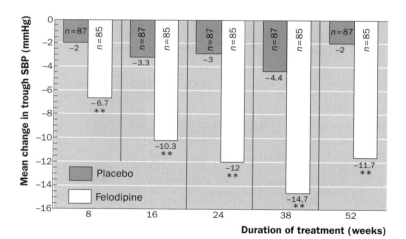

Fig. 1.1 Mean trough SBP reduction (compared with baseline) in patients randomized to felodipine- extended-release (ER) (hatched bars) or placebo (open bars) according to duration (in weeks) of treatment. **Statistically significant differences from placebo ($P < 0.01$). Data at week 52 include the last observation carried forward in those subjects who concluded their participation prematurely. Source: Black *et al.* (2001).

Comment

As already discussed above, the lower stages of BP have recently received increased attention. This study is timely and is designed to investigate whether lowering BP is both possible and beneficial in elderly patients with stage 1 systolic hypertension.

Indeed, the results showed that pharmacological treatment is effective, safe, well tolerated, and associated with beneficial effects on left ventricular hypertrophy (LVH) and quality of life irrespective of age, gender, or race/ethnicity of the patients. The superiority of active treatment was observed in all analyses, as well as in comparisons of regimens across response rates and the prevalence of controlled hypertension.

Although the sample size in the present study was too small to detect a difference in clinical events between treatments, there was a significant difference in both the prevalence and incidence of LVH, a strong predictor of future CV morbidity and mortality among hypertensive patients. Notably, the 22% prevalence of LVH at baseline among the enrolled subjects with stage 1 systolic hypertension in this study suggests that target-organ changes are present in a substantial proportion of patients who often currently go untreated.

However, outcomes studies are still needed to determine whether drug treatment of hypertension in this range prevents CV events; furthermore, its cost-effectiveness also needs to be determined.

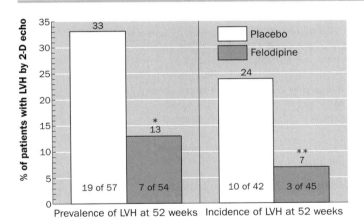

Fig. 1.2 Prevalence (left) and incidence (right) of LVH by echocardiogram after 52 weeks of treatment with felodipine-extended release (ER) (hatched bars) or placebo (open bars). $*P = 0.014$; $**P = 0.005$. The denominator in the prevalence calculation includes all patients who (1) took at least 1 dose of blinded study medication, (2) had baseline measurements, and (3) had at least 1 echocardiogram after beginning study medication. The denominator in the incidence calculation includes only those who did not have LVH at baseline. Source: Black et al. (2001).

Abandoning diastolic blood pressure – isolated systolic hypertension rules OK

Introduction

Traditionally, we have based our antihypertensive treatment on DBP as previous epidemiological studies had used DBP as a means of predicting CV risk. Such an approach was also reinforced by a number of therapeutic trials which showed benefits in treating hypertension defined on the basis of elevated DBP. At the same time, SBP was considered to be a natural and innocuous effect of increased stiffness of the aorta caused by aging.

However, more evidence is now emerging showing that DBP has the least predictive value. Only recently has our focus turned back to SBP, and lately pulse pressure is becoming fashionable as the better predictor of CV outcome, especially in the older patient. This is due in part to a reappraisal of the early studies and the emergence of new insights into the pathophysiological significance of increased arterial stiffness and its influence on BP components, particularly SBP and pulse pressure.

By the early 1990s, many major multi-centre clinical trials had shown the beneficial effects of antihypertensive therapy on morbidity and mortality in elderly hypertensives, predominantly by systolic hypertension. These included the UK Medical Research Council (MRC) trial of treatment of hypertension in older adults, the Swedish Trial in Older Patients with Hypertension (STOP-Hypertension) and the Systolic Hypertension in the Elderly Program (SHEP) trials, which played a major part in changing our perspective of the risk:benefit ratio of treatment of systolic hypertension.

Until we perform trials that evaluate the effects of different antihypertensive agents on the pulse pressure, we will continue to target SBP reduction as the primary therapeutic goal.

Predominance of isolated systolic hypertension among middle-aged and elderly US hypertensives: analysis based on National Health and Nutrition Examination Survey (NHANES) III.

Franklin SS, Jacobs MJ, Wong ND, L'Italien GJ, Lapuerta P. *Hypertension* 2001; **37**(3): 869–74.

BACKGROUND. Multiple clinical and observational studies in the elderly have demonstrated that elevated SBP is a more potent predictor of adverse CV outcomes than elevated DBP and that treating ISH in the elderly reduces risk of CVD events. Despite the strength of these observational and intervention studies, only about one quarter of hypertensive individuals are being treated to goal.

INTERPRETATION. Contrary to previous perceptions, ISH was the major subtype of uncontrolled hypertension in subjects of ages 50–59 years. It comprised 87% frequency for subjects in the sixth decade of life, and required greater reduction in SBP in these subjects to reach treatment goal compared with subjects in the younger group. Better awareness of this middle-aged and older high-risk group and more aggressive anti-hypertensive therapy is necessary to address this treatment gap.

Comment

The purpose of the present study was to examine patterns of systolic and diastolic hypertension by age in the nationally representative National Health and Nutrition Examination Survey (NHANES) III and to determine when treatment and control efforts should be recommended. Percentage distribution of three BP subtypes (ISH, combined systolic/diastolic hypertension, and isolated diastolic hypertension) was categorized for uncontrolled hypertension (untreated and inadequately treated) in two age groups (ages < 50 and ≥ 50 years).

Overall, ISH was the most frequent subtype of uncontrolled hypertension (65%). Most subjects with hypertension (74%) were ≥ 50 years of age, and of this untreated older group, nearly all (94%) were accurately staged by SBP alone, in contrast to subjects in the untreated younger group who were best staged by DBP. Furthermore, most subjects (80%) in the older untreated and the inadequately treated groups had ISH and required a greater reduction in SBP than in the younger groups (-13.3 and -16.5 mmHg *versus* -6.8 and -6.1 mmHg, respectively; $P = 0.0001$) to attain a SBP treatment goal of < 140 mmHg.

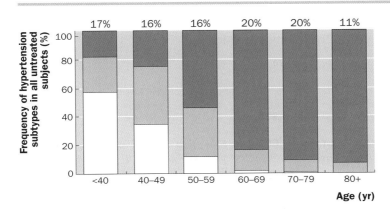

Fig. 1.3 Frequency distribution of untreated hypertensive individuals by age and hypertension subtype. Numbers at the tops of bars represent the overall percentage distribution of all subtypes of untreated hypertension in that age group. ■, ISH (SBP ≥ 140 mmHg and DBP < 90 mmHg); ▨, SDH (SBP ≥140 mmHg and DBP ≥ 90 mmHg); □, IDH (SBP < 140 mmHg and DBP ≥ 90 mmHg). Source: Franklin *et al.* (2001).

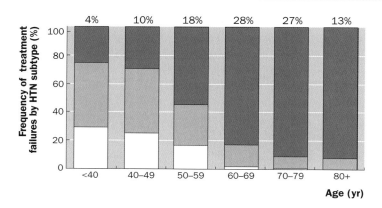

Fig 1.4 Frequency distribution of hypertensive individuals classified as inadequately treated by age and hypertension (HTN) subtype. Numbers at tops of bars represent overall percentage distribution of all subtypes of inadequately treated hypertension in that age group. ■, ISH (SBP ≥140 mmHg and DBP < 90 mmHg); ■, SDH (SBP ≥ 140 mmHg and DBP ≥ 90 mmHg); □, IDH (SBP < 140 mmHg and DBP ≥ 90 mmHg). Source: Franklin *et al.* (2001).

Prognostic value of systolic and diastolic blood pressure in treated hypertensive men.

Benetos A, Thomas F, Bean K, Gautier S, Smulyan H, Guize L. *Arch Intern Med* 2002 **162**(5): 577–81.

BACKGROUND. In the past few years, the importance of SBP has been emphasized, especially in older subjects, and more recently it has been proposed that DBP values could be the best predictor of CV risk in younger subjects and SBP or pulse pressure in older subjects.

INTERPRETATION. In hypertensive men treated in clinical practice, SBP is a good predictor of CVD and CHD risk. DBP, which remains the main criterion used by most physicians to determine drug efficacy, appears to be of little value in determining CV risk. Evaluation of risk in treated individuals should take SBP rather than DBP values into account.

Comment

In this analysis of 4714 hypertensive men who had a standard health check-up between 1972 and 1988, their risks of CVD and CHD mortality were assessed for a

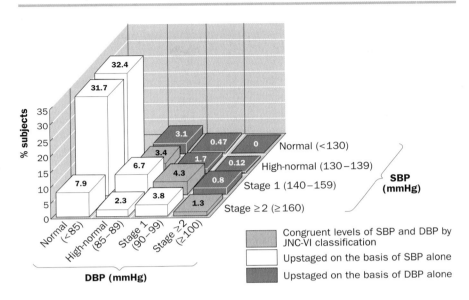

Fig 1.5 Percentages of NHANES III participants ≥ 50 years of age with untreated high-normal BP and hypertension classified into each Sixth Joint National Committee on Prevention, Detection, Evaluation and Treatment of High Blood Pressure (JNC-VI) SBP and DBP category after eliminating subjects with congruent normal SBP and DBP. Source: Franklin *et al.* (2001).

mean period of 14 years. After adjustment for age and associated risk factors, treated subjects presented an increased risk for CVD mortality (risk ratio [RR], 1.66; 95% confidence interval [CI], 1.04–2.64) and for CHD mortality (RR, 2.35; 95% CI, 1.03–5.35) compared with controlled subjects. After adjustment for age, associated risk factors and DBP, and compared with subjects with SBP under 140 mmHg, the RR for CVD mortality was 1.81 (95% CI, 1.04–3.13) in subjects with SBP between 140 and 160 mmHg and 1.94 (95% CI, 1.10–3.43) in subjects with SBP over 160 mmHg. By contrast, after adjustment for SBP levels, CVD risk was not associated with DBP. Compared with subjects with DBP under 90 mmHg, RR for CVD mortality was 1.17 (95% CI, 0.80–1.70) in subjects with DBP between 90–99 mmHg and 1.03 (95% CI, 0.67–1.56) in subjects with DBP over 100 mmHg. Similar results were observed for CHD mortality.

Risks of untreated and treated isolated systolic hypertension in the elderly: meta-analysis of outcome trials.

Staessen JA, Gasowski J, Wang JG, *et al. Lancet* 2000; **355**(9207): 865–72.

BACKGROUND. Previous meta-analysis of outcome trials in hypertension has not specifically focused on ISH or they have explained treatment benefit mainly as a function of the achieved DBP reduction. This study was undertaken to overview trials quantitatively and to further evaluate the risks associated with SBP in treated and untreated older patients with ISH.

INTERPRETATION. Drug treatment is justified in older patients with ISH whose SBP is 160 mmHg or higher. Absolute benefit is larger in men, in patients aged 70 or more and in those with previous CV complications or wider pulse pressure. Treatment prevented stroke more effectively than coronary events. However, the absence of a relationship between coronary events and SBP in untreated patients suggests that the coronary protection may have been underestimated.

Comment

In eight trials 15 693 patients with ISH were followed up for 3.8 years (median). They found that in untreated patients SBP was a more accurate predictor of mortality and CV complications than DBP. After correction for regression dilution bias, a 10 mmHg increase in SBP was significantly and independently correlated with increases by nearly 10% in the risk of all fatal and non-fatal complications, except for coronary events. DBP, on the other hand, was inversely correlated with total and CV mortality. At any given level of SBP, the risk of death rose with lower DBP and therefore also with greater pulse pressure. Active treatment reduced total mortality by 13% (95% CI 2–22, $P = 0.02$), CV mortality by 18%, all CV complications by 26%, stroke by 30%, and coronary events by 23%. The number of patients to treat for 5 years to prevent one major CV event was lower in men (18 *vs* 38), at or above age 70 (19 *vs* 39), and in patients with previous CV complications (16 *vs* 37). Although the patients were selected with a low DBP, further lowering of DBP did not produce harm without any evidence of a J-curve phenomenon in this meta-analysis.

The findings on the role of SBP as a risk factor may have important clinical implications. The target level of BP to be reached by antihypertensive drug treatment should, in older patients, be based on systolic rather than on diastolic BP. However, why antihypertensive treatment apparently provided less protection against coronary complications than against stroke remains unclear.

Treatment of isolated systolic hypertension is most effective in older patients with high-risk profile.

Ferrucci L, Furberg CD, Penninx BW, *et al. Circulation* 2001; **104**: 1923–6.

BACKGROUND. **Although present guidelines suggest that treatment of hypertension is more effective in patients with multiple risk factors and higher risk of CV events, this hypothesis was never verified in older patients with systolic hypertension.**

INTERPRETATION. Treatment of systolic hypertension is most effective in older patients who, because of additional risk factors or prevalent CVD, are at higher risk of developing a CV event. These patients are prime candidates for antihypertensive treatment.

Comment

This study has shown that treating ISH in older patients is especially effective in those with a high absolute risk of developing a CV event. Using data from the SHEP, the global CV risk score was calculated according to the American Heart Association Multiple Risk Factor Assessment Equation (derived from the Framingham study) in 4453 persons of age ≥ 60 and ISH. Treating the high-risk older adult was four times more effective in preventing heart attack, stroke and heart failure than treating those with lower levels of risk. In addition, the 'numbers needed to treat' (NNTs) to prevent one CV event over 4.5 years were progressively smaller according to higher CV risk quartiles. In participants with baseline CV disease, the NNTs were similar to those estimated for CV disease-free participants in the highest-risk quartile. These suggested that patients at the high end of the spectrum of CV risk may already be affected by subclinical CV disease and that the multiple risk factors equation should be used to forecast the risk of developing future CV events and hence to target the patients in whom the antihypertensive treatment is most effective.

Additional comment

Increasing data points towards the importance of SBP, which is a far better predictor of CV and stroke risk, even if corrected for underlying DBP. To quote one famous epidemiologist: 'one sometimes wishes that Nikolai Korotkov did not describe the 4th and 5th (diastolic) sounds …' for measuring BP. Indeed, undeserved clinician bias towards DBP treatment goals and an irrational physician fear of aggressive DBP lowering have contributed to poor SBP control. Perhaps a society for the abolishment of measurement of DBP is urgently needed.

The available data are convincing and 2001 has seen a new analysis using data from NHANES III indicating that, contrary to previous perceptions, ISH was the most common form of uncontrolled hypertension in the USA. Of all hypertensives receiving inadequate or no treatment, 65% had ISH, 21% had SDH, and 14% had IDH. Most subjects with hypertension (74%) were aged > 50 years, and of this untreated older group, 94% were accurately staged by SBP alone, in contrast to subjects in the untreated younger group, who were best staged by DBP. In the over 60's, ISH accounted for 87% of hypertension.

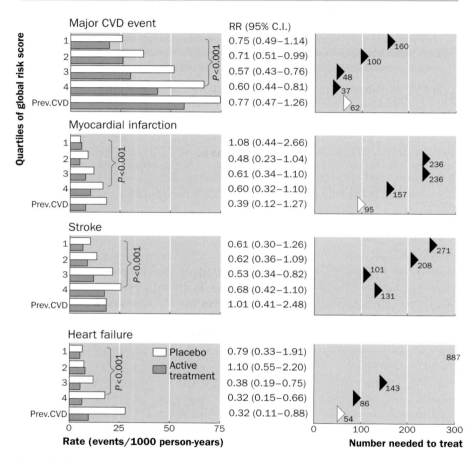

Fig. 1.6 For each type of CVD event, the bars on the left indicate rates of new events according to quartiles of global risk score. The fifth group of bars in each panel shows data for subjects with prevalent CVD at baseline. Values reported in the middle column are relative risks (and 95% CIs) of developing an event over the follow-up for active treatment compared with placebo. The right column reports estimates of the NNT to prevent one event according to strata of global risk. NNTs could not be computed in strata with RR ≥ 1. Source: Ferrucci *et al.* (2001).

In the study by Ferrucci *et al.*, treating ISH in older patients was especially effective in those with a high absolute risk of developing a CV event. Indeed, the NNTs to prevent one CV event over 4.5 years are progressively smaller according to higher CV risk quartiles. Some clinicians (erroneously) have several reasons for not aggressively treating hypertension in elderly adults who have multiple risk factors, in view of concerns about possible drug interactions, the belief that little can be done to alter the natural progression of blood vessel disease, or worry that lowering BP could be more risky than beneficial.

Antihypertensive drug therapy in older patients.
Wang JG, Staessen JA. *Curr Opin Nephrol Hypertens* 2001; **10**(2): 263–9.

BACKGROUND. Elevated pulse pressure is an important CV risk factor in the elderly, and it remains to be determined whether this can be reversed.

INTERPRETATION. Absolute treatment benefit is greater in men, in patients aged 70 years or more, and in those with previous CV complications or greater pulse pressure.

Comment

In the recently published comparative trials, BP gradients largely accounted for most, if not all, of the differences in outcome. In hypertensive patients, calcium-channel blockers may offer greater protection against stroke than against MI, resulting in an overall CV benefit similar to that provided by older drug classes. The hypothesis that angiotensin-converting enzyme inhibitors (ACEIs) or alpha-blockers might influence outcome over and beyond that expected on the basis of their BP lowering effects still remains to be proven.

Elevated pulse pressure is an important CV risk factor in the elderly, and it remains to be determined whether this can be reversed. Drug treatment is justified in older patients with isolated systolic hypertension whose SBP is 160 mmHg or higher on repeated measurement. Absolute benefit is greater in men, in patients aged 70 years or more, and in those with previous CV complications or greater pulse pressure. In the recently published comparative trials BP gradients largely accounted for most, if not all, of the differences in outcome. In hypertensive patients, calcium-channel blockers may offer greater protection against stroke than against MI, resulting in an overall CV benefit similar to that provided by older drug classes. The hypothesis that angiotensin-converting enzyme inhibitors or alpha-blockers might influence outcome over and beyond that expected on the basis of their BP lowering effects still remains to be proven.

New risk classification by SBP

Systolic blood pressure and mortality.
Port S, Demer L, Jennrich R, Walter D, Garfinkel A. *Lancet* 2000;
355(9199): 175–80.

BACKGROUND. **The current systolic blood-pressure threshold for hypertension treatment is 140 mmHg for all adults. WHO and the International Society of Hypertension have proposed that normal pressure be lower than 130 mmHg with an optimum pressure of less than 120 mmHg. These recommendations are based largely on the assumption that CV and overall mortality depend in a strictly increasing manner on SBP. The Framingham study was instrumental in establishing this viewpoint. Data were reassessed from that study to find out whether the relationship is strictly increasing or whether there is a threshold.**

INTERPRETATION. The Framingham data contradict the concept that lower pressures imply lower risk and the idea that 140 mmHg is a useful cut-off value for hypertension for all adults. There is an age-dependent and sex-dependent threshold for hypertension. A substantial proportion of the population who would currently be thought to be at increased risk are, therefore, at no increased risk.

Comment
See below

Elevated systolic blood pressure as a cardiovascular risk factor.
Kannel WB. *Am J Cardiol* 2000; **85**(2): 251–5.

BACKGROUND. **Most clinical trials have also used DBP as the benchmark measure. Recently, however, the importance of SBP has become regarded as equal to, if not greater than, that of DBP in the treatment of hypertension.**

INTERPRETATION. The health community needs to be re-educated to consider the importance of systolic and DBP in assessing appropriate management strategies for hypertensive patients.

Comment
This paper reviewed the evolution of attitudes toward the treatment and diagnosis of hypertension. The review highlights a perplexing historical oddity. For nearly a century, the treatment and diagnosis of hypertension have been based on DBP levels. However, the belief that DBP is a better predictor of the CV risk associated with hypertension is a misconception. In fact, as many clinical trials and popula-

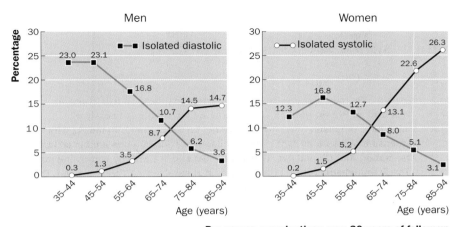

Per person examinations over 30 years of follow-up

Fig. 1.7 Prevalence of isolated systolic and DBP by age and sex in the Framingham Heart Study. Source: Kannel (2000).

tion-based studies have shown, systolic pressure is the prime causal factor of hypertension and its adverse CV sequelae.

Contrary to previous interpretation, re-analysis of 18-year data from the Framingham Heart Study using a mathematical rather than a biostatistical approach shows that the relationship between SBP and either all-cause or CV mortality is not strictly linear in the Framingham data. Instead, the risk appeared relatively stable up to the 70th percentile of values for a given sex and age, and then increased sharply after the 80th percentile.

In the analysis by Port *et al.*, the mortality risk was independent of SBP for all pressures below a given threshold for a person of a given age and sex. This threshold was typically at the 70th percentile of systolic pressure, whilst beyond the 80th percentile there was a sharp increase in the risk of death. For example, a man at 45 years of age might be considered hypertensive with a systolic pressure of 140 mmHg, but by the time he is 74, because of the natural increase in systolic pressures over time, he could maintain a systolic pressure of 160 and have no greater risk than the man of similar age with a pressure of 120 mmHg. Once he reached a pressure above the 80% percentile for his age and sex, however, his risk would rise sharply.

Obviously, the paper by Port *et al.* would have important implications for the treatment of patients. Current recommendations use 140 mmHg as a threshold for treatment for both sexes and all ages.

In the review article by Kannel, changing attitudes about the relative importance of systolic compared to diastolic hypertension are highlighted, and described as a

Table 1.6 Risk classification by SBP

Category	Increase above background	Range
Normal	None	Systolic pressure <70th percentile
High normal	Slight	Systolic pressure between 70th and 80th percentiles
Hypertension	Rapidly increasing	Systolic pressure <80th percentile

Source: Port *et al.* (2000).

'perplexing historical oddity'. Many clinical trials and population-based studies have shown that systolic pressure is the prime causal factor of hypertension and its adverse CV sequelae.

Isolated systolic hypertension leads to target organ damage

Similar effects of isolated systolic and combined hypertension on left ventricular geometry and function: the LIFE Study.
Papademetriou V, Devereux RB, Narayan P, *et al. Am J Hypertens* 2001; **14**(8 Pt 1): 768–74.

BACKGROUND. Elevated SBP either isolated or combined with elevated DBP has long been recognized as a strong contributor to the development of target organ disease and CV complications. Numerous studies have shown that left ventricular (LV) hypertrophy is a strong and independent predictor of CV events

INTERPRETATION. The present results add support to the concept that SBP is a stronger determinant than diastolic pressure of cardiac target organ damage in hypertension.

Comment

The purpose of this study was to assess LV structural and functional changes in patients with ISH and evidence of electrocardiographic LVH and compare them to similar patients with combined SDH (CSDH), recruited from the same population. Echocardiograms of 143 patients with ISH were compared to 808 patients with CSDH. The results clearly demonstrated that, LV wall thickness, dimension, and LV mass indexed for either body surface area or height as well as measures of systolic and diastolic function were virtually identical in ISH and CSDH groups despite substantial and significant differences of 12 mmHg in mean and 18 mmHg in DBP. There was no difference in the distribution of concentric remodelling, eccentric or concentric LVH patterns between the two groups, suggesting similar pathologic effects of these two patterns of hypertension despite a substantial between-group difference in mean and diastolic arterial pressure. These findings strongly suggest a greater role for systolic than mean and especially, DBP in the development of LV target organ abnormalities. Further analysis to relate ISH and its associated abnormalities to prognosis will be needed at the end of the Losartan Intervention For Endpoint Reduction in Hypertension (LIFE) trial.

Cardiac and vascular remodelling in older adults with borderline isolated systolic hypertension: the ICARe Dicomano Study.

Pini R, Cavallini MC, Bencini F, *et al. Hypertension* 2001; **38**: 1372–6.

BACKGROUND. Although borderline ISH, defined as a BP of 140 to 159 ≤ 90 mmHg, is a proven CV risk factor, the major clinical trials on treatment of ISH have used a cut-off of 160 mmHg. Moreover, no data exist on the CV modifications associated with borderline ISH. Therefore, the present study was undertaken to analyse the cardiac and vascular characteristics of subjects with borderline ISH compared with subjects with diastolic (essential) hypertension or ISH.

INTERPRETATION. In this study of an older population, individuals with borderline ISH had a similar prevalence of left ventricular hypertrophy and carotid atherosclerosis to subjects with diastolic hypertension, despite lower systolic and mean pressures. Among BP values, pulse pressure was the single or strongest independent predictor of CV remodelling.

Comment

The study included 135 untreated subjects (95 diastolic hypertension, 87 borderline ISH and 43 ISH; age ≥ 65 years) who underwent extensive clinical examination, echocardiography, carotid ultrasonography and applanation tonometry. The results showed that subjects with borderline ISH demonstrated the same cardiac and vascular abnormalities (LV mass, atherosclerotic plaques and carotid cross-sectional area and stiffness index) as those of patients with diastolic (essential) hypertension, despite lower systolic and mean BP. Moreover, borderline ISH patients exhibited comparable prevalences of ischaemic heart disease and cerebrovascular events as those of patients with diastolic (essential) hypertension or ISH. The present study also supports previous observations that pulse pressure is a stronger predictor of CV disease than SBP. Thus, based on these observations and previous studies, older patients with borderline ISH may be especially likely to benefit from antihypertensive treatment.

The J curve – still present?

Introduction

It has been well established that antihypertensive treatments reduce CV events in subjects with high BP. The issue of how far BP should be lowered to achieve the greatest benefit, in terms of reduced CV morbidity and mortality, has been a matter of scientific controversy. In addition, concerns have been expressed that too vigorous reduction in BP may be associated with increased CV events – the so-called J-curve concept. The reports of a J-shaped relationship have come from longitudinal cohort studies of treated hypertensive patients or clinical trial data on antihypertensive treatment groups and, in some trials, control groups. Interpretation of such results has varied.

Indeed, the presence of a J curve in the relationship between BP and CV and stroke risk has been hotly debated. Many studies have claimed the existence of a J curve, with an equal number disputing its existence. The concept of a J curve was thought to particularly apply to the elderly, whereby reduced BP (presumably due to overtreatment) would reduce perfusion to (diseased) coronary and cerebral arteries, resulting in an excess of myocardial infarctions (MI) and strokes especially in hypertensive patients with a history of MI. However, even those clinical trials specifically designed to consider only elderly populations tended to confine themselves to the study of patients between the ages of 65–74, and none looked at groups older than 84 who may be greater risk. Some researchers have considered that the increased risk in patients with low BP is independent of treatment and may be attributed to confounding factors related to comorbid conditions or pulse pressure.

J-shaped relation between blood pressure and stroke in treated hypertensives.

Vokó Z, Bots ML, Hofman A, *et al. Hypertension* 1999; **34**: 1181–5.

BACKGROUND. **Although two clinical trials have investigated the optimal target BP level in treated hypertensive patients, it is still a question whether the risk of stroke continues to decrease the further BP is reduced in hypertensive patients.**

INTERPRETATION. Hypertension and ISH are strong risk factors for stroke in the elderly. The increased stroke risk in the lowest stratum of BP in treated hypertensive patients may indicate that the therapeutic goal of 'the lower the better' is not the optimal strategy in the elderly.

Comment

The objective of this study was to investigate the relationship between hypertension and risk of stroke in the elderly. The study was performed within the framework of the Rotterdam Study, a prospective population-based cohort study. The risk of

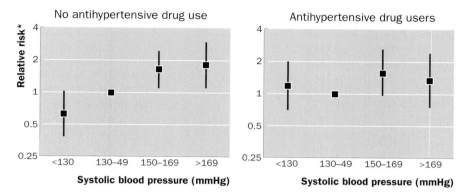

Fig. 1.8 Association between SBP and risk of first-ever stroke, according to antihypertensive treatment. Reference category is the second lowest category of SBP. Values are plotted on logarithmic scale. *Adjusted for age, gender, smoking habit, diabetes mellitus, ankle-to-arm index, minor vascular events (intermittent claudication, angina pectoris, history of coronary revascularization procedure), myocardial infarction, atrial fibrillation, and typical and atypical transient ischaemic attack. Source: Vokó *et al.* (1999).

first-ever stroke was associated with hypertension (relative risk, 1.6; 95% CI, 1.2 to 2.0) and with ISH (relative risk, 1.7; 95% CI, 1.1 to 2.6). There is a continuous increase in stroke incidence with increasing BP in non-treated subjects. In treated subjects, a J-shaped relationship between BP and the risk of stroke was also found. In the lowest category of DBP, the increase of stroke risk was statistically significant compared with the reference category.

This report from the Rotterdam Study describes the presence of a 'J-shaped' curve among elderly subjects treated for hypertension, with an increase in stroke risk at the lowest systolic and diastolic pressures. Whilst there was a continuous increase in the stroke incidence among non-treated subjects as BPs rose, there was also a J-shaped relationship between BP and the risk of stroke among those receiving treatment.

Blood pressure and mortality during an up to 32-year follow-up.

Strandberga TE, Salomaab VV, Vanhanena HT, Pitkälää K. *J Hypertension* 2001; **19**: 35–9.

BACKGROUND. Elevated BP is an established risk factor of CVD, but there is a constant debate as to whether the association is continuous or with a threshold.

INTERPRETATION. During a truly long-term follow-up, the relationship between SBP and mortality was initially flat up to 131–140 mmHg although a linear relationship is suggested in men with other CV risk factors.

Comment

In 1960, the study recruited 3267 initially healthy 30–45-year-old male business executives, whose baseline BP was related to mortality during up to 32 years of follow-up.

During the follow-up, there were 701 deaths, 33.4% of them due to coronary heart disease, 7.0% to stroke, 6.0% to other CVDs and 29.1% to cancer. The mortality risk starts to increase from 140–150 mmHg systolic and 86–90 mmHg diastolic BP (Korotkoff's 4th phase), whereafter the risk is consistently higher with systolic than diastolic BP (with the chosen cut-off points). Multivariate analyses confirm the results by showing that the risk increase is not significant until 141–150 mmHg systolic pressure. Furthermore, the results suggest, but do not prove, that BP is linearly associated with long-term mortality only in the presence of other risk factors. The association is J- or even U-shaped in men without other CV risk factors, that is, mortality seems to be higher at 110 mmHg than between 111–150 mmHg systolic BP and rises again thereafter.

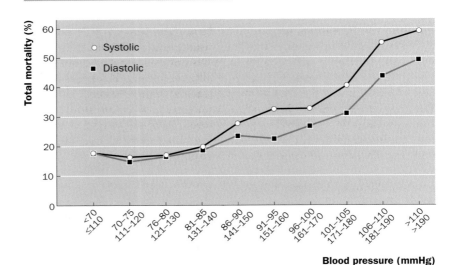

Fig. 1.9 Crude total mortality (701 deaths) according to systolic and diastolic BP (Korotkoff's 4th phase) at baseline in 3267 initially healthy men. Source: Strandberga *et al.* (2001).

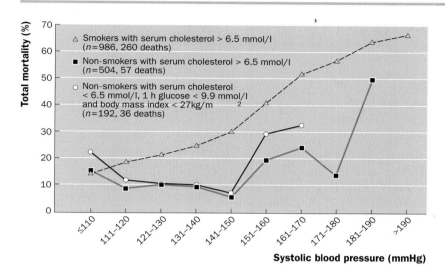

Fig. 1.10 Total mortality according to SBP and stratified by baseline risk factor status.
Source: Strandberga *et al.* (2001).

There were few limitations in this study. First, there was no strict protocol planned in 1960 and only one baseline BP measurement is available; at the time Korotkoff's 4th phase was used instead of 5th phase for diastolic BP. Secondly, the effects of antihypertensive treatment on the results are unclear. Thirdly, the study population was highly selected, i.e. middle-aged men of the highest social class thus reducing the generalizability of the results. Fourthly, the power of the study, with a total of 701 deaths, is not enough to definitely prove that the shapes of the mortality curves are statistically different. For these reasons, further research to confirm the findings with even larger and more representative populations is needed.

Twenty-four-hour ambulatory BP in the Hypertension Optimal Treatment (HOT) study.

Mancia G, Omboni S, Parati G, et al. J Hypertens 2001; **19**(10): 1755–63.

B A C K G R O U N D. The Hypertension Optimal Treatment (HOT) study showed that when antihypertensive treatment reduces diastolic BP well below 90 mmHg, there can be a further reduction of CV events, particularly myocardial infarction, with no evidence of a J-shaped curve at lower pressures. Office measurement, however, gives no information about BP outside the office. This paper describes a HOT substudy in which patients underwent both office measurement and 24-h ambulatory BP monitoring (ABPM).

INTERPRETATION. In the HOT study, treatment reduced not only office but also ambulatory BP throughout the 24 hours. The reduction was less marked for ambulatory than for office BP.

Comment

Given the demographic and clinical similarities between the patients involved in the ABPM substudy and those recruited in the HOT study as a whole, the two novel findings interpreted above can allow two suggestions to be made: (1) the HOT study regimen provided adequate BP control not only at the office but also throughout the 24-h dosage interval; (2) aggressive reduction of office BP was not associated with an excessive drop in BP throughout the day and night. As pointed out in the paper, this may have accounted for the lack of any J-curve phenomenon (possibly by avoiding vital organ underperfusion) and/or the benefit seen when the reduction in office BP by treatment was more marked. However, extrapolation from the present data to the entire HOT study requires caution.

Hypertension in the Very Elderly Trial (HYVET): protocol for the main trial.
Bulpitt C, Fletcher A, Beckett N, *et al. Drugs & Aging* 2001; **18**(3): 151–64.

BACKGROUND. A number of trials and meta-analyses have demonstrated clear benefits of BP reduction in patients aged <80 years with regard to the reduction in stroke and CV events. However, most intervention trials to date have either excluded or not recruited sufficient patients aged ≥ 80 years to determine whether there is a significant benefit from treatment in this age group.

INTERPRETATION. The Hypertension in the Very Elderly Trial (HYVET) pilot recruited 1283 patients aged ≥ 80 years and showed the feasibility of performing such a trial in this age group. It was a Prospective Randomized Open Blinded End-Points design but the main trial has additional pharmaceutical sponsorship to run a double-blind trial. Therefore, the main trial is a randomized, double-blind, placebo-controlled trial designed to assess the benefits of treating very elderly patients with hypertension. It compares placebo with a low dose diuretic (indapamide sustained release 1.5 mg daily) and additional ACEI (perindopril) therapy if required. As in the pilot trial, the primary end-point is stroke events (fatal and non-fatal) and the trial is designed to determine whether a 35% difference occurs between placebo and active treatment. The main objective will be achieved with 90% power at the 1% level of significance. Secondary outcome measures will include total mortality, CV mortality, cardiac mortality, stroke mortality and skeletal fracture. A total of 2100 patients aged ≥ 80 years are to be recruited and followed up for an average of 5 years. Entry BP criteria after 2 months of a single-blind placebo run-in period are a sustained sitting SBP of 160–199 mmHg and a DBP of 90–109 mmHg. The standing SBP must be > 140 mmHg.

Comment

A meta-analysis of intervention trials that recruited patients aged ≥ 80 years has suggested a benefit in terms of stroke reduction but has also raised the possibility of an increase in total mortality (i.e. J-curve phenomenon). The benefit to risk ratio therefore needs to be clearly established before recommendations can be made for treating very elderly patients with hypertension. The HYVET pilot recruited 1283 patients aged ≥ 80 years and showed the feasibility of performing such a trial in this age group.

Risk scoring systems and predictive models in hypertensive patients

Introduction

The availability of effective antihypertensive therapies provides a rationale to develop risk prediction models based on BP that can contribute to the development of risk assessment/management guidelines. An individual's overall CV risk is complex and multifaceted, requiring tailored treatment strategies and a simple risk scoring system would encourage more widespread screening in primary health care. One commonly used scoring system is the Framingham score which gives a 10-year CV and stroke risk. However, one frequent criticism of the Framingham risk score is that it applies to white, middle-aged men and women from a small USA town. Questions therefore arise as to whether the Framingham score applies to other countries and ethnic groups, or even to multiethnic patient populations. These issues will be highlighted below.

Development of predictive models for long-term cardiovascular risk associated with systolic and diastolic blood pressure.

Glynn RJ, L'Italien GJ, Sesso HD, Jackson EA, Buring JE. *Hypertension* 2002; **39**: 105–10.

BACKGROUND. Most existing risk prediction models have not considered the joint contribution of SBP and DBP to CV risk, and some suggest that there are thresholds below which further reductions of BP yield no additional benefit.

INTERPRETATION. These predictive models may be useful for risk estimation associated with hypertension in similar populations and may also be used to infer the benefits of antihypertensive therapy.

Comment

The present study used two large cohorts from the Physicians' Health Study and the Women's Health Study (of middle-aged patients with no prior CVD) to develop gender-specific risk prediction models with continuous values of both SBP and DBP in one model. The findings have corroborated the prognostic importance of SBP in the subsequent development of CVD, while also suggesting that DBP may contribute independent information. The data also showed that lower levels of BP predicted lower event rates with no evidence of a plateau or a J-shaped curve. As suggested by the authors, the model can be used to infer the clinical benefit of anti-hypertensive regimens that target the various stages of hypertension. However, it should be noted that evidence is accumulating to support the use of pulse pressure as a more important predictor in older populations and in those with prevalent disease.

Elevated midlife blood pressure increases stroke risk in elderly persons. The Framingham Study.
Seshadri S, Wolf PA, Beiser A, *et al. Arch Intern Med* 2001; **161**: 2343–50.

BACKGROUND. Stroke risk predictions are traditionally based on current BP. The potential impact of a subject's past BP experience (antecedent BP) is unknown.

INTERPRETATION. Antecedent BP contributes to the future risk of ischaemic stroke. Optimal prevention of late-life stroke will likely require control of midlife BP.

Comment

The use of antecedent or past BP instead of current BP to predict future stroke risk is novel and interesting. A previous study has shown midlife BP is predictive of the degree of carotid stenosis (a direct precursor of atherothrombotic stroke) in elderly persons.

This study assessed the incremental impact of antecedent BP in predicting the 10-year risk of completed initial ischaemic stroke for 60-, 70-, and 80-year-old subjects as a function of their current BP (at baseline), recent antecedent BP (average of readings at biennial examinations 1–9 years before baseline), and remote antecedent BP (average at biennial examinations 10–19 years earlier), with adjustment for smoking and diabetes mellitus.

The principal findings were that antecedent BP increased the future risk of ischaemic stroke even after adjusting for current BP levels. The effect was robust, consistent in both sexes, evident at baseline ages 60 and 70 years, demonstrable for all BP components (SBP, DBP and pulse pressure) evaluated, and significant in hypertensive and non-hypertensive subjects. While this is not entirely surprising given the continuum of risk, the data strongly suggest that midlife BP levels continue to affect the future risk of stroke not only over a short span, such as 5 years, but over more prolonged periods, up to 30 years. Hence, the importance of a past BP elevation as a potentially modifiable risk factor for the prevention of stroke in this group should not be overlooked.

The traditional analyses of the benefits of BP control at a given age use estimates of the 5-year (or 10-year) absolute risk of adverse events and may therefore under-estimate the long-term risk reduction achievable with adequate BP control in midlife. Emphasizing the long-term adverse effects of midlife BP elevations may serve to motivate middle-aged adults to become aware of and address their elevated BP levels.

A score for predicting risk of death from CV disease in adults with raised BP, based on individual patient data from randomized controlled trials.

Pocock SJ, McCormack V, Gueyffier F, Boutitie F, Fagard RH, Boissel JP.
BMJ 2001; **323**(7304): 75–81.

B A C K G R O U N D . **To create a risk score for death from CVD that can be easily used.**

I N T E R P R E T A T I O N . The risk score is an objective aid to assessing an individual's risk of CVD, including stroke and CHD. It is useful for physicians when determining an individual's need for antihypertensive treatment and other management strategies for CV risk.

Comment

This new risk scoring system was derived from an analysis of eight major random-ized controlled trials of antihypertensive drugs with mortality data. The paper proposes a 'more quantitative and discriminating' risk scoring system tailored to hypertensives to assess an individual's risk for all CV diseases, specifically stroke, as well as CHD risk.

Using 16 baseline factors available in each of the eight trials, Pocock *et al.* (inves-tigators for the Individual Data Analysis of Antihypertensive Intervention Trials [INDANA]) fitted a multivariate Cox proportional hazards model based on eleven risk factors (age, sex, SBP, total cholesterol, height, serum creatinine, cigarette smoking, diabetes mellitus, left ventricular hypertrophy, history of stroke and his-tory of myocardial infarction) and five interactions from the total of 1639 patients who died from over 47 088 participants in the eight trials. They subsequently con-verted the Cox model to an integer score and assigned different scores to individual risk factors based on an additive point system in which points are added to an individual's score for each factor, according to its association with risk.

In their meta-analysis antihypertensive treatment appeared to have more of an effect on preventing fatal stroke than fatal coronary disease (relative risk reduction with antihypertensive drugs 36.6% for stroke, 11.0% for CHD. The risk scores were designed to predict an individual's risk of death within 5 years. Age, sex and smoking status, as the three strongest predictors of CV risk, account for some of the largest numerical scores. Stroke risk is highlighted in the system. Other risk factor scores are also weighted by gender – for example, serum total cholesterol concentration is assigned more points in men than in women, because the link between cholesterol and mortality is stronger in men, while the converse is true for diabetes and smoking, both of which carried a higher risk for women. The effect of antihypertensive treatment could be assigned a score of –2.

Antihypertensive treatment reduced the score. The five-year risk of death from CVD for scores of 10, 20, 30, 40, 50, and 60 was 0.1%, 0.3%, 0.8%, 2.3%, 6.1%, and 15.6%, respectively. Age and sex distributions of the score from the two UK trials enabled individual risk assessment to be age and sex specific. Risk prediction models are also presented for fatal CHD, fatal stroke, and all cause mortality. The only other methodology that combines risks of stroke and CHD in its overall risk assessment is the Framingham algorithm. However, unlike the methodology proposed by Pocock *et al.* which was drawn from both European and North American population data, Framingham used risk and mortality numbers from a cohort of people from one US state only.

A key message to take from their analysis and scoring system is that an individual's overall CV risk is complex and multifaceted, requiring tailored treatment strategies and a simple risk scoring system would encourage more widespread screening in primary health care.

CHD risk prediction group. Validation of the Framingham coronary heart disease prediction scores: results of a multiple ethnic groups investigation.
D'Agostino RB Sr, Grundy S, Sullivan LM, Wilson P. *JAMA* 2001; **286**(2): 180–7.

B A C K G R O U N D . **The Framingham Heart Study produced sex-specific CHD prediction functions for assessing risk of developing incident CHD in a white middle-class population. Concern exists regarding whether these functions can be generalized to other populations. The objective of this paper is to test the validity and transportability of the Framingham CHD prediction functions.**

I N T E R P R E T A T I O N . The sex-specific Framingham CHD prediction functions perform well among whites and blacks in different settings and can be applied to other ethnic groups after recalibration for differing prevalences of risk factors and underlying rates of CHD events.

Comment

The Framingham risk score for the prediction of CHD assigns a risk score based on weighted risks, including sex, age, BP, LDL, HDL, total cholesterol, smoking and diabetes status. As highlighted above, one frequent criticism of the Framingham risk score is that it applies to white, middle-aged men and women, from a small USA town. Questions therefore arise as to whether the Framingham score applies to other countries and ethnic groups, or even to multiethnic patient populations (as seen in Birmingham, England).

This paper by D'Agostino *et al.* suggests that the Framingham CHD prediction scoring system can also be used in different ethnic groups but some recalibration of the Framingham formulas may be necessary in populations with higher or lower rates of specific risk factors. They applied the Framingham equation to the Athero-sclerosis Risk in Communities Study (ARIC, including African Americans 1987–1988), the Physicians' Health Study (1982), the Honolulu Heart Program (HHP, including Japanese Americans 1980–1982), the Puerto Rico Heart Health Program (including Hispanics 1965–1968), the Strong Heart Study (including American Indians 1989–1991) and the Cardiovascular Heath Study (1989–1990) and concluded that the Framingham functions generally produced similar risk pre-diction scores as those devised from the individual cohort data, particularly among white men and women in other studies, and among black men in the ARIC cohort. Nevertheless, among women in the ARIC cohort, relative risks for elevated BP were somewhat higher.

Some quirks were apparent. For example, smoking in the Japanese American men in the HHP study did not appear to convey the same degree of risk as it did in the Framingham cohort. Likewise, cholesterol abnormalities and smoking in the Cardiovascular Heath Study cohort were associated with lower relative risk than in the Framingham study. Among Native Americans in the Strong Heart Study, cholesterol and diabetes appeared to convey different degrees of risk.

The ethnic groups in general where the Framingham formula did not work quite as well were those in which there was more diabetes and hypertension.

BP levels and absolute CHD mortality risk in different populations

The relation between blood pressure and mortality due to coronary heart disease among men in different parts of the world. Seven Countries Study research group.
van den Hoogen PC, Feskens EJ, Nagelkerke NJ, Menotti A, Nissinen A, Kromhout D. *N Engl J Med* 2000; **342**(1): 1–8.

BACKGROUND. Elevated BP is known to be a risk factor for death from CHD. However, it is unclear whether the risk of death from CHD in relation to BP varies among populations.

INTERPRETATION. Among the six populations we studied, the relative increase in long-term mortality due to CHD for a given increase in BP is similar, whereas the absolute risk at the same level of BP varies substantially. If the absolute risk of CHD is used as an indication for antihypertensive therapy, these findings will have major implications for treatment in different parts of the world.

Comment

The Seven Countries Study included 12 761 men enrolled between 1958 and 1964, who were between 40 and 59 years of age at baseline, and who resided in one of the following countries: the United States, Finland, the Netherlands, Italy, Greece, the former Yugoslavia, and Japan. To increase the study's statistical power, the 16 cohorts in these countries were pooled into six populations: the United States, Mediterranean southern Europe, Finland, southern Europe, rural Serbia, and Japan. Only 56 men were lost to follow-up over the 25 years. Now with 25 years of follow-up, this study suggests that while the relative risk of CHD death associated with a given increment in BP is similar for all the populations studied, the absolute risk at a given BP varies very widely.

At SBPs and DBPs of about 140 and 85 mmHg respectively, 25-year rates of age-standardized CHD mortality varied by a factor of more than 3 among the populations. For example, at those BPs mortality rates in the US and northern Europe were high at approximately 70 deaths per 10 000 person-years, whereas they were much lower in Japan and Mediterranean southern Europe at approximately 20 deaths per 10 000 person-years. At the same time, the relative increase in 25-year CHD mortality for a given increment in BP was similar among the populations. The overall unadjusted relative risk of death due to CHD was 1.17 for every increment of 10 mmHg in SBP, 1.13 per 5 mmHg elevation in diastolic pressure, and 1.28 for each of these increments after adjustment for within-subject variability in BP.

A previous report from the Seven Countries Study has also shown differences between populations in the absolute risk of death at similar serum cholesterol levels. These differences could not be explained by age or smoking status, for which the investigators were able to control, thus implying the importance of other

Table 1.7 Baseline characteristics and age-standardized 25-year CHD mortality of men in six regions

Region	Number (n)	Total cholesterol (mmol/l ± SD)	High BP (%)*	Smoking (%)	CHD mortality at 25 years**
United States	2416	6.19 ± 1.16	25.5	59.4	73
Northern Europe	2377	6.51 ± 1.32	29.8	66.6	100
Mediterranean Southern Europe	2516	5.17 ± 1.08	17.3	59.2	22
Inland Southern Europe	2870	5.28 ± 1.08	27.5	59.3	46
Serbia	981	4.24 ± 0.83	15.7	56.1	41
Japan	871	4.25 ± 0.91	16.2	74.5	17

* defined as a systolic BP of ≥ 160 mmHg, a diastolic BP of ≥ 95 mmHg, or both.
** age-standardized mortality (number per 10 000 person-years).

Source: van den Hoogen *et al.* (2000).

Table 1.8 Relative risk of CHD death associated with hypertension

Population	25-year mortality from CHD		Relative risk (95% CI)**
	Normotensives*	Hypertensives*	
United States	60	116	2.06 (1.57–2.70)
Northern Europe	81	153	2.14 (1.69–2.71)
Mediterranean southern Europe	18	44	2.68 (1.69–4.26)
Inland southern Europe	41	59	1.61 (1.20–2.16)
Serbia	35	76	3.08 (1.73–5.48)
Japan	14	44	2.85 (1.18–6.88)
Total	46	97	2.13 (1.85–2.45)

* age-standardized mortality (number per 10 000 person-years).
** multivariate-adjusted for within-subject variability.

Source: van den Hoogen *et al.* (2000).

factors such as genetic predisposition or dietary patterns. These factors are known to vary greatly between the countries studied.

Risk factors, atherosclerosis and cardiovascular disease among Aboriginal people in Canada: the Study of Health Assessment and Risk Evaluation in Aboriginal Peoples (SHARE-AP).

Anand SS, Yusuf S, Jacobs R, *et al. Lancet* 2001; **358**(9288): 1147–53.

BACKGROUND. Little is known about the rates of CVD, atherosclerosis, and their risk factors among Canada's Aboriginal people. To establish the relative prevalence of risk factors, atherosclerosis and CVD, we undertook a population-based study among people of Aboriginal and European ancestry in Canada.

INTERPRETATION. A significant proportion of Aboriginal people live in poverty that is associated with high rates of CVD and CVD risk factors. Improvement of the socioeconomic status of Aboriginal people might be a key to reduce CVD in this group.

Comment

An increased prevalence of CVD and atherosclerosis among Aboriginal peoples in Canada appears to be associated with significantly higher rates of risk factors and lower socioeconomic status, compared to European Canadians.

The SHARE-AP compared CVD and atherosclerosis rates, as well as conven-

Table 1.9 CVD risk factors in Aboriginals compared to European Canadians

Risk factor	Aboriginals	European Canadians
Men smoking	39%	20%
Women smoking	42%	13%
New diabetes	12%	6%
Impaired glucose tolerance	14%	12%

Source: Anand *et al.* (2001).

tional and new CVD risk factors, in 301 Aboriginals between 35 and 75 years old with those in 326 Canadians of European descent.

Risk factors, such as smoking, glucose intolerance, obesity and hypertension, all of which lead to higher CVD and atherosclerosis rates, were higher. Poverty, unemployment, and other societal-level CVD risk factors were also higher in this group, compared to Europeans.

Management of hypertensive patients

Introduction

Hypertension is the second most common reason for an outpatient visit in the United States, accounting for approximately 30 million visits a year. However, only 29% of people with hypertension had their BP controlled to < 140/90 mmHg. The reasons for the epidemic of uncontrolled hypertension are unclear and several explanations have been considered. The high proportion of people with untreated hypertension is typically attributed to a lack of access to health care, treatment non-compliance, and social or economic factors within different racial and ethnic groups. The intensity and costs of medical therapy and polypharmacy can also relate to BP control. Improvement of its management will require an understanding of the patient characteristics and treatment factors associated with uncontrolled hypertension. Equally important, physician's adherence to treatment guidelines must not be overlooked when investigating poor BP control. Furthermore, a multi-disciplinary approach to hypertension management is gaining in popularity and as we shall see a physician/nurse team with the initiation of rapid titration programme of antihypertensive medications in patients with raised office BP can result in a significant long-term BP control as assessed by home BP measurements.

Improved hypertension management and control: results from the health survey for England 1998.

Primatesta P, Brookes M, Poulter NR. *Hypertension* 2001; **38**(4): 827–32.

BACKGROUND. A survey in 1994 showed that among the 20% of the adult English population who were identified as hypertensive, approximately 30% had their BPs controlled to < 160 mmHg SBP and < 95 mmHg DBP. The 1998 Health Survey for England data update the 1994 findings in light of new thresholds and targets for treatment outlined in recent national and international guidelines. This cross-sectional survey is analysed to describe the prevalence, awareness, treatment and control of hypertension in a random, nationally representative sample of 11 529 English adults (≥ 16 years) living in non-institutional households in 1998 and to compare these rates with those from 1994.

INTERPRETATION. The 1998 data suggest that improved detection, greater use of non-pharmacological measures, and increased use of > 1 antihypertensive agent per patient would produce greater success in achieving target levels. This could lead to major reductions in fatal and non-fatal CV events.

Comment

The observations of the previous study are echoed by the 1998 Health Survey for England data which suggest that improved detection, greater use of non-pharmacological measures, and increased use of > 1 antihypertensive agent per patient would produce greater success in achieving target levels. This survey found that 20% and 37% of adults were hypertensive according to the old (SBP ≥ 160 mmHg or DBP ≥ 95 mmHg) and new (SBP ≥ 140 mmHg or DBP ≥ 90 mmHg) definitions, respectively. Corresponding values in 1994 were 20% and 38%. Treatment and control rates among hypertensive adults (new definition) improved from 26% to 32% and from 6% to 9%, respectively, although 60% of those on treatment received only one antihypertensive drug in both years.

Characteristics of patients with uncontrolled hypertension in the United States.

Hyman DJ, Pavlik VN. *N Engl J Med* 2001; **345**(7): 479–86.

BACKGROUND. Treatment of hypertension is one of the most common clinical responsibilities of US physicians, yet only one fourth of patients with hypertension have their BP adequately controlled.

INTERPRETATION. Most cases of uncontrolled hypertension in the United States consist of isolated, mild systolic hypertension in older adults, most of whom have access to health care and relatively frequent contact with physicians.

Comment

Using data from the third National Health and Nutrition Examination Survey, Hyman and Pavlik reviewed over 16 000 adults aged 25 years or older and found that 27% of the surveyed population had high BP, and almost one-third of these patients were unaware of their condition, while 17% were aware of, but not being treated for, their elevated BP. An additional 29% were being treated for hypertension that remained uncontrolled. Notably, people with uncontrolled hypertension, including those who were unaware of their disease, or who were aware, but untreated or ineffectively treated – typically had only mild elevations in SBP, and a DBP under 90 mmHg. Older people, men and non-Hispanic blacks were more likely to have uncontrolled hypertension.

Predictors of uncontrolled hypertension in ambulatory patients.

Knight EL, Bohn RL, Wang PS, Glynn RJ, Mogun H, Avorn J. *Hypertension* 2001; **38**: 809–14.

BACKGROUND. Hypertension remains poorly controlled in the United States. Improvement of its management will require an understanding of the patient characteristics and treatment factors associated with uncontrolled hypertension.

INTERPRETATION. Multivariate analysis revealed several independent predictors of poor control: older age, multi-drug regimens, lack of knowledge by the patient of their target SBP, and a report of antihypertensive drug side effects. Patients with angina had a higher likelihood of adequate BP control. Fewer than 40% of the treated patients studied had a mean BP 140/90 mmHg, and specific patient-related factors appear to predict poor control. Some of these may be amenable to modification. Further identification of patients at risk of poor control can lead to targeted interventions to improve management.

Comment

The authors are to be praised for conducting such comprehensive investigations on the predictors of poor BP control. Knight *et al.* report a study of 525 hypertensive patients in three different healthcare systems over a 1-year period. Only 39% of patients had mean BP < 140/90 mmHg during the study period; about half had stage 1 hypertension (mean SBP 140 to 159 mmHg and/or mean DBP 90 to 99 mmHg), and 12% had stage 2 or greater hypertension (SBP > 160 mmHg and/or DBP > 100 mmHg). Several independent predictors of poor control were identified: older age, multi-drug regimens, lack of knowledge by the patient of their target SBP, and a report of antihypertensive drug side effects. Many of these factors may be amenable to improvement.

Interestingly, in the present study, no specific medications were associated with poorer *versus* better BP control on multivariate analysis. Moreover, although the study sample included a large number of diabetic patients, diabetes was not associated with better control despite published recommendations suggesting that these patients should be particularly well controlled, with a target of < 130/85 mmHg. Equally important to point out is that despite the proven benefit of antihypertensive therapy in the older age group, older patients are still treated less aggressively compared with younger patients.

A systematic review of predictors of maintenance of normotension after withdrawal of antihypertensive drugs.

Nelson M, Reid C, Krum H, McNeil J. Am J Hypertens 2001; **14**(2): 98–105.

BACKGROUND. The identification and treatment of hypertension in the general community has contributed to the reduction in strokes and coronary heart disease observed during the past 30 years. However, concerns have arisen that some patients may be receiving unnecessary antihypertensive drug therapy leading to wasted resources and the potential for adverse drug effects. Once therapy has been started, treating physicians have difficulty in selecting patients for withdrawal and have concerns regarding patient safety and their own legal liability.

INTERPRETATION. On the basis of this information, a trial of withdrawal of antihypertensive medication might be recommended for patients who have mildly elevated, uncomplicated BP that is well controlled on a single agent, and who are motivated and likely to accept lifestyle changes.

Comment

This study reviews and consolidates information from published studies to identify known predictors of the successful maintenance of normotension after antihypertensive drug withdrawal. The predictors were identified by determining the proportion of subjects with various baseline characteristics who remained normotensive while off medication for at least 12 months. From these data, a clinical algorithm was developed to help identify patients in whom antihypertensive drug withdrawal might be considered.

The analysis indicated that if antihypertensive medication is withdrawn from selected patients with mild-to-moderate hypertension, then approximately 42% of these patients are likely to remain normotensive for periods in excess of 12 months. The most consistent predictors identified were BP (lower pre-treatment, on treatment and after withdrawal), nature of pharmacotherapy (fewer agents and lower dose), and preparedness to accept dietary intervention (weight and sodium reduction). This may assist primary care physicians in achieving successful withdrawal of antihypertensive therapy among selected hypertensive patients who are willing to undertake lifestyle changes.

Multidisciplinary approach to hypertension

Rapid adjustment of antihypertensive drugs produces a durable improvement in blood pressure.
Canzanello VJ, Jensen PL, Hunder I. *Am J Hypertens* 2001; **14**: 345–50.

BACKGROUND. Antihypertensive drugs are often initiated and adjusted over a period of weeks to months. It is not clear whether the time and inconvenience of this approach is necessary. The authors studied whether or not drug adjustment over several days in the context of a physician–nurse team could produce a durable BP benefit according to home BP measurements.

INTERPRETATION. The results suggest that a clinically significant lowering of BP can often be achieved over several days and maintained for up to 1 year. Increased use of rapid drug titration, a physician–nurse team approach, and self-BP measurement at prescribed intervals have the potential to improve BP control rates and reduce the expense and inconvenience associated with the treatment of hypertension.

Comment

Increasing evidence suggests that nurse management of hypertension, working to clear methodology and protocols confers better management of hypertension, especially since only about 37–50% of treated hypertensives have BPs controlled to the recommended level of 140/90 mmHg. Nevertheless many cardiovascular risk factors occur in clusters, and a multidisciplinary approach towards cardiovascular risk factor management may be more appropriate, with efforts to stop smoking, treat hypertension and hyperlipidaemia, psychological management, etc. Easy access to clinicians to deal with problems or complications is also crucial.

The model of a nurse-managed hypertension clinic is not new but this study examined the use of rapid dosage titration at the Mayo Clinic's Short-term Hypertension Care Clinic, a specialist nurse-managed, physician-supervised treatment centre, providing unique and creative methods to treat and control hypertension. Of the 60 patients studied, 16 were referred to the clinic to confirm satisfactory BP control and had no changes made in their medication. The other group of 44 patients had uncontrolled hypertension and required the initiation or titration of antihypertensive drug therapy. Most of the patients whose drug regimen changed while at the clinic did not require further changes over the 12 months of follow-up. The control rate (BP < 140/90 mmHg) for patients in the second group at the latest follow-up was 75%.

Canzanello *et al.* suggest that a significant reduction in BP can be achieved within days, and maintained in the long-term by the combined use of rapid dose adjustment of antihypertensive medications, a physician/nurse team approach, and home BP monitoring. Further study is needed to assess whether such creative approach is cost-effective.

Discontinuation of antihypertensive drugs due to adverse events: a systematic review and meta-analysis.

Ross SD, Akhras KS, Zhang S, Rozinsky M, Nalysnyk L. *Pharmacotherapy* 2001; **21**(8): 940–53.

BACKGROUND. When choosing antihypertensive agents for patients with essential hypertension, practitioners are well advised to follow current evidence-based guidelines. These recommendations are driven primarily by evidence of efficacy and safety. Little is known about the likelihood of drug discontinuation, yet these considerations should factor into treatment decisions regarding patients with long-term conditions such as essential hypertension.

INTERPRETATION. This systematic review suggests that the frequency of discontinuation due to adverse events (DAEs) in monotherapy antihypertensive trials varies across drug classes and should be considered when choosing drugs for patients with essential hypertension.

Comment

The objective of this study was to quantify the frequency of discontinuation of antihypertensive agents (according to the class of the agents) DAEs from a meta-analysis of all of the randomized, controlled, monotherapy trials since 1990 of oral antihypertensive agents in patients with essential hypertension. A total of 190 studies met inclusion criteria. The highest frequency of discontinuations due to DAEs occurred with calcium channel blockers (CCBs) (6.7%) and alpha-adrenergic blockers (6.0%); the lowest with diuretics and angiotensin receptor blockers (each 3.1%). Only in CCBs studies was the frequency of DAEs greater in treated patients than in patients receiving placebo, but the difference was not significant.

It should be noted that, however, these data only apply to those patients with essential hypertension who are otherwise well and are receiving single-agent antihypertensive therapy. Nevertheless, the message is clear and further study greatly needed to support considerations of drug toxicity and impact on quality of life in selection of drug therapy, especially for chronic asymptomatic conditions such as hypertension.

Physician's adherence to guidelines – a reminder!

Physician-related barriers to the effective management of uncontrolled hypertension.

Oliveria SA, Lapuerta P, McCarthy BD, L'Italien GJ, Berlowitz DR, Asch SM. *Arch Intern Med* 2002; **162**: 413–20.

BACKGROUND. Primary care physicians may not be aggressive enough with the management of hypertension. The purpose of this study was to identify barriers to

primary care physicians' willingness to increase the intensity of treatment among patients with uncontrolled hypertension.

INTERPRETATION. Our findings suggest that an important reason why physicians do not treat hypertension more aggressively is that they are willing to accept an elevated systolic BP (SBP) in their patients. This has an important impact on public health because of the positive association between SBP and CV disease.

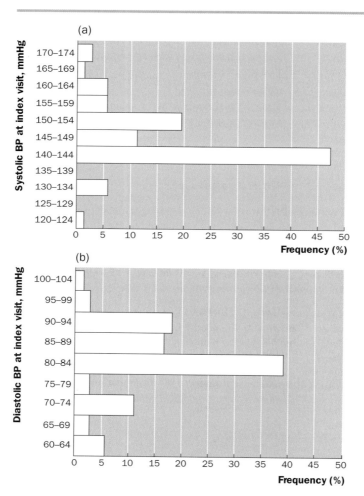

Fig. 1.11 (a), SBP for 72 patients with no initiation or change of hypertension medication. (b), DBP for 72 patients with no initiation or change of hypertension medication. Reasons given for no initiation or change in hypertension included satisfactory BP response, DBP reading was satisfactory, or only borderline hypertension. Source: Oliveria *et al.* (2001).

Comment

This is a descriptive survey study that sampled 270 patient visits in a large mid-western health system in the US to identify patients with uncontrolled hypertension. The treating primary care physicians were asked to complete a survey about the patient visit with a copy of the office notes attached to the survey (response rate, 86%). The results showed that at 93% of these visits, SBP values were ≥ 140 mmHg, which is above the cut-off point recommended by Sixth Joint National Committee on Prevention, Detection, Evaluation and Treatment of High Blood Pressure (JNC VI) guidelines, and 35% were ≥ 150 mmHg. Surprisingly, most physicians reported that 150 mmHg was the lowest SBP at which they would start treatment to patients, compared with 91 mmHg for DBP, despite being aware of the guideline's recommendations. Furthermore, the findings also suggested that physicians focus on diastolic pressures instead of ISH.

It is of note that much effort having been directed to patients' factors in treatment adherence, this study should prompt the focus on a physician's adherence to guidelines recommendations if we are to improve patient outcomes.

Patients' adherence to treatment guidelines

Patient-reported adherence to guidelines of the Sixth Joint National Committee on Prevention, Detection, Evaluation and Treatment of High Blood Pressure.

Cheng JWM, Schwartz AM. *Pharmacotherapy* 2001; **21**(7): 828–41.

BACKGROUND. Despite its prevalence, the NHANES III data indicate that 35% of those with hypertension are unaware of their condition and, even more disturbing, optimal BP control (< 140/90 mmHg) occurs in only 27% of hypertensive patients. This is particularly disappointing as it has been 30 years since the Joint National Committee on Prevention, Detection, Evaluation and Treatment of High Blood Pressure (JNC) published its first treatment guidelines based on research.

INTERPRETATION. Compliance with JNC VI guidelines has decreased over time, and patient adherence to drug therapy is suboptimal. Continuing-education efforts to reinforce optimal BP management are necessary.

Comment

The objective of this study was to compare antihypertensive drug compliance with treatment guidelines established by the JNC VI, and to identify patient adherence to antihypertensive drugs and factors affecting prescribing patterns. The authors studied patients filling prescriptions in community pharmacies in the metropolitan New York area. This enabled them to acquire a large number of patients with a wide

Table 1.10 Factors that may result in suboptimal BP control

Inappropriate antihypertensive agent may be selected (side effects, cost, multiple dosing)
Non-adherence to drug therapy (as polypharmacy, lifelong drug regimen require)
Inadequate follow-up by health care professionals
Inadequate or submaximal dose
Ineffective dissemination of information and updated national treatment guidelines to health care providers
Lack of patient education or information about disease and medication
Failure to dose in accordance with duration of action of each medication
Inappropriate use, or lack of use, of diuretics
Inappropriate drug combinations
Patient non-compliance with medication regimen
Patient non-compliance with dietary sodium restriction
Concomitant medications, including non-steroidal anti-inflammatory drugs

variety of medical problems, and factors affecting adherence to treatment guidelines were assessed.

The results showed that 61% of patients had their BP in control during the time of the study, based on a one-time BP measurement, but only 37% of patients claimed to be consistently compliant with their drugs. Only 6% of patients stated that they understood why they were prescribed specific antihypertensive agents; 45% knew what their BP was at the time of their diagnosis of hypertension. The most prescribed class of antihypertensive agents was angiotensin-converting enzyme inhibitors, followed by diuretics and beta-blockers. Over the study period, compliance with JNC VI guidelines decreased significantly from 85% to 64% ($P < 0.05$).

This study has re-emphasized the importance of a patient's understanding of disease in determining the compliance with antihypertensive therapy. However, data on other factors which potentially influence a patient's adherence to treatment guidelines were not assessed, such as appropriateness of agents selected, side effects of medications, inadequate dose titration, optimal physician follow-up, etc.

How well can blood pressure be controlled? Progress report on the Systolic Hypertension in Europe Follow-Up Study (Syst-Eur 2).

Thijs L, Staessen JA, Beleva S, *et al. Curr Control Trials Cardiovasc Med* 2001; **2**(6): 298–306.

B A C K G R O U N D . The randomized, double-blind, placebo-controlled Systolic Hypertension in Europe trial (Syst-Eur 1) proved that BP lowering therapy starting with nitrendipine reduces the risk of CV complications in elderly patients with ISH. In an attempt to confirm the safety of long-term antihypertensive therapy based on a dihydropyridine, the Syst-Eur patients remained in open follow-up after the end of

Syst-Eur 1. This paper presents the second progress report of this follow-up study (Syst-Eur 2). It describes BP control and adherence to study medications.

INTERPRETATION. Substantial reductions in systolic BP may be achieved in older patients with ISH with a treatment strategy starting with the dihydropyridine calcium channel blocker, nitrendipine, with the possible addition of enalapril and/or hydrochlorothiazide.

Comment

This paper described BP control and compliance with study medications in 3516 older patients with ISH who are being followed in Syst-Eur 2. After the end of Syst-Eur 1 all patients, treated either actively or with placebo, were invited either to continue or to start antihypertensive treatment with the same drugs as previously used in the active treatment arm. In order to reach the target BP (sitting SBP < 150 mmHg), the first line agent, nitrendipine, could be associated with enalapril and/or hydrochlorothiazide. At the last available follow-up visit, 74% of the patients had reached a systolic BP level below the target of 150 mmHg and an additional 14% achieved a systolic pressure below 160 mmHg. SBP/DBP at entry in Syst-Eur 2 averaged 160/83 mmHg in the former placebo group and 151/80 mmHg in the former active-treatment group. SBP/DBP in the patients previously randomized to placebo or active treatment had decreased by 16/5 mmHg and 7/5 mmHg, respectively. The main results of the Syst-Eur 2 study will be reported in the year 2002.

The 'Birmingham Hypertension Square' for the optimum choice of add-in drugs in the management of resistant hypertension.

Lip GYH, Beevers M, Beevers DG. *J Hum Hypertens* 1998; **12**(11): 761–3.

BACKGROUND. To assist in the rational selection of antihypertensive treatment, the authors have developed the 'Birmingham Hypertension Square' for 'add-in' antihypertensive therapy (Fig. 1.12).

INTERPRETATION. After choosing a logical first-line drug, the possible second-line agents are immediately adjacent, as indicated by the arrows. Third-line drugs can be chosen in similar fashion. The phenylalkylamine calcium channel blocker (CCB), verapamil, has not been incorporated into this concept, and the combination of verapamil and a beta-blocker may even be dangerous. Instead, verapamil is a useful alternative to beta-blockers when the latter are contra-indicated because of the side effect profile or asthma.

Comment

An easy to use aid for effective antihypertensive combination therapy in resistant hypertension is offered.

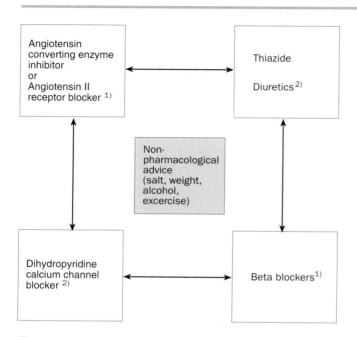

Fig. 1.12 The 'Birmingham Hypertension Square' for the optimum choice of add-in drugs in the management of resistant hypertension. Suppression of the renin–angiotensin-system (RAS) (first-line drugs in young; ACEIs first-line in diabetes mellitus). Activation of the renin–angiotensin-system (first-line in elderly and Afro-Caribbean). Source: Lip *et al.* (1998).

Baseline characteristics and early blood pressure control in the CONVINCE Trial.

Black HR, Elliot WJ, Neatson JD, *et al. Hypertension* 2001; **37**(1): 12–18.

BACKGROUND. BP control rates around the world are suboptimal. Part 2 of the NHANES III indicates that only 27.4% of hypertensive Americans aged 18 to 74 years have a BP of < 140/90 mmHg. The present study aims to assess BP control during the first 2 years and to describe the baseline characteristics of patients enrolled in the Controlled ONset Verapamil INvestigation of Cardiovascular Endpoints (CONVINCE) Study, an international clinical trial that compares outcomes in hypertensive patients randomized to initial treatment with either controlled-onset extended-release verapamil or the investigator's choice of atenolol or hydrochlorothiazide.

INTERPRETATION. These data suggest that the control of SBP is more difficult than the control of DBP. The US national goal of having 50% of hypertensives with a BP of < 140/90 mmHg may be achievable if a forced titration strategy is used. Interested investigators, free care and medications, and well-educated subjects may make the attainment of such a goal easier in the CONVINCE study than in the general population.

Comment

The CONVINCE Study provides an excellent opportunity to examine the extent of BP control in a clinical trial in which forced titration of antihypertensive medication is recommended whenever the BP is ≥ 140/90 mmHg. At randomization, only 20% of the 16 602 subjects had controlled hypertension, but the proportion increased to ~85% during forced titration of antihypertensive medications and then levelled off at ~70% during 2.5 years of follow-up. Compared with other recent hypertension trials, CONVINCE has the highest proportion of enrolled subjects with controlled BPs. At 12 months after randomization, the Antihypertensive and Lipid-Lowering treatment to prevent Heart Attack Trial (ALLHAT) Research Group reported that only 53% achieved SBP of < 140 mmHg; the corresponding value for CONVINCE is 71.4%. The LIFE Study reported that only 25.8% had a SBP of < 140 mmHg at 12 months. Though the excellent attainment rate to target BP level in the CONVINCE study could be explained by employment of a forced

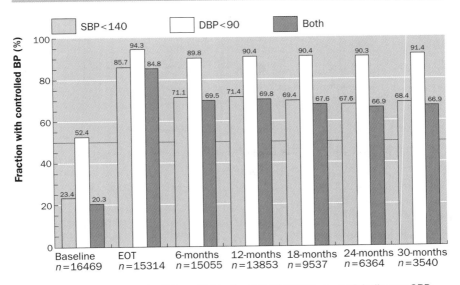

Fig. 1.13 BP control (< 140/90 mmHg) in the CONVINCE Study. SBP indicates SBP; DBP, DBP; Both, both SBP and DBP. Source: Black *et al.* (2001).

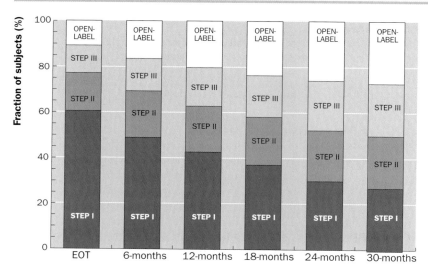

Fig. 1.14 Distribution of treatment regimens in the CONVINCE Study. Step I indicates COER-verapamil or HCTZ or atenolol; Step II, COER-verapamil plus HCTZ or atenolol plus HCTZ; Step III, Step IV plus another antihypertensive drug (ACEI is recommended); and open-label, any regimen not including blinded COER-verapamil, HCTZ or atenolol. Source: Black *et al.* (2001).

titration strategy and well-trained healthcare providers in the clinical trial setting, there was no evidence in the data presented and discussion in the article to suggest that the provision of free care and medications has any influence on the attainment rate to target BP level.

Gender and age effects in clinical trials

Elderly hypertensives respond to non-pharmacological measures to lower BP at least as well as younger patients and there is some evidence that salt restriction is more effective than in younger patients. For mild to moderate hypertension, drug therapy should not be introduced until about 3 months of non-pharmacological manoeuvres including salt restriction, alcohol moderation, weight control and increased exercise.

Antihypertensive therapy is indicated and clearly beneficial in people aged 60 years or more, when BP averages are > 160 mmHg systolic and > 90 mmHg diastolic. There is no firm evidence to guide policy for SBPs 140–159 mmHg and DBPs < 90 mmHg (borderline ISH). However, treatment is advised when there are CV complications or evidence of target organ damage.

From the most recent WHO/ISH and British Hypertension Society guidelines, there appears to be little argument against the older hypertensive patients having increased risks of CV and cerebrovascular disease and benefits of active treatment. However, some caution should be taken in treating the older patient with risks of orthostatic hypotension and other side effects. There is no compelling evidence to dismiss the use of a particular class of drug in the over 60s but common sense and care for concomitant diseases in these patients is paramount.

Gender and age effects on the ambulatory blood pressure and heart rate responses to antihypertensive therapy.
White WB, Johnson MF, Black HR, Elliott WJ, Sica DA. *Am J Hypertens* 2001; **14**(12): 1239–47.

BACKGROUND. Demographics such as gender and age may play an important role in a patient's clinical response to antihypertensive therapy. However, the influence of such individual characteristics on response to treatment is not routinely evaluated in clinical hypertension trials.

INTERPRETATION. Both gender and age were significant determinants of the response to controlled-onset, extended-release (COER)-verapamil. The antihypertensive effect of verapamil is greater in women than in men and in older patients compared with younger patients.

Comment

Meta-analyses were performed on three prospective randomized, double-blind, placebo-controlled trials with COER-verapamil in patients with mid-stage I to stage III essential hypertension. The aim was to assess potential differences in the 24-h antihypertensive response to treatment with the (COER) calcium antagonist, verapamil in men *versus* women and older *versus* younger patients with hypertension. The findings are really not unexpected as it is well established that the metabolisms (pharmacokinetic and pharmacodynamic differences) of a particular drug are influenced by a variety of factors; age and gender are the two obvious confounders. The fact is that clinical trials with antihypertensives generally are not designed to detect or to account for potential differences among various subpopulations. This report only serves as a reminder to researchers in the field. Whether these pharmacokinetic and pharmacodynamic differences affect CV outcomes with antihypertensive therapy is one of the many hypotheses being assessed in the CONVINCE trial. Further evaluation of differences in response to treatment between men and women and between older and younger patients may help to identify whether specific antihypertensive regimens may offer therapeutic advantages in these populations.

Placebo effect revisited

Evaluation of the placebo effect and reproducibility of blood pressure measurement in hypertension.

Asmar R, Safar M, Queneau P. *Am J Hypertens* 2001; **14**(6 Pt 1): 546-52.

BACKGROUND. **Pharmacologic studies in hypertension often describe BP reductions in placebo control groups. This placebo effect is currently debated, as it seems to be related to BP measurement methods and as a regression to the mean phenomenon may lead to misinterpretation. Furthermore, data on pulse pressure are lacking. This study was designed to evaluate the placebo effect on BP and to differentiate it from regression to the mean.**

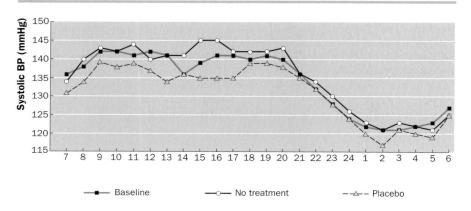

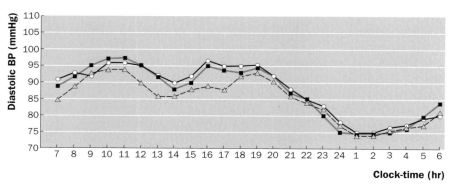

Clock-time (hr)

Fig. 1.15 Mean hourly values and circadian variations of ambulatory SBP and DBP recorded at baseline, after 1 month without treatment and after 1 month of placebo in the total population. Source: Asmar *et al.* (2001).

INTERPRETATION. This study conclusively shows the effect of placebo in mild-to-moderate hypertension on both clinic and ambulatory systolic, diastolic and mean BP in which it has been shown to differ from the regression to the mean phenomenon. This effect was not observed for pulse pressure or heart rate.

Comment

Considering that the primary reason for misinterpretation in identifying the placebo effect is its differentiation from the time effect or regression to the mean phenomenon, and that most studies that have analysed the placebo effect were not designed in any manner to allow for this differentiation, this study was appropriately designed to evaluate the effect of placebo on clinic and ambulatory BP measurements, also including pulse pressure (PP). The major findings of this study are the following: 1) in hypertensive patients, there is a placebo effect that differs from the regression to the mean phenomenon; 2) this effect is independent of the BP measurement method used, inasmuch as similar results were obtained with both clinic and ABPM; and 3) the placebo effect is observed for SBP, DBP and MAP but not for PP or HR. These findings highlight the need for control groups in trials on hypertension. In the absence of a comparison with placebo-treated patients to delineate the role of a placebo effect in the therapeutic effect of antihypertensive drugs, the therapeutic evaluation may overestimate the pharmacologic effect of the medication and lead to an inappropriate use of the treatment.

2

Risk factors

Alcohol

Introduction

Fairly good evidence suggests that alcohol probably has a causal relationship to hypertension. Nevertheless, this relationship needs to be carefully examined in relation to the quality of the available data, and the many possible confounding factors that may exaggerate or attenuate the relationship, if true.

Hypertension is a very common condition and it would be hard to believe that all (or even most) hypertensives have a drink problem. Hypertension is also likely to be multifactorial and many confounding factors may actually influence the relationship between alcohol and hypertension. Furthermore, not all studies examining the relationship between alcohol and hypertension have been overtly positive. Some consideration would also be needed to other adverse effects of alcohol on other systems, including the heart (arrhythmias, alcoholic cardiomyopathy, etc.), the liver (alcoholic hepatitis, cirrhosis, etc.) and the nervous system (peripheral neuropathy and other neurological sequelae).

When advising patients about alcohol consumption, it is important to take each individual's characteristics onto consideration. There will be a number of people who should be advised to abstain completely, especially those who are problem drinkers and people who already manifest alcohol-related pathologies. Other patients, such as those with congestive cardiac failure or cardiac arrhythmias should be advised to drink sparingly. People with hypertension and possibly angina should be also advised to drink in moderation only.

Mechanisms

Three mechanisms have been proposed for the rise in blood pressure (BP) associated with alcohol. First, there is an 'acute effect' of alcohol seen in some of the alcohol loading studies; second, there is a 'delayed pressor effect' which is seen after two or more days of regular drinking; and finally, there may be a 'withdrawal related effect' in alcoholics or heavy drinkers.

Alcohol initially has an acute vasodilator effect, as shown by reduced forearm vascular reactivity to noradrenaline, but it also exerts a central pressor effect that overcomes the peripheral dilator effects. It has been proposed that repeated small increases in plasma noradrenaline following regular alcohol consumption overtime will subsequently result in a sustained increase in BP.

Table 2.1 Factors that may influence the relationship between alcohol and BP.

Factor	Evidence	Comment
ETHNICITY	Studies performed in many countries and races: • USA-white, black and oriental. • Japan: oriental. • Australia: white and aboriginal. • India: Indian. • Europe: white. • Hawaii: oriental.	• All show a positive relationship between alcohol and BP. • Racial differences are found: eg. orientals lack expression of aldehyde dehydrogenase therefore have hypotensive effect after acute alcohol consumption. • Black people may have weaker relationship between alcohol and BP.
GENDER	• Studies show different patterns of association between alcohol and BP in men and women. • Some studies have shown weaker relationship in women compared to men (refs 26, 18, 28). • Others demonstrate J or U-shaped relationship in women (refs 4, 5).	• Differences may be due to smaller numbers of women in these studies. • Also the numbers of heavy drinking females is lower than heavy drinking males in most studies.
AGE	• When results stratified according to age, then relationship between alcohol and BP appears to be stronger in older people.	• Differences may be due to higher baseline BP in older population. • Also metabolic differences may occur in older people.
OBESITY	• When stratified according to adiposity, then the relationship of alcohol and BP remains.	• BP increases with obesity. • High alcohol intake associated with increased incidence of obesity.
SMOKING	• When smoking taken into account the relationship between alcohol and BP still remains.	• Smoking has negative relationship with alcohol. • Smoking has positive association with alcohol intake. • Therefore smoking may lead to underestimation of relationship between alcohol and BP.
PHYSICAL ACTIVITY	• Some studies show no effect of exercise on relationship between alcohol and BP.	• Physically inactive subjects have higher incidence of hypertension. • Alcohol consumption higher in those taking part in regular physical activity.
TYPE OF BEVERAGE	• Different studies looked at populations in which the predominant drink consumed were different e.g. beer, wine, saki, spirits.	

Table 2.1 (*Continued*)

Factor	Evidence	Comment
PATTERNS OF DRINKING	• Studies suggest that acute effects of alcohol consumption appear to be more important than chronic effects.	
STRESS	• Some studies found that stress increased the BP/alcohol relationship while others did not.	• Stress may predispose to hypertension. • Stress may predispose of alcoholism.

Finally, at the cellular level, there is some evidence that alcohol influences smooth muscle cell ion transport and contractility by increasing intracellular calcium concentration, thus resulting in a pressor effect on BP.

Alcohol consumption and coronary heart disease risk

 Moderate alcohol consumption and risk of coronary heart disease among women with type 2 diabetes mellitus.
Solomon CG, Hu FB, Stampfer MJ, *et al. Circulation* 2000; **102**(5): 494–9.

BACKGROUND. **Moderate alcohol consumption is associated with reduced risk for coronary heart disease (CHD) in generally healthy populations. This study assessed prospectively the association between moderate alcohol intake and CHD risk in women with type 2 diabetes mellitus (DM), a group at high risk for cardiovascular disease (CVD).**

INTERPRETATION. Although potential risks of alcohol consumption must be considered, these data suggest that moderate alcohol consumption is associated with reduced CHD risk in women with diabetes and should not be routinely discouraged.

Comment

Women in the Nurses' Health Study who reported a diagnosis of DM at 30 years of age were studied. There were 295 CHD events occurred during a total of 39 092 person-years of follow-up from 1980 to 1994. Odds ratios derived from logistic regression were used to estimate relative risks (RRs) for CHD as a function of usual alcohol intake, with adjustment for potential confounders. Compared with diabetic

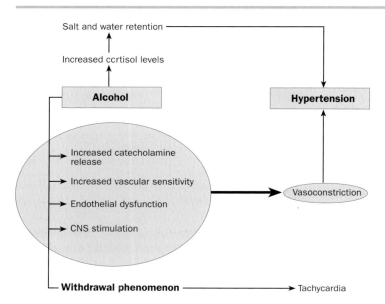

Fig. 2.1 Possible mechanisms for the pressor effect of alcohol. Source: Lip *et al.* (1999).

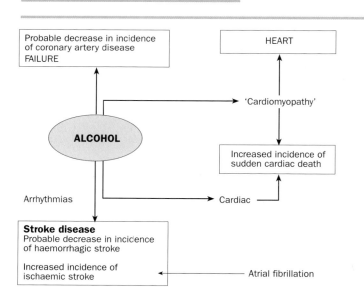

Fig. 2.2 Alcohol and cardiovascular disease. Source: Lip *et al.* (1999).

women reporting no alcohol intake, the age-adjusted RR for non-fatal or fatal CHD among diabetic women reporting usual intake of 0.1 to 4.9 g ($<$ 0.5 drinks) of alcohol daily was 0.74 (95% confidence interval (CI) 0.56 to 0.98), and among those reporting usual intake $\geq$ 5 g/day, it was 0.48 (95% CI 0.32 to 0.72) (*P*-value for trend $<$ 0.0001). Inverse associations between alcohol intake and CHD risk remained significant in multivariate analysis adjusting for several other coronary risk factors (0.1 to 4. 9 g/d: RR 0.72 [95% CI 0.54 to 0.96]; $\geq$ 5 g/day: RR 0.45 [0.29 to 0.68]).

Alcohol consumption and risk of CHD by diabetes status.

Ajani UA, Gaziano JM, Lotufo PA, *et al. Hypertension* 2000; **102**(5): 500–5.

BACKGROUND. **An inverse association between moderate alcohol consumption and CHD has been observed in several epidemiological studies. To assess whether a similar association exists among diabetics, this study examined the relationship between light to moderate alcohol consumption and CHD in men with and without DM in a prospective cohort study.**

INTERPRETATION. The study suggests that light to moderate alcohol consumption is associated with similar risk reductions in CHD among diabetic and non-diabetic men.

Comment

In this study, a total of 87 938 US physicians (2790 with diagnosed DM) who participated in the Physicians' Health Study and were free of myocardial infarction, stroke, cancer or liver disease at baseline were followed for an average of 5.5 years for death with CHD as the underlying cause. During 480 876 person-years of follow-up, 850 deaths caused by CHD were documented: 717 deaths among non-diabetic men and 133 deaths among diabetic men. Among men without diabetes at baseline, the RR estimates for those reporting rarely/never, monthly, weekly, and daily alcohol consumption were 1.00 (referent), 1.02, 0. 82, and 0.61 (95% CI 0.49 to 0.78; *P* for trend $<$ 0.0001) after adjustment for age, aspirin use, smoking, physical activity, body mass index, history of angina, hypertension and high cholesterol. Among men with diabetes at baseline, the RR estimates were 1.00 (referent), 1.11, 0.67, and 0.42 (95% CI 0.23 to 0.77; *P*-value for trend = 0.0019).

Alcohol consumption and the incidence of hypertension: the Atherosclerosis Risk in Communities Study.

Fuchs FD, Chambless LE, Whelton PK, Nieto FJ, Heiss G. *Hypertension* 2001; **37**(5): 1242–50.

BACKGROUND. **A close relationship between alcohol consumption and hypertension has been established, but it is unclear whether there is a threshold level for this**

association. In addition, it has infrequently been studied in longitudinal studies and in black people.

INTERPRETATION. Consumption of ≥ 210 g alcohol per week is a risk factor for hypertension in free-living North American populations, independent of race, gender, age and other risk factors for hypertension. The consumption of low to moderate amounts does not appear to increase substantially the risk of hypertension in whites, whereas it is associated with an increased risk of hypertension in black men.

Comment

This study involved 8334 participants (45–64 years of age at baseline and free of hypertension and CHD) of the Atherosclerosis Risk in Communities (ARIC) Study who had their BPs ascertained after 6 years of follow-up. Alcohol consumption was assessed by dietary interview. Those who consumed large amounts of ethanol (≥ 210 g per week) had an increased risk of hypertension, with black men having the highest adjusted odds ratio (OR), 2.31 (95% CI: 1.11 to 4.86). Systolic BP (SBP) and diastolic BP (DBP) were higher in black men who consumed low to moderate amounts of alcohol compared with the non-consumers but not in the three other race-gender strata. Models with polynomial terms of alcohol exposure suggested a non-linear association in white and black men. Higher levels of consumption of all types of alcoholic beverages were associated with a higher risk of hypertension for all race-gender strata. The consumption of alcohol in amounts ≥ 210 g per week is an independent risk factor for hypertension in free-living North American populations. The consumption of low to moderate amounts of alcohol also appears to be associated with a higher risk of hypertension in black men. Further race-specific studies on the alcohol and hypertension relationship are warranted. In the interim, we should view with caution the health effects of a low to moderate intake of ethanol in blacks.

Additional comment

Alcohol access can lead to hypertension, and acute ingestion can precipitate arrhythmias such as atrial fibrillation. More chronic excessive alcohol consumption can lead to a dilated cardiomyopathy, which is partly reversible with abstinence. No difference in the protective effects by the type of alcoholic beverage, suggesting alcohol itself is the protective factor.

Nevertheless, light to moderate alcohol consumption has been associated with a lower risk for CHD in men and women. The Nurses' Health Study and the Physicians' Health Study prospectively investigated the relationship between moderate alcohol intake and CHD risk in women and men, respectively, suffering from type 2 diabetes, which is associated with a three-fold increase in CHD risk.

In the Nurses' Health Study, 5103 nurses diagnosed with diabetes mellitus and free of CHD at baseline, who filled out a questionnaire about their usual alcohol consumption and were analysed during an average follow-up of 14 years.

Table 2.2 Association of alcohol consumption with RR for CHD in diabetic women (NHS)

Indicators	No alcohol	Daily alcohol 0.1–4.9g*	Daily alcohol ≥ 5g
% of study subjects	58.1%	26.4%	15.5%
CHD cases	204	65	26
RR for CHD**	1.0	0.72	0.45

* One 12-oz can of beer = 12.8g of alcohol; one 4-oz wine = 11.0g; one standard drink of spirits = 14.0g.
** Adjusted for age, time period, body mass index (BMI), parental history of myocardial infarction (MI), hypertension, hypercholesterolemia, menopausal status and hormone use, aspirin-, multivitamin-, and vitamin E supplement use, and physical activity level.

Source: Fuchs *et al.* (2001).

Table 2.3 Frequency of alcohol consumption and CHD mortality and incident CHD risk in diabetics

Indicator	rarely	monthly	weekly	daily
Enrolment cohort	799	396	986	609
Cases CHD mortality	799	396	986	609
RR CHD mortality*	1.00	1.11	0.67	0.42
Randomized cohort	128	86	172	124
Cases incident CHD	33	21	39	27
RR incident CHD*	1.00	0.84	0.75	0.66

*Adjusted for age, randomized treatment assignment, smoking, physical activity, BMI, parental history of MI, personal history of angina, hypertension, and hypercholesterolemia.

Source: Fuchs *et al.* (2001).

Table 2.4 Frequency of alcohol consumption and CHD mortality and incident CHD risk in non-diabetics

Indicator	rarely	monthly	weekly	daily
Enrolment cohort	14091	9757	39542	21758
Cases CHD mortality	166	83	267	201
RR CHD mortality*	1.00	1.02	0.82	0.61
Randomized cohort	3105	2336	10498	5275
Cases incident CHD	314	204	900	409
RR incident CHD*	1.00	0.94	0.90	0.67

*Adjusted for age, randomized treatment assignment, smoking, physical activity, BMI, parental history of MI, personal history of angina, hypertension, and hypercholesterolaemia.

Source: Fuchs *et al.* (2001).

Age-adjusted rates of CHD were significantly lower in women who reported moderate alcohol intake than in those who reported drinking no alcohol, even after adjustments for other CHD risk factors these RRs remained statistically significant.

In the paper from Fuchs *et al.*, based on data from the ARIC study, there was an increased risk of hypertension in those who consumed large amounts of ethanol (≥ 210 g per week) compared with those who did not consume alcohol over the 6 years of follow-up, with an adjusted odds ratios (95% CI) of 1.2 (0.85 to 1.67) for white men, 2.02 (1.08 to 3.79) for white women, and 2.31 (1.11 to 4.86) for black men. At low to moderate levels of alcohol consumption (1 to 209 g per week), the adjusted odds ratios (95% CI) were 0.88 (0.71 to 1.08) in white men, 0.89 (0.73 to 1.09) in white women, 1.71 (1.11 to 2.64) in black men and 0.88 (0.59 to 1.33) in black women. Higher levels of consumption of all types of alcoholic beverages were associated with a higher risk of hypertension for all race-gender strata. Thus, the consumption of alcohol in amounts ≥ 210 g per week is an independent risk factor for hypertension in free-living North American populations.

In the Physicians' Health Study, a total of 87 938 US physicians (enrolment cohort), 2790 of whom were diabetic, were asked about the frequency of their alcohol consumption. In a subanalysis, 21 852 of the enrolment cohort physicians (510 with diabetes) were subsequently randomized to assess the RR for CHD incidence in association with alcohol consumption for an average follow-up of 12 years (randomized cohort). The enrolment cohort was followed for CHD mortality only.

During an average follow-up of 5.5 years, low-to-moderate consumption of alcohol was associated with a decreased risk of CHD mortality in men with diabetes, just as it is among men without diabetes.

In patients with type 2 diabetes, increasing levels of HDL cholesterol, increased fibrinolytic activity and decreased platelet aggregation with alcohol intake could be possible explanations for the inverse relationship between alcohol consumption and CHD risk. Furthermore, moderate alcohol intake (less than two drinks per day) might lower BP and fasting insulin levels in women.

Prior alcohol consumption and mortality following acute myocardial infarction.

Mukamal KJ, Maclure M, Muller JE, Sherwood JB, Mittleman MA. *JAMA* 2001; **285**(15): 1965–70.

BACKGROUND. Studies have found that individuals who consume one alcoholic drink every 1–2 days have a lower risk of a first acute myocardial infarction (AMI) than abstainers or heavy drinkers, but the effect of prior drinking on mortality after AMI is uncertain.

INTERPRETATION. Self-reported moderate alcohol consumption in the year prior to AMI is associated with reduced mortality following infarction.

Comment

The objective of this study was to determine the effect of prior alcohol consumption on long-term mortality among early survivors of AMI. The studied cohort included a total of 1913 adults hospitalized with AMI recruited into the Prospective Inception Cohort study between 1989 and 1994. Of the 1913 patients studied, 47% were abstained from alcohol, 36% consumed less than seven alcoholic drinks per week, and 17% consumed seven or more alcoholic drinks per week. Patient groups who consumed less or more than seven drinks week had a lower all-cause mortality rate compared with abstainers. After adjusting for propensity to drink and other potential confounders, increasing alcohol consumption remained predictive of lower mortality for less than seven drinks per week. The association was similar for total and cardiovascular mortality, among both men and women, and among different types of alcoholic beverages.

Moderate alcohol consumption and risk of heart failure among older persons.

Abramson JL, Williams SA, Krumholz HM, Vaccarino V. *JAMA* 2001;
285(15): 1971–7.

BACKGROUND. Heavy consumption of alcohol can lead to heart failure, but the relationship between moderate alcohol consumption and risk of heart failure is largely unknown.

INTERPRETATION. Increasing levels of moderate alcohol consumption are associated with a decreasing risk of heart failure among older persons. This association is independent of a number of confounding factors and does not appear to be entirely mediated by a reduction in MI risk.

Comment

The purpose of this study was to determine whether moderate alcohol consumption predicts heart failure risk among older persons, independent of the association of moderate alcohol consumption with lower risk of MI. A prospective cohort of 2235 non-institutionalized elderly persons (free of heart failure at baseline) was

Table 2.5 All-cause mortality after MI by level of alcohol consumption

End-point	Abstainers	Patients consuming < 7 drinks/week	Patients consuming ≥ 7 drinks/week
All-cause mortality (deaths per 100 person-years)	6.3	3.4	2.4

Source: Abramson *et al.* (2001).

studied (maximum follow-up of 14 years). The results revealed increasing alcohol consumption in the moderate range was associated with decreasing heart failure rates. For persons consuming no alcohol (50.0%), 1 to 20 oz (40.2%), and 21 to 70 oz (9.8%) in the month prior to baseline, crude heart failure rates per 1000 years of follow-up were 16.1, 12.2, and 9.2, respectively. After adjustment for confounding factors, the RR of heart failure for those consuming no alcohol, 1 to 20 oz, and 21 to 70 oz in the month prior to baseline was 1.00 (referent), 0.79 (95% CI, 0.60–1.02), and 0.53 (95% CI, 0.32–0.88) (P for trend = 0.02).

Again, a prior history of moderate alcohol use was associated with lower mortality after an MI; in another, moderate alcohol consumption related to a decreased risk of congestive heart failure (CHF). Previous studies in the general population have shown lower rates of non-fatal MI and CHD mortality among individuals consuming one alcoholic drink every 1–2 days compared to abstainers or heavier drinkers.

Mukamal et al. prospectively studied 1913 patients hospitalized for MI, where 896 (47%) described themselves as abstainers, 696 (36%) had less than seven drinks per week, and 321 (17%) consumed more than seven drinks per week. Both groups who reported drinking had lower all-cause mortality compared with abstainers; those consuming 7 or less drinks had a hazard ratio of 0.55 (95% CI 0.43–0.71), while seven or more drinks was associated with a hazard ratio of 0.38 (0.25–0.55), with a P value of < 0.001.

Even after adjustment, the association between increasing alcohol consumption and lower mortality remained, with a hazard ratio of 0.79 (0.60–1.03) for the under seven drinks per week group, and 0.68 (0.45–1.05, p = 0.01) for the seven drinks and over group. The association remained across all patient groups and all beverage types.

Abramson et al. studied 2235 elderly individuals who were free of CHF at baseline: 50% reported no alcohol consumption, 40.2% reported drinking 1–20 oz of alcohol, and 9.8% reported drinking 21–70 oz. Over the study period, 281 first CHF events occurred, 28 of which were fatal. Increasing alcohol consumption in this moderate range was associated with decreasing heart failure rates; crude heart failure rates per 1000 years of follow-up were 16.1 for those drinking no alcohol, 12.2 for the 1–20 oz group, and 9.2 among those drinking 21–70 oz.

Table 2.6 Relative risk of heart failure* by alcohol consumption in the month prior to baseline

End-point	No alcohol (referent)	1–20 oz alcohol	21–70 oz alcohol
Adjusted risk of heart failure	1.00	0.79 (0.60–1.02)	0.53 (0.32–0.88)

*adjusted for age, sex, race, education, angina, history of MI and diabetes, MI during follow up, pulse pressure, BMI, and current smoking

Source: Abramson et al. (2001).

Women: time for a drink, 'light, not heavy'

Prospective study of moderate alcohol consumption and risk of hypertension in young women.
Thadhani R, Camargo CA, Stampfer MJ, et al. Arch Intern Med 2002; **162**: 569–74.

BACKGROUND. **Heavy alcohol consumption is associated with an increased risk of hypertension. However, the effect of moderate alcohol consumption; the specific effects of wine, beer, and liquor; and the pattern of drinking in relation to risk of hypertension among young women are unclear.**

INTERPRETATION. The association between alcohol consumption and risk of chronic hypertension in young women follows a J-shaped curve, with light drinkers demonstrating a modest decrease in risk and more regular heavy drinkers demonstrating an increase in risk.

Comment

This new analysis of the Nurses' Health Study showed that women who regularly consume light alcoholic drinks appear to protect themselves from developing chronic hypertension, but heavy drinking increases the risk.

Thadhani *et al.* prospectively reviewed the association between alcohol consumption and subsequent development of hypertension in 70 891 women from the sponsored study who were 25 to 42 years of age and normotensive at the time the study began. The women were followed for 8 years, and during this time, 4188 cases of incident hypertension (5.9%) were reported. After adjustment for multiple covariates, the association between alcohol consumption and hypertension followed a J-shaped curve. Women whose alcohol consumption averaged 0.25 to 0.50 drinks a day had the greatest decrease (14%) in their risk of developing chronic hypertension; women who consumed an average of more than 2 drinks a day had the greatest increase in risk (31%). Exclusion of past drinkers yielded similar results.

Compared to non-drinkers, the risks of developing hypertension based on the average number of drinks consumed per day are categorized as follows:

0.25 or less   = 4% lower risk of hypertension
0.26 to 0.5 drinks   = 14% lower risk of hypertension
0.51 to 1 drink   = 8% lower risk of hypertension
1.01 to 1.5 drinks   = equivalent risk of hypertension
1.51 to 2 drinks   = 20% increased risk of hypertension
>2 drinks   = 31% increased risk of hypertension.

Salt sensitivity and cardiovascular mortality

Introduction

It is generally accepted that salt, and an individual's particular reaction to it, plays an important role in the development of high BP and subsequent adverse health effects. Several studies have shown that individuals whose BP is responsive to changes in sodium balance and extracellular fluid volume status (i.e. salt sensitive) are at increased risk of cardiovascular (CV) death, even if they are normotensive. However, the mechanisms of a salt sensitivity and the heterogeneity of this effect are far from being completely understood. Salt sensitivity is more prevalent in certain groups, including the elderly, African Americans, diabetics, first-degree relatives of hypertensives, and those with a family member who is salt-sensitive. Salt sensitivity is present in 30% of normotensive and over 50% of hypertensive persons.

Salt sensitivity is also linked to target-organ effects, such as an increased risk of left ventricular hypertrophy, endothelial dysfunction, proteinuria, and a blunted decline in nocturnal BP. There is also clear evidence to support a strong relationship between obesity hypertension, sodium sensitivity and insulin resistance.

Salt sensitivity, pulse pressure, and death in normal and hypertensive humans.
Weinberger MH, Fineberg NS, Fineberg SE, Weinberger M. *Hypertension* 2001; **37**(2 suppl): 429–32.

BACKGROUND. Although factors such as age, BP, and its responsiveness to changes in sodium balance and extracellular fluid volume status (salt sensitivity) are associated with an increased risk of end-organ disease and CV events in hypertensive subjects, no such relationship with mortality has been demonstrated for salt sensitivity in normotensive subjects.

INTERPRETATION. These observations provide unique evidence of a relationship between salt sensitivity and mortality that is independent of elevated BP.

Comment

This study adds to a growing body of evidence that suggests salt, and an individual's susceptibility to it, plays an important role in the development of hypertension and subsequent adverse health effects. In this study, the salt sensitivity or resistance status of BP was ascertained in 596 subjects (normo or hypertensive) about 27 years ago. Of the overall cohort, 338 were found to be salt sensitive and 123 had died. As expected, age, gender, BMI, and all measures of BP including SBP, DBP, mean arterial pressure, and pulse pressure, were associated with significantly increased mortality. However, when survival curves were examined, normotensive salt-sensitive subjects aged > 25 years when initially studied were found to have a cumulative mortality similar to that of hypertensive subjects, whereas salt-resistant normotensive subjects had increased survival.

From their earlier studies, Weinberger *et al.* noted that salt sensitivity is more common in certain groups. These include the elderly, African Americans, first-degree relatives of hypertensives, and those with a family member who is salt-sensitive. The condition is also linked to different end-organ effects than is hyper-

Table 2.7 Risk factors and associated odds ratios for CV death

Risk factor	Odds ratio	P value
Age	1.06	<0.001
Female gender	0.34	<0.005
Pulse pressure	1.06	<0.001
Salt sensitivity	2.17	<0.003

Source: Weinberger *et al.* (2001).

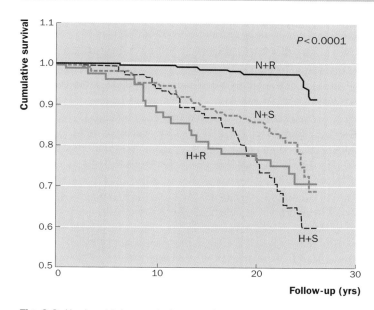

Fig. 2.3 Kaplan–Meier survival curves for normotensive salt-resistant subjects (N+R), normotensive salt-sensitive subjects (N+S), hypertensive salt-resistant subjects (H+R), and hypertensive salt-sensitive subjects (N+S) over the follow-up period. As noted, only the N+R group had an increased survival. Source: Weinberger *et al.* (2001).

tension. These include an increased risk of left ventricular hypertrophy, proteinuria and a blunted decline in nocturnal BP. Among the individuals who were deemed salt-sensitive in their initial study, there was a significantly greater rise in BP with age and time, compared to salt-resistant subjects. The observation suggests that salt-sensitivity in normotensives may presage an increased risk for age-related hypertension. If this turns out to be the case, it is possible that intervention in susceptible individuals, by reducing salt intake, could prevent or delay the subsequent age-related increase in BP, the development of hypertension, and the increased risk of CV events and death.

However, testing for salt-sensitivity remains cumbersome and mass screening is not practicable. Nevertheless, such findings from this study remind the general public with a simple message: people with normal BP should stick to the daily-recommended sodium of < 2400 mg! The benefit will be even greater if they reduce their salt intake to 1500 mg a day, as was shown in the Dietary Approaches to Stop Hypertension (DASH)-Sodium study. In that study, the lower the sodium intake, the lower the BP level.

Sodium sensitivity and cardiovascular events in patients with essential hypertension.
Morimoto A, Uzu T, Fujii T, *et al. Lancet* 1997; **350**(9093): 1734–7.

BACKGROUND. In patients with sodium-sensitive hypertension, glomerular pressure is increased and microalbuminuria, a marker of glomerular hypertension, is a predictor of CV events. Similarly, the lack of a nocturnal decrease in BP in these patients is also associated with an increased risk of CV events.

INTERPRETATION. Cardiovascular events occurred more frequently in patients with sodium-sensitive hypertension. Sodium sensitivity is an independent CV risk factor in Japanese patients with essential hypertension.

Comment

It was hypothesised in this study that sodium sensitivity might be the common factor in those patients who experienced CV events. The study retrospectively analysed 350 patients with essential hypertension who had had sodium sensitivity measured in the clinic. The definition of sodium sensitivity was a 10% or greater difference in BP on low-sodium or high-sodium diets. The results revealed 62 patients with sodium sensitive and 94 non-sodium sensitive. Left-ventricular hypertrophy was found more frequently in the sodium-sensitive group than in the non-sodium-sensitive group (38 *vs* 16%; $P < 0.01$), whereas significantly fewer patients in this group smoked (23 *vs* 42%; $P < 0.05$). There were 17 CV events in the sodium-sensitive group and 14 in the non-sodium-sensitive group. The rate of total, non-fatal and fatal CV events was 2.0 per 100 patient-years in the non-sodium-sensitive group and 4.3 per 100 patient-years in the sodium-sensitive group. Cox's proportional-hazards model identified sodium sensitivity ($P < 0.01$), mean arterial pressure ($P < 0.01$), and smoking ($P < 0.01$) as independent CV risk factors.

Additional comment

Weinberger *et al.* ascertained BP salt sensitivity or resistance status in 430 normal and 278 hypertensive subjects more than 25 years ago, where 338 were found to be salt sensitive. With follow-up data on 596 of the original study cohort, 123 subjects had died. As expected, age, gender, BMI, and all measures of BP, including SBP, DBP, mean arterial pressure and pulse pressure, were associated with significantly increased mortality. However, for the first time, salt sensitivity of BP was found to be associated with increased mortality even in individuals who had normal BP.

According to survival curves, normotensive salt-sensitive subjects who were 25 years or older at the time of the initial study had a cumulative mortality that was similar to that of hypertensive patients, whereas salt-resistant normotensive subjects demonstrated a significantly increased survival ($P < 0.001$).

The paper Weinberger *et al.* parallels the earlier study by Morimoto *et al.*, who found that CV events were twice as common among salt-sensitive hypertensives compared to salt-resistant hypertensives.

Salt-sensitive hypertension more common in thyroid disorders

Influence of short-time application of a low sodium diet on blood pressure in patients with hyperthyroidism or hypothyroidism during therapy.
Marcisz C, Jonderko G, Kucharz EJ. *Am J Hypertens* 2001; **14**(10): 995–1002.

BACKGROUND. Hyperthyroidism or hypothyroidism are commonly associated with altered BP. Restriction of sodium in the diet produces a decrease in BP in some individuals. It is also well known that hormones other than thyroid affect BP. The present study was designed to evaluate the influence of a low sodium diet on BP in patients with hyperthyroidism or hypothyroidism during therapy.

INTERPRETATION. The high incidence of salt-sensitive BP was found only in untreated hypothyroid patients. In addition, in hypothyroid patients the application of a low sodium diet led to a lower increase in plasma renin activity in subjects with salt-sensitive BP than in individuals with salt-resistant BP. Therefore, different mechanisms are responsible for BP elevation in patients with hyperthyroidism or hypothyroidism.

Comment

Systolic hypertension occurs in one third of all people with hyperthyroidism, and in one-fifth of people with hypothyroidism, although increased BP is due to different physiological effects of the abnormal thyroid hormone levels. The above study was designed to evaluate the effect of a short-term application of a low sodium diet on BP in patients with hyperthyroidism or hypothyroidism with simultaneous determination of plasma renin activity, aldosterone, arginine vasopressin and atrial natriuretic peptide levels.

Patients with hypertension and hypothyroidism appear to be particularly sensitive to salt intake. The paper by Marcisz *et al.* looked at 75 people with hyperthyroidism, 31 people with hypothyroidism and 37 healthy controls. BP, changes in plasma volume, serum aldosterone, atrial natriuretic peptide (ANP), vasopressin levels and plasma renin activity were measured after 3 days on a normal sodium diet and after another 3 days on a sodium-reduced diet. Although SBP was elevated in both hyper- and hypothyroid patients, mean arterial BP was higher only in the untreated hypothyroid patients. Salt sensitivity was found in about one quarter of healthy controls and hyperthyroid patients, and this proportion remained constant during thyroid therapy in the latter group. More than half of the hypothyroid patients were salt sensitive at the start of the study, but this proportion dropped to 35% after medications normalized thyroid hormone levels. Measurements of plasma renin and aldosterone levels appeared to reflect some degree of salt sensitivity, predominantly in the hypothyroid patients.

Renal endothelin ETA/ETB receptor imbalance differentiates salt-sensitive from salt-resistant spontaneous hypertension.

Rothermund L, Luckert S, Koßmehl P, Paul M, Kreutz R. *Hypertension* 2001; **37**: 275–80.

BACKGROUND. It is unclear why a subgroup of patients with essential hypertension develops salt-sensitive hypertension with progression of target organ damage (TOD) over time.

INTERPRETATION. Activation of the renal endothelin (ET) system together with an increased ETA/ETB receptor ratio may contribute to the development and progression of salt-sensitive spontaneous hypertension (SS-SH).

Comment

There are abundant experimental data indicating that the ET system plays an important role in the pathogenesis of salt-sensitive hypertension and the hypertensive TOD in this disease. This is an interesting experimental study on the role of the renal ET system (including ETA and ETB receptor regulation) in the stroke-prone spontaneously hypertensive rat (SHRSP) model of salt-sensitive spontaneous hypertension (SS-SH) compared with the spontaneously hypertensive rat (SHR) model of salt-resistant spontaneous hypertension (SR-SH). Both strains were studied after either sham-operation on a normal diet (Sham) or after unilateral nephrectomy and high NaCl loading (NX-NaCl) with 4% NaCl in diet for 6 weeks. The study indeed demonstrated that activation of the renal ET system in conjunction with an increased ETA/ETB receptor ratio contributes to decreased urinary Na^+ and to higher susceptibility to the development of SS-SH and kidney damage in SHRSP-NX-NaCl compared with SR-SS in the SHR-NX-NaCl model. However, whether this unfavourable imbalance of renal ETA/ETB receptor ratio may also be involved in the progression of salt-sensitive hypertension in other experimental models and ultimately in patients with salt-sensitive hypertension remains to be investigated. In this regard, ETA receptor antagonism may become a promising new approach in the pharmacological treatment of salt-sensitive hypertension.

Cognitive function and hypertension

Introduction

The importance of looking at elderly groups continues to increase as the population ages, especially in the developed countries. Many of us agreed the beneficial effects of treating hypertension in elderly individuals and the relatively small number 'needed-to-treat' to avert an acute cerebrovascular event. Since the risk of developing dementia increases at least nine-fold after a stroke, it seems plausible that risk factors for stroke could also influence the development of dementia or decline in cognitive function. A putative link between dementia and hypertension has long been suspected, even if large scale testing of the hypothesis has not, until now, been carried out. Indeed, a longitudinal study of nearly 1000 elderly Swedish men has shown an inverse relationship between DBP at age 50, and cognitive function at age 70. The Study on COgnitive and Prognosis in the Elderly (SCOPE) is the first major clinical trial to consider the impact of hypertension, and its adequate control, on dementia and cognitive function.

Hypertension linked to impaired cognitive function in the elderly

Cognitive performance in hypertensive and normotensive older subjects.

Harrington F, Saxby BK, McKeith IG, Wesnes K, Ford GA. *Hypertension* 2000; **36**(6): 1079–82.

BACKGROUND. Longitudinal studies suggest that hypertension in midlife is associated with cognitive impairment in later life. Cross-sectional studies are difficult to interpret because BP can change with onset of dementia and the inclusion of subjects on treatment and with hypertensive end-organ damage can make analysis difficult.

INTERPRETATION. Hypertension in older subjects is associated with impaired cognition in a broad range of areas in the absence of clinically evident TOD.

Comment

In about 40% of elderly people who develop cognitive impairment or dementia, the problem is related to vascular changes subsequent to hypertension. In this paper, mild to moderate hypertension in older subjects is associated with impaired cognition in a broad range of areas in the absence of clinically evident target organ damage. These subjects were found to perform slower and less accurately than normotensive people in cognitive tests. As hypertension seems to be associated with impaired cognition, it raises the possibility that antihypertensive therapy could possibly prevent or delay cognitive decline. Indeed, the Syst-Eur Vascular Dementia project in 1998, for example, reported a 50% decline in the incidence of dementia in elderly patients taking the calcium channel blocker nitrendipine.

Whilst several previous studies have found a link between hypertension and cognitive impairment, the effect of increasing BP on cognitive performance in older men and women without cerebrovascular disease has not yet been investigated. In this study, of 107 moderately hypertensive (BP 164/89) and 116 normotensive individuals (BP 131/74), mean age 76, without cerebrovascular disease

Table 2.8 Results of cognitive assessment battery in hypertensive and normotensive groups

Ms (%)	Hypertensive	Normotensive	P
Simple reaction time	346 (100)	318 (56)	<0.05
Choice reaction time	510 (75)	498 (72)	0.08
Number vigilance accuracy	99.2 (2.5)	99.9 (0.9)	<0.01
Memory scanning reaction time	867 (243)	789 (159)	<0.01
Immediate word recognition			
Reaction time	947 (261)	886 (192)	<0.05
Accuracy	88.8 (11)	89.3 (9.7)	0.68
Delayed word recognition			
Reaction time	937 (230)	856 (184)	<0.05
Accuracy	83.5 (16)	87.9 (9.8)	<0.01
Picture recognition			
Reaction time	952 (184)	894 (137)	<0.01
Accuracy	88 (13)	89.1 (10.4)	0.29
Spatial memory			
Reaction time	1390 (439)	1258 (394)	<0.01
Accuracy	64 (32)	79 (20)	<0.0001

Data are mean SD.

Source: Harrington *et al.* (2000).

or any vascular risk factors, the hypertensive group performed slower in all tests – simple reaction time, immediate and delayed word recognition time, picture recognition time, number vigilance, special memory, and memory scanning – except choice reaction time.

In addition, hypertensive subjects performed less accurately compared to normotensives. The 10% decrement observed in hypertensives is approximately two or three times greater in patients suffering from mild dementia.

Hypertension may directly affect cognitive function by a number of different mechanisms:

- asymptomatic cerebrovascular disease, e.g. multiple small strokes, which might have been increasingly prevalent in the hypertensive group, can lead to dementia.
- certain brain lesions have been associated with hypertension and impaired cognitive function
- hypertension has been found to influence cerebral autoregulation and blood flow, which suggests psychomotor impairment might be directly triggered by elevated BP.
- the apolipoprotein E allele, which has been associated with both CVD and dementia, suggests a genetic link between hypertension and cognitive function.

Study on Cognitive and Prognosis in the Elderly (SCOPE): baseline characteristics.

Hansson L, Lithell H, Skoog I, et al. Blood Press 2000; **9**: 146–151.

BACKGROUND. The Study on COgnition and Prognosis in the Elderly (SCOPE) is a multi-centre, prospective, randomized, double-blind, parallel-group study. The primary objective of SCOPE is to assess the effect of the angiotensin II type 1 (AT1) receptor blocker, candesartan cilexetil 8-16 mg once daily, on major cardiovascular events in elderly patients (70-89 years of age) with mild hypertension (DBP 90-99 and/or SBP 160-179 mmHg). A total of 4964 patients from 15 participating countries are being followed for a minimum of 2 years.

INTERPRETATION. The mean age of the patients at enrolment was 76 years, the ratio of male to female patients was approximately 1:2, and 52% of patients were already being treated with an antihypertensive agent at enrolment. The majority of patients (88%) were educated to at least primary school level. At randomization, mean sitting BP values were SBP 166 mmHg and DBP 90 mmHg, and the mean Mini Mental State Examination (MMSE) score was 28. Previous CVD in the study population included myocardial infarction (4%), stroke (4%) and atrial fibrillation (4%). Men, more often than women, had a history of previous MI, stroke and atrial fibrillation. A greater percentage of men were smokers (13% vs 6% in women) and had attended university (11% vs 3% of women). Of the randomized patients, 21% were 80 years of age. In this age group smoking was less common (4% vs 10% for 70-79-year-olds) and fewer had attended university (4% vs 7% for 70-79-year-olds). The incidence of MI was similar in both age groups. However, stroke and atrial fibrillation had occurred approximately twice as frequently in the older patients. The patients' mean age at baseline was similar in the participating countries, and most countries showed the approximate 1:2 ratio for male to female patients. There was also little inter-country variation in terms of mean SBP, DBP or MMSE score. However, there was considerable regional variation in the percentage of patients on therapy prior to enrolment.

Comment

SCOPE is particularly interesting for a variety of reasons. Firstly, it is the first major study of antihypertensive therapy on major cardiovascular events in a really elderly population (79–89 years of age). Secondly, it is targeting those with mild hypertension i.e. with SBP of 160–179 mmHg and/or DBP of 90–99 mmHg. Thirdly, it is the first major study to consider the effect on major CV events – rather than simply on BP levels – of one of the angiotensin II receptor blockers. But perhaps of most interest of all are the secondary objectives of the study – to test the hypothesis that antihypertensive therapy can prevent cognitive decline (as measured by the MMSE) and dementia, and to assess the effect of therapy on total mortality, MI, stroke, renal function and hospitalization. If the SCOPE study does prove a definitive causal link between hypertension in the elderly and dementia by showing a positive correlation between degree of BP control and cognitive function, there will undoubtedly be an increase in demand for treatment from the consumer. More importantly, it will provide yet another incentive to treat elderly hypertensives.

Hormone replacement therapy

Introduction

Recent large prospective randomised studies, the Heart and Estrogen-progestin Replacement Study (HERS) and the Estrogen Replacement and Atherosclerosis (ERA) trial have failed to confirm the observations from several large epidemiological surveys which showed a clear benefit of hormone replacement therapy (HRT) in the prevention of CHD. Few arguments had been raised to try to explain the discrepancy. One of these arguments was the bias in patient selection theory that woman on HRT might have been healthier and taken a greater interest in modifying CV risks. Some have also argued that a single, relatively short clinical trial may not reliably predict long-term benefit, especially when so much *a priori* evidence suggests that estrogen should be beneficial. Hence, several more randomized clinical trials are currently underway.

SBP increases in both sexes with age, but before middle age, SBP among women is typically lower than in men; afterwards, both SBP and DBP generally become higher among women. However, an association between HRT and hypertension in postmenopausal women reported in the 1970s and 1980s prompted many physicians to consider high BP as a contraindication to HRT. Cross-sectional studies, however, reported similar or even lower SBP and DBPs in postmenopausal women taking HRT and those not taking HRT. Of note, neither of the two large randomized trials of HRT and secondary prevention of CVD – the HERS and the ERA trial – included BP. The Nurses' Health Study, which included more than 70 000 postmenopausal women, also did not study BP. In the Baltimore Longitudinal Study on Aging (BLSA), HRT may suppress the increase in SBP often seen in women after menopause, especially in older women and those with higher BMI.

Hormone replacement therapy and longitudinal changes in blood pressure in postmenopausal women.

Scuteri A, Bos AJ, Brant LJ, Talbot L, Lakatta EG, Fleg JL. *Ann Intern Med* 2001; **135**(4): 229–38.

BACKGROUND. The incidence of hypertension in postmenopausal women exceeds that in age-matched men. Longitudinal studies relating HRT to BP changes are sparse.

INTERPRETATION. Postmenopausal women taking HRT have a smaller increase in SBP over time than those not taking HRT. This difference is intensified at older ages.

Comment

The aim of this study was to investigate the association between HRT and longitudinal changes in BP in postmenopausal women.

The BLSA was a prospective study of community-dwelling volunteers from Baltimore and Washington. This paper examined BPs over time in 225 healthy, normotensive postmenopausal women with a mean age of about 64 years, followed for about 5 years. Of these, 77 used both oestrogen and progestin, and 149 used neither. Blood pressure, as well as other lifestyle variables and CV risk factors were measured at baseline and every 2 years thereafter. They found SBP was similar between users and non-users at baseline, at about 133 and 132 mmHg respectively. Over time, though, average SBP increased less among users than non-users (mean 7.6 mmHg, compared to a rise of 18.7 mmHg in non-users). None of the available variables that might influence blood pressure (BMI, total and HDL cholesterol levels, smoking, alcohol intake, physical activity, or family history of CVD) influenced this relationship. In addition, the smaller increase in SBP over time in HRT users was more evident at older age. Finally, HRT use did not affect DBP; values did not change significantly over time in either group. However, additional longitudinal studies are needed to confirm these observations.

HRT – has the bubble burst?

Postmenopausal hormone therapy and risk of stroke: the Heart and Estrogen-progestin Replacement Study (HERS).

Simon JA, Hsia J, Cauley JA, *et al. Circulation* 2001; **103**(5): 638–42.

BACKGROUND. Observational studies have shown that postmenopausal hormone therapy may increase, decrease, or have no effect on the risk of stroke. To date, no clinical trial has examined this question.

Table 2.9 Hormone replacement therapy and risk of various stroke outcomes

Outcome	Relative hazard	95% CI
Non-fatal stroke	1.18	0.83–1.66
Fatal stroke	1.61	0.74–3.55
TIA	0.90	0.57–1.42
Any stroke or TIA	1.09	0.84–1.43

Source: Simon *et al.* (2001).

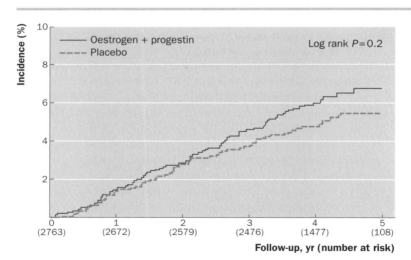

Fig. 2.4 Kaplan–Meier estimate of cumulative incidence of stroke events. Number of women observed at each year of follow-up and still free from stroke events is provided in parentheses; lines become thinner when this number drops below half of the cohort. Log-rank *P* value is 0.20. Source: Simon *et al.* (2001).

INTERPRETATION. Hormone therapy with conjugated equine oestrogen and progestin had no significant effect on the risk for stroke among postmenopausal women with coronary disease.

Comment

The aim of this study was to investigate the relationship between oestrogen plus progestin therapy and risk of stroke among postmenopausal women.

Heart and Estrogen/progestin Replacement Study (HERS) research group

Randomized trial of estrogen plus progestin for secondary prevention of coronary heart disese in postmenopausal women.
Hulley S, Grady D, Bush T, *et al. JAMA* 1998; **280**(7): 605–13.

BACKGROUND. Observational studies have found lower rates of CHD in postmenopausal women who take oestrogen than in women who do not, but this potential benefit has not been confirmed in clinical trials.

INTERPRETATION. During an average follow-up of 4.1 years, treatment with oral conjugated equine oestrogen plus medroxyprogesterone acetate did not reduce the overall rate of coronary heart disease CHD events in postmenopausal women with established coronary disease. The treatment did increase the rate of thromboembolic events and gallbladder disease. Based on the finding of no overall CV benefit and a pattern of early increase in risk of CHD events, we do not recommend starting this treatment for the purpose of secondary prevention of CHD. However, given the favourable pattern of CHD events after several years of therapy, it could be appropriate for women already receiving this treatment to continue.

Comment

For many years, HRT has been promoted as being crucial for the prevention of CVD. Much of these data are based upon cross-sectional or cohort analyses, which have been criticized for a 'healthy cohort' effect. Only recently have well-conducted randomized placebo-controlled trials shown that HRT is not cardioprotective. The HERS trial also suggested that HRT use may be associated with an increase in cardiac events in the first year amongst patients with existing coronary artery disease.

Recent new data from the HERS trial show no effect of HRT on the risk of stroke or transient ischaemic attack (TIA) among postmenopausal women with established heart disease. The objective of this HERS paper was to determine if oestrogen plus progestin therapy alters the risk for CHD events in postmenopausal women with established coronary disease.

HERS was the first randomized trial to show no overall effect of HRT treatment in 2763 women, who were randomly assigned to take conjugated equine oestrogen plus progestin, or placebo over 4.1 years of follow up. There was an apparent early increase in risk with treatment compared to placebo, followed later by a protective effect.

In the overall group, 149 women, or about 5%, had 165 strokes. Of these, 85% were ischaemic, and resulted in 26 deaths. Analysis showed no significant association between HRT and the risk of non-fatal stroke, fatal stroke or TIA. By the end of the study, about 7% of women taking HRT had had a fatal or non-fatal stroke, compared to 5% in the placebo group, but this difference was not statistically significant.

Effects of estrogen replacement on the progression of coronary-artery atherosclerosis.

Herrington DM, Reboussin DM, Brosnihan KB, *et al. N Engl J Med* 2000; **343**(8): 522–9.

BACKGROUND. Heart disease is a major cause of illness and death in women. To understand better the role of oestrogen in the treatment and prevention of heart disease, more information is needed about its effects on coronary atherosclerosis and the extent to which concomitant progestin therapy may modify these effects.

INTERPRETATION. Neither oestrogen alone nor oestrogen plus medroxyprogesterone acetate affected the progression of coronary atherosclerosis in women with established disease. These results suggest that such women should not use oestrogen replacement with an expectation of CV benefit.

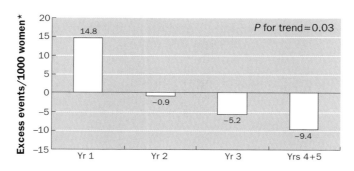

*Compared to placebo

Fig. 2.5 Excess CHD events by year in HERS among women taking oestrogen plus progestin therapy. *P* = 0.05 compared to placebo. Source: Herrington *et al.* (2001).

Comment

The National Heart, Lung, and Blood Institute funded ERA trial, like HERS, was a secondary prevention trial. The study examined whether unopposed conjugated equine oestrogen or oestrogen plus medroxyprogesterone acetate (MPA) would affect progression of coronary artery atherosclerosis in 309 women with angiographically verified coronary disease. After baseline angiography, women were randomized to receive 0.625 mg of conjugated oestrogen per day, 0.625 mg of conjugated oestrogen plus 2.5 mg of MPA per day, or placebo and were followed for a mean of 3.2 years. Follow-up angiography revealed that women in the two hormone treatment groups had essentially the same rate of progression of coronary disease as the placebo group. There were also no differences among numerous secondary angiographic outcomes. These data are consistent with the results of the HERS that showed no overall effect of oestrogen plus MPA on the risk of clinical CV events in women with established heart disease. Since similar results were seen in both the unopposed oestrogen and the oestrogen plus MPA groups, these data suggest that the null effect in HERS was not a function of the use of MPA.

On the basis of these results, women with heart disease should not use conjugated oestrogen, alone or in combination with MPA, with an expectation of CV benefit.

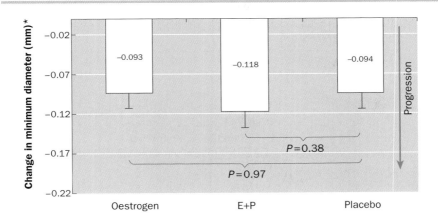

*After covariate adjustment

Fig. 2.6 Change in mean minimum coronary diameter (adjusted for pre-specified covariates) by treatment arm among 248 women in the ERA trial. E + P = oestrogen plus progestin. Source: Herrington *et al.* (2001).

Obesity and hypertension

Introduction

Obesity, no doubt, is a complex medical problem. While the main cause of death is CV related, CVD is merely part of the obesity-related morbidity, physically as well as psychosocially. The prevalence of obesity or of being overweight has reached an epidemic level in developed countries while the rest of the developing world is catching up.

Obesity is associated with a pre-clinical manifestation of cardiovascular disease, which is prognostically relevant. Obese individuals have a relative risk for the development of hypertension that is three times that of lean subjects, and risk estimates from the Framingham Heart Study suggest that 78% of hypertension in men and 65% in women can be directly ascribed to obesity. However, the complex mechanisms linking obesity and hypertension remain poorly understood. For example, increasing evidence suggests that activation of the sympathetic nervous system plays a key role in obesity hypertension. Obese subjects often have increased plasma and urine norepinephrine and other indirect measures of sympathetic activation.

In the Framingham Heart Study, obesity was an independent predictor of echocardiographic left ventricular hypertrophy (LVH) with a 51% increase in the risk of LVH in women and a 47% increase in men for every 2 kg/m^2 increment in BMI. As we will see in one of the studies below, obesity is the strongest determinant of increased left ventricular mass (LVM); its effects on LVM are additive to those of age, hypertension and diabetes.

Most obese hypertensives will ultimately need medication for BP reduction. Given the fact that obesity is frequently part of a complex metabolic syndrome with coexisting dyslipidaemia, insulin resistant diabetes and other obesity-related medical problems, the choice of antihypertensive agent must take all these factors into account; for example α-adrenergic blocker may have a positive metabolic effect by improving insulin sensitivity and lipid metabolism as well as lowering SBP and DBP. Indeed, although prolonging life is important, quality of life is equally crucial in these patients.

Although both hypertension and obesity are risk factors for cardiovascular disease and death, obese hypertensive patients actually have better clinical outcomes than those who are lean, despite having fewer metabolic abnormalities. Population studies have suggested, for example, that over a 10-year period, lean hypertensives may face upwards of a 20% increase in mortality or clinical events. Studies designed to investigate the differences between obese and lean subjects could potentially reveal important mechanistic factors that would help further our understanding in the pathophysiology of disease in the obese. This will be elicited in two of the studies below.

Obesity and hypertension: a growing problem.

Pickering TG. *J Clin Hypertens* 2001; **3**(4): 252–4.

BACKGROUND. The prevalence of obesity has increased markedly in the US and other countries in the past 20 years: in 1978, one quarter of Americans were overweight, as defined by a BMI of 25–30 kg/m^2, and in 1990, one-third were overweight – a 33% increase.

INTERPRETATION. There is no simple solution to the epidemic of obesity. Its origin lies in our culture and society, and is epitomized by the suburban mall, with its drive-through fast-food restaurants. Dealing with it will require action at several levels: policy, education and incorporation of a team approach to patient care that involves dieticians and health educators. However, most physicians often feel that there is little they can do about it, but then obesity is too big a problem to ignore.

Comment

This paper gives details account of the current epidemic in obesity from children to the adolescents and adults in the US. There is evidence that American children are less physically active today than in the past, both at home and at school. Between 1984 and 1990, the percentage of high school students enrolled in physical education classes declined substantially. The long-term consequences of adolescent obesity are already clear. About 25% of obese children between the ages of 5 and 11 have elevated BP, and the Bogalusa Heart Study showed that overweight adolescents are eight times more likely than lean adolescents to have hypertension as adults. Despite varying definitions of obesity, the findings are quite consistent and indicate that childhood obesity results in a relative risk of about 1.5 for all-cause mortality and 2.0 for CHD mortality. The implication of these studies is that the incidence of new cases of CVD is almost certainly going to increase in the next few years, as the plaques now incubating in our overweight adolescents finally mature. Surveys have shown that more than two-thirds of all Americans are trying to lose or maintain weight, but only 20% of those trying to lose weight are using the recommended combination of calorie restriction and exercise of more than 150 minutes per week.

The worldwide obesity epidemic.

James PT, Leach R, Kalamara E, Shayeghi M. *Obes Res* 2001; **9**(suppl 4): 228S–33S.

BACKGROUND. The recent World Health Organization (WHO) agreement on the standardized classification of overweight and obese, based on BMI, allows a comparable analysis of prevalence rates worldwide for the first time.

INTERPRETATION. In Asia, however, there is a demand for a more limited range for normal BMIs (i.e. 18.5–22.9 kg/m^2) rather than 18.5–24.9 kg/m^2) because of the high prevalence of comorbidities, particularly diabetes and hypertension. In children, the International Obesity Task-Force age-, sex-, and BMI-specific cut-off points are increasingly being used. BMI data is currently being evaluated globally as part of a new millennium analysis of the Global Burden of Disease. WHO is analysing data in terms of 20 or more principal risk factors contributing to the primary causes of disability and lost lives in the 191 countries within the WHO. The prevalence rates for overweight and obese people are different in each region, with the Middle East, Central and Eastern Europe and North America having higher prevalence rates. In most countries, women show a greater BMI distribution with higher obesity rates than do men. Obesity is usually now associated with poverty, even in developing countries. Relatively new data suggest that abdominal obesity in adults, with its associated enhanced morbidity, occurs particularly in those who had lower birth weights and early childhood stunting. Waist measurements in nationally representative studies are scarce but will now be needed to estimate the full impact of the worldwide obesity epidemic.

Prevalence of the metabolic syndrome among US adults. Findings from the Third National Health and Nutrition Examination Survey.

Ford ES, Giles WH, Dietz WH. *JAMA* 2002; **287**: 356–9.

BACKGROUND. The Third Report of the National Cholesterol Education Program Expert Panel on Detection, Evaluation, and Treatment of High Blood Cholesterol in Adults (ATP III) highlights the importance of treating patients with the metabolic syndrome to prevent cardiovascular disease. Limited information is available about the prevalence of the metabolic syndrome in the United States, however.

INTERPRETATION. These results from a representative sample of US adults show that the metabolic syndrome is highly prevalent. The large numbers of US residents with the metabolic syndrome may have important implications for the health care sector.

Comment

The recently released ATP III report drew attention to the importance of the metabolic syndrome and provided a working definition of this syndrome for the first time. The metabolic syndrome as defined by ATP III is (3 of the following abnormalities): waist circumference > 102 cm in men and > 88 cm in women; serum triglycerides level of ≥ 150 mg/dl (1.69 mmol/l); HDL- cholesterol level of < 40 mg/dl (1.04 mmol/l) in men and < 50 mg/dl (1.29 mmol/l) in women; BP of ≥ 130/85 mmHg; or serum glucose level of ≥ 110 mg/dl (6.1 mmol/l). The data was derived from 8814 men and women aged 20 years or older from the Third National Health and Nutrition Examination Survey (NHANES III) 1988–1994, a cross-sectional health survey of a nationally representative sample of the non-

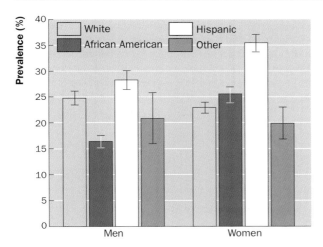

Fig. 2.7 Age-adjusted prevalence of the metabolic syndrome among 8814 US adults aged at least 20 years, by sex and race or ethnicity. NHANES III 1988-1994 data are presented as percentage (SE). Source: Ford *et al.* (2002).

institutionalized civilian US population. The results showed that ~22% of US adults (24% after age adjustment) have the metabolic syndrome. The unrelenting increase in the prevalence of obesity in the United States suggests that the current prevalence of the metabolic syndrome is now very likely higher than that estimated from 1988–1994 NHANES III data. However, limited information is available about the prevalence of the metabolic syndrome on the other side of the Atlantic. Because the implications of the metabolic syndrome for health care are substantial, we should seek to establish the prevalence of this condition.

Treatment of obesity hypertension and diabetes syndrome.

Zanella MT, Kohlmann O Jr, Ribeiro AB. *Hypertension* 2001; **38**(3 Pt 2): 705–8.

BACKGROUND. **Obesity has been shown to be an independent risk factor for CHD. The insulin resistance associated with obesity contributes to the development of other cardiovascular risk factors, including dyslipidaemia, hypertension and type 2 diabetes.**

INTERPRETATION. Diuretics and beta-blockers are reported to reduce insulin sensitivity and increase triglyceride levels, whereas calcium channel blockers (CCBs) are metabolically neutral and angiotensin-converting enzyme inhibitors (ACEIs) increase insulin sensitivity. For the high-risk hypertensive diabetic patients, ACE inhibition has proven to confer additional renal and vascular protection. Because hypertension and glycaemic control are very important determinants of cardiovascular outcome in obese diabetic hypertensive patients, weight reduction, physical exercise, and a combination of antihypertensive and insulin sensitisers agents are strongly recommended to achieve target BP and glucose levels. However, pharmacological treatment should take into account the effects of the antihypertensive agents on insulin sensitivity and lipid profile.

Comment

The coexistence of hypertension and diabetes increases the risk for macrovascular and microvascular complications, thus predisposing patients to cardiac death, CHF, CHD, cerebral and peripheral vascular diseases, nephropathy and retino-pathy. Both non-pharmacological and pharmacological treatments for the obese hypertensives with diabetic syndrome were discussed in detail with emphasis on antidiabetic therapy, ACEIs, diuretics, beta-blockers and CCBs. Because the BP targets are difficult to achieve in these patients, weight reduction, physical exercise, and a combination of several antihypertensive and antidiabetic agents are usually necessary.

Body weight reduction increases insulin sensitivity and improves both blood glucose and BP control. Diuretics and beta-blockers are reported to reduce insulin sensitivity and increase triglyceride levels, whereas CCBs are metabolically neutral and ACEIs increase insulin sensitivity.

For the high-risk hypertensive diabetic patients, ACE inhibition has proven to confer additional renal and vascular protection. Metformin therapy also improves insulin sensitivity and has been associated with decreases in cardiovascular events in obese diabetic patients. Antihypertensive treatment in diabetics decreases cardiovascular mortality and slows the decline in glomerular function.

Choice of drug treatment for obesity-related hypertension: where is the evidence?

Sharma AM, Pischon T, Engeli S, Scholze J. *J Hypertens* 2001; **19**(4): 667–74.

BACKGROUND. Hypertension and obesity are common medical conditions independently associated with increased cardiovascular risk. Many large epidemiological studies have demonstrated associations between BMI and BP and there is evidence to suggest that obesity is a causal factor in the development of hypertension in obese individuals.

INTERPRETATION. This paper reviews the theoretical reasons for the differential use of the major classes of antihypertensive agents in the pharmacological management of obesity-related hypertension and also considers the potential role of anti-obesity agents.

Comment

All hypertension management guidelines consider weight reduction as a first step in the management of increased BP in obese individuals. Weight reduction may be achieved by behaviour modification, diet and exercise, or by the use of anti-obesity medications. However, the long-term outcomes of weight management programmes for obesity are generally poor, and most hypertensive patients will require antihypertensive drug treatment. Some classes of antihypertensive agents may have potentially unwanted effects on some of the metabolic and haemodynamic abnormalities that link obesity and hypertension, yet most hypertension guidelines fail to provide specific advice on the pharmacological management of obese patients. This may be because there are currently no studies examining the efficacy of specific antihypertensive agents in reducing mortality in obese hypertensive patients.

Lean versus obese hypertensives

Antihypertensive effect of alpha- and beta-adrenergic blockade in obese and lean hypertensive subjects.
Wofford MR, Anderson DC Jr, Brown CA, Jones DW, Miller ME, Hall JE.
Am J Hypertens 2001; **14**(7 Pt 1): 694–8.

BACKGROUND. **Several potential mechanisms have been proposed to explain the increased prevalence of hypertension in obese people, including metabolic abnormalities such as insulin resistance, abnormalities of the kidney resulting in increased sodium and water reabsorption, activation of the renin–angiotensin system, and activation of the sympathetic nervous system. Increasing evidence suggests that activation of the sympathetic nervous system plays a key role in obesity hypertension.**

INTERPRETATION. The results indicate that BP is more sensitive to adrenergic blockade in obese than in lean hypertensive patients and suggest that increased sympathetic activity may be an important factor in the maintenance of hypertension in obesity.

Comment

The purpose of this study was to compare the responses to adrenergic blockade in obese and lean hypertensive patients using 12-h ambulatory BP monitoring (ABPM) to detect changes in heart rate and BP and thus determine the contribution of the adrenergic system in mediating hypertension in obese (BMI $28 \geq$ kg/m^2) and lean (BMI < 25 kg/m^2). Participants were given doxazosin (alpha-adrenergic blocker) during the first week, with atenolol (beta-adrenergic blocker) added in the second week; all patients underwent a second ABPM session one month later. The effect of treatment on the mean arterial BP could be summarised in the histogram below. The baselines BP of obese and lean hypertensive patients were not significantly

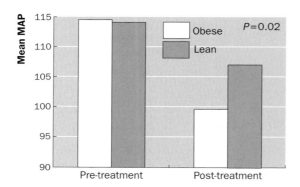

Fig. 2.8 Mean arterial pressures in obese and lean patients before and after treatment with doxazosin and atenolol. Source: Wofford *et al.* (2001).

different and there was no significant difference in heart rate after 1 month of adrenergic blockade. The results suggest that increased adrenergic activity may contribute to obesity hypertension. However, this does not imply that adrenergic blockade is the ideal antihypertensive therapy for obese patients. It is of note that beta-blockers can adversely affect the metabolic profile, causing weight gain, dyslipidemia and insulin resistance whereas alpha-adrenergic blocker lowers SBP and DBP and may have a positive metabolic effect by improving insulin sensitivity and lipid metabolism. It is therefore important that future studies should test the effectiveness of adrenergic blockers in correcting the metabolic abnormalities associated with obesity as well as in reducing BP. Additional studies are also needed to evaluate the quantitative importance of the sympathetic nervous system and other mechanisms of obesity hypertension in humans.

Contrasting clinical properties and exercise responses in obese and lean hypertensive patients.

Weber MA, Neutel JM, Smith DH. *J Am Coll Cardiol* 2001; **37**(1): 169–74.

BACKGROUND. **Although lean hypertensive patients have fewer metabolic abnormalities than obese hypertensive patients, paradoxically they appear to have a poorer cardiovascular prognosis. This may be related the differences in activity of the renin–angiotensin and sympathetic nervous systems at rest or during exercise between lean and obese hypertensive patients.**

INTERPRETATION. Compared with obese hypertensive patients, cardiovascular properties in lean hypertensive patients are more dependent on catecholamines and the renin system. The different neuroendocrine responses to dynamic stimuli in lean and obese patients also might help to explain the disparity in their cardiovascular outcomes.

Comment

Despite frequent association of their metabolic abnormalities with adverse cardio-vascular events, obese hypertensive patients actually have better clinical outcomes than those who are lean. The findings of this study emphasise the differences between lean and obese types of hypertension in neuroendocrine response to exercise that may contribute to the differing cardiovascular properties and outcomes

Table 2.10 Changes in plasma norepinephrine in response to standing, and renin and epinephrine in response to treadmill exercise

Measure	Lean hypertensive patients	Obese hypertensive patients	P value
Plasma norepinephrine in response to standing	55%	22%	<0.05
Increase in renin in response to treadmill exercise	145%	65%	<0.01
Increase in epinephrine in response to treadmill exercise	500%	200%	<0.05

Source: Weber *et al.* (2001).

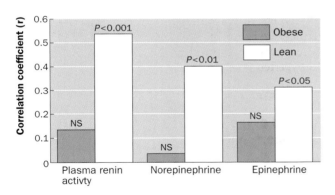

Fig. 2.9 Correlation coefficients for the relations between LVMI and plasma renin activity or plasma concentrations of norepinephrine and epinephrine in obese and lean hypertensive patients. The r values are significant by univariate analysis for each of the variables in the lean patients; however, by multivariate analysis, only the plasma renin activity and norepinephrine relations remain in the model. Source: Weber *et al.* (2001).

and thus may have implications for different therapy between the two groups. Study results showed that, compared with the lean normotensive subjects, both lean and obese hypertensives had greater left ventricular mass index (LVMI) values, but on multivariate analysis, LVMI correlated significantly with plasma renin activity and plasma norepinephrine in the lean, but not the obese, hypertensive patients. Arterial compliance, measured by the ratio of stroke volume to pulse pressure, was also reduced in the lean hypertensive patients, and the ratio correlated significantly with plasma norepinephrine. It is possible, therefore, that arterial stiffening may be a characteristic of lean hypertension that distinguishes it from obese hypertension. Interestingly, the obese hypertensive group also had a reduced sympathetic and renin system response both on standing and exercise even in comparison to the lean normotensive controls. Thus, for obese hypertensives, although seemingly at higher baseline risk, the sympathetic system and renin system are stimulated far less

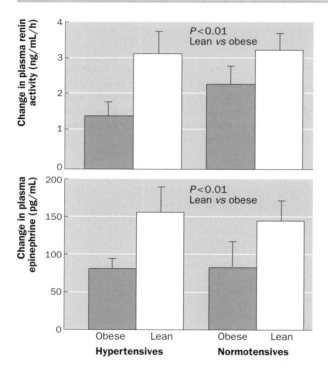

Fig. 2.10 Changes in plasma renin activity and in plasma norepinephrine (PNE) concentrations during treadmill testing in obese and lean hypertensive patients and normotensive volunteers. By two-way analysis of variance, the differences between the obese and lean patients were significant, but not the differences between hypertensive patients and normotensive subjects Source: Weber *et al.* (2001).

during stress and so confer cardioprotection. In contrast, the increased activity of the sympathetic and renin-angiotensin systems in the lean hypertensives, not only raise BP, but also have direct pathologic effects on the vascular systems. Accordingly, the underlying mechanism of hypertension in obesity appears to be mainly increased plasma volume and thus response is better with a diuretic. This is supported by data from Systolic Hypertension in the Elderly (SHEP), where the best outcomes with diuretic therapy were among those with a BMI of 30, considered the threshold of obesity. Those with a BMI between 20 and 25 – otherwise an ideal measure – had a higher death rate and a higher incidence of events than the obese group. The lean hypertensive, on the other hand, might fare better with an ACE inhibitor, angiotensin receptor blocker, or a beta-blocker.

The importance of age and obesity on the relation between diabetes and left ventricular mass.

Kuperstein R, Hanly P, Niroumand M, Sasson Z. *J Am Coll Cardiol* 2001; **37**(7): 1957–62.

B A C K G R O U N D . Epidemiological studies demonstrate a general rise of LVM with aging, but whether this phenomenon is independent or a function of coexisting diseases that accompany the aging process is unclear. Although obesity, hypertension and diabetes often coexist and increase in prevalence with age, studies of LVM in diabetics have been reported in mostly non-obese populations, and with little regard to the age-hypertension-obesity interactions and effects on LVM.

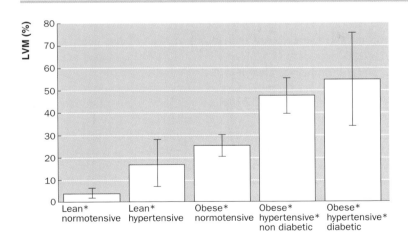

Fig. 2.11 Prevalence of LVH according to obesity, hypertension, and diabetes (*n* = 875). Source: Kuperstein *et al.* (2001).

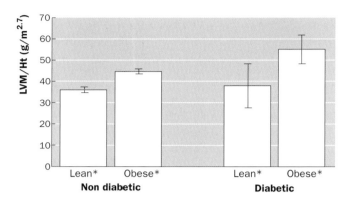

Fig. 2.12 Interaction of obesity with diabetes on left ventricular mass corrected for height 2.7 (LVM/Ht2.7), excluding coronary artery disease patients (*n* = 818). Source: Kuperstein *et al.* (2001).

INTERPRETATION. Age, obesity, hypertension and diabetes are all independent determinants of LVM. The magnitude of the effect of diabetes on LVM is mainly consequent to a significant interaction of diabetes with obesity and age.

Comment

In this study the authors meticulously analysed the impact of age, obesity, hypertension, coronary artery disease (CAD), and DM on LVM in a large cohort of a mainly obese patient population. They found that obesity was the strongest predictor of LVM (calculated using the Devereux formula and corrected for height 2.7 [VM/Ht]) in this population, and its effects on LVM were additional to the clear and independent effects of age, CAD and hypertension. Diabetes is also an independent predictor of LVM, but its effects are magnified through significant interactions with obesity and increasing age. As diabetic subjects are usually older and obese, these interactions explain most of the increase in LVM in this population. It is of note that more than 90% of the patients studied were Caucasians, and thus the findings cannot be extrapolated to African-Americans, a population with a high prevalence of obesity-diabetes-hypertension. However, the inclusion of a large number of obese and hypertensive subjects allowed an analysis of the effects of DM on LVM in relation to these most commonly associated factors.

Effect of obesity on endothelium-dependent, nitric oxide-mediated vasodilation in normotensive individuals and patients with essential hypertension.

Higashi Y, Sasaki S, Nakagawa K, Matsuura H, Chayama K, Oshima T.
Am J Hypertens 2001; **14**(10): 1038–45.

BACKGROUND. Several studies have shown that hypertension and obesity are associated with an altered form of endothelial nitric oxide (NO) release. It has been postulated that the hypertension- and obesity-induced cardiovascular complications may contribute to abnormal NO production.

INTERPRETATION. The findings suggest that obesity and hypertension are independently involved in abnormal endothelium-dependent vasodilation by attenuated nitric oxide production.

Comment

The purpose of this study was to determine the interdependent and independent effects of hypertension and obesity on endothelial function in humans. The study evaluated the forearm blood flow response to endothelium-dependent vasodilation evoked by acetylcholine and endothelium-independent vasodilation evoked by isosorbide dinitrate in four groups: lean and obese normotensive individuals and lean and obese hypertensive patients without a history of smoking, hypercholesterolemia, diabetes mellitus and renal dysfunction. The results demonstrated that endothelium-dependent, NO-mediated vasodilation is impaired to a similar degree in obese normotensive individuals and lean hypertensive patients, and impaired to a greater extent in patients with obesity and high BP. Multivariate regression analysis revealed that obesity and high BP contribute independently to the impairment of endothelium-dependent vasodilation in the brachial artery. These observations are in keeping with previous studies demonstrating that endothelium-dependent forearm vasodilation is impaired in obesity and hypertension. However, in this study, there was no significant difference in the degree of insulin resistance or hyperinsulinemia between lean hypertensive patients and lean normotensive individuals and between obese hypertensive patients and obese normotensive individuals. Such findings suggest that insulin resistance or hyperinsulinemia may not always play important roles in hypertension.

One important finding of this study was that the combination of obesity and hypertension has additive effects on endothelium-dependent vasodilation. Therefore, it is important to control not only BP but also body weight in patients with obesity and hypertension.

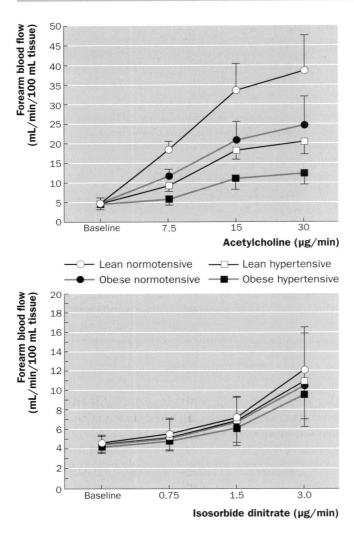

Fig. 2.13 Line graphs show the forearm blood flow responses to acetylcholine (top) and isosorbide dinitrate (bottom) in lean and obese normotensive individuals and lean and obese hypertensive patients. Source: Higashi *et al.* (2001).

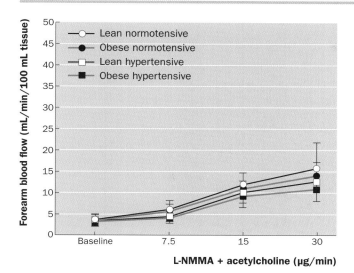

Fig. 2.14 Line graphs show the forearm blood flow response to acetylcholine in the presence of L-NMMA in lean and obese normotensive individuals and lean and obese hypertensive patients. L-NMMA = NG-monomethyl-L-arginine. Source: Higashi *et al.* (2001).

Serum aldosterone changes during hyperinsulinemia are correlated to body mass index and insulin sensitivity in patients with essential hypertension.

Haenni A, Reneland R, Lind L, Lithell H. *J Hypertens* 2001; **19**: 107–12.

B ACKGROUND . **Essential hypertension is characterized by peripheral insulin resistance and hyperinsulinaemia. However, the relationship of insulin resistance, free fatty acids, aldosterone and electrolytes (sodium, potassium, calcium, magnesium) in patients with essential hypertension is still unclear. The objective of this study is to measure the effects of hyperinsulinaemia on serum electrolyte status and associated hormones, and on serum free fatty acid (FFA) concentrations, in patients with essential hypertension.**

I NTERPRETATION . Hypertensive patients with normal BMI and a more pronounced glucose uptake showed a larger serum potassium decline and lowered aldosterone concentrations during induced euglycemic hyperinsulinemia. Insulin-resistant patients showed a less pronounced reduction in FFAs during hyperinsulinemia. The observations in the present study may indicate that alterations in aldosterone and FFA metabolism might be linked to the insulin resistance metabolic syndrome.

Comment

This is a physiological study carried out in patients with untreated essential hypertension. The results showed a significant association between BMI, insulin-mediated glucose infusion rate and changes in circulating aldosterone concentrations during induced euglycemic hyperinsulinaemia. Interestingly, hypertensive patients with normal BMI and greater glucose disposal showed a larger serum potassium decline and a more pronounced aldosterone decrease not explained by plasma renin activity. By contrast, insulin-resistant patients showed a less pronounced reduction in FFA during hyperinsulinaemia. These observations were supported by previous studies that plasma aldosterone was associated with visceral obesity, fasting insulin concentrations and insulin resistance as measured by glucose tolerance tests. The observations in the present study may indicate that alterations in aldosterone and FFA metabolism might be linked to the insulin resistance metabolic syndrome.

Familial dyslipidemic hypertension syndrome: familial combined hyperlipidemia and the role of abdominal fat mass.

Keulen ET, Voors-Pette C, de Bruin TW. *Am J Hypertens* 2001; **14**(4 Pt 1): 357–63.

B A C K G R O U N D . **Familial combined hyperlipidaemia (FCHL) is the most frequent genetic lipid abnormality in humans, with a 5- to 10-fold increased risk of early myocardial infarction. Familial combined hyperlipidaemia has been proposed as the leading cause of dyslipidaemia in familial dyslipidemic hypertension (FDH).**

I N T E R P R E T A T I O N . In FCHL, age, waist circumference, and hyperlipidemia are predictors of SBP. Visceral adipose tissue strongly contributes to the high prevalence of dyslipidemic hypertension in FCHL families. Reduction of visceral fat should be tested as a potential therapeutic intervention for hyperlipidaemia and hypertension in FCHL individuals.

Comment

Hyperlipidaemia, hypertension, and a positive family history of CAD combined, occur as a separate entity: FDH. It is very likely that the presence of both hyperlipidaemia and hypertension in FCHL families contribute to high risk of early CAD. The present study not only ties FDH and FCHL together as specific hypertensive entities, but also suggests that a common mechanism is responsible for the pathogenesis of dyslipidaemia as well as hypertension in FCHL. The mechanism could be free fatty acid flux from visceral adipose tissue, or an indirect mechanism inducing increased adipose tissue mass, or through lipoprotein abnormalities and insulin resistance. Further genetic and metabolic studies are awaited, as this may have future implications for pathogenesis and treatment.

Effects of atorvastatin on early recurrent ischemic events in acute coronary syndromes. The MIRACL Study: a randomized controlled trial.

Schwartz GG, Olsson AG, Ezekowitz MD, *et al. JAMA.* 2001; **285**: 1711–18.

BACKGROUND. Patients experience the highest rate of death and recurrent ischemic events during the early period after an acute coronary syndrome, but it is not known whether early initiation of treatment with a statin can reduce the occurrence of these early events.

INTERPRETATION. For patients with acute coronary syndrome (ACS), lipid-lowering therapy with atorvastatin, 80 mg/d, reduces recurrent ischaemic events in the first 16 weeks, mostly recurrent symptomatic ischaemia requiring rehospitalization.

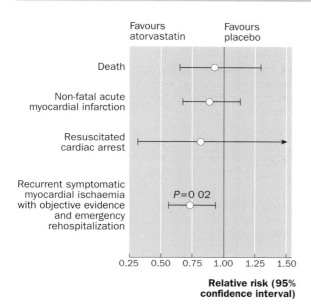

Fig. 2.15 Risk ratio plot. Death, non-fatal AMI and resuscitated cardiac arrest were not significantly reduced in the atorvastatin group compared with the placebo group. Recurrent symptomatic myocardial ischemia with objective evidence and requiring urgent rehospitalization was significantly reduced in the atorvastatin group compared with the placebo group (relative risk, 0.74; 95% CI 0.57–0.95). Source: Schwartz *et al.* (2001).

Comment

The results of the Myocardial Ischaemia Reduction with Aggressive Cholesterol Lowering (MIRACL) study suggest that patients with ACS should be on this treatment before leaving hospital, irrespective of baseline levels of low-density lipoprotein-cholesterol. By adopting such an approach, the study managed to reduce the incidence of the composite end-point (from 17.4% to 14.8%; $P = 0.048$) of death, non-fatal infarction, resuscitated cardiac arrest, and recurrent symptomatic myocardial ischaemia with new objective symptoms requiring emergency rehospitalization among the 3086 patients enrolled. However, it is unknown whether a lower dose of atorvastatin, or of any other statin, could have produced the same degree of benefit. There are at least three other clinical trials that are currently under way that will expand our knowledge of the effects of statins early on after an acute coronary event.

Part II

Hypertension and co-existing conditions

3

Stroke

Stroke: the 'paradox' and vascular rectivity

Introduction

The association between increasing blood pressure (BP) and stroke occurrence is well established and many trials have shown that antihypertensive agents reduce stroke incidence by about 40% whereas the prevention of ischaemic heart disease was much less effective. It is also not well understood why stroke is predominantly 'thromboembolic' rather than haemorrhagic. It might be possible that most haemorrhagic stroke is a consequent of a 'thromboembolic' event. Indeed, the pathophysiological mechanisms whereby hypertension leads to stroke are not entirely clear. Hypertension may directly cause mechanical damage to the endothelium with subsequent atherosclerotic plaque formation that persists even after the systemic BP has been lowered to non-hypertensive levels by medications, and thus predisposing to thromboembolic formation. In addition, the presence of a hypercoagulable state may precipitate an acute cardiovascular (CV) event or exacerbate such event during the acute stage. Furthermore, CV hyperreactivity which reflects increased underlying sympathetic nervous system activation and manifests as excessive BP or heart rate responses to psychological stressors may also contribute to elevations in BP, thicker carotid atherosclerosis, and increased risk of coronary artery disease as well as stroke. Such issues will be discussed in the following articles.

Abnormal haemorheology, endothelial function and thrombogenesis in relation to hypertension in acute (ictus < 12 h) stroke patients: the West Birmingham Stroke Project.

Lip GYH, Blann AD, Farooqi IS, Zarifis J, Sagar G, Beevers DG. *Blood Coagulation and Fibrinolysis* 2001; **12**: 307–15.

BACKGROUND. While the blood vessels are exposed to high pressures in hypertension, the main complications of hypertension (stroke and myocardial infarction) are paradoxically thrombotic rather than haemorrhagic.

INTERPRETATION. This study of hypertension and haemostasis in acute stroke has demonstrated clear abnormalities of haemorheology, endothelial dysfunction, platelet activation and thrombogenesis, which do not appear to be affected by the height of the BP or the presence of hypertension. This is despite the known hypercoagulable state found in hypertension and the relationship of haemostatic abnormalities to vascular complications.

Comment

The aim of the present study was to investigate abnormalities of haemorheology (plasma viscosity, fibrinogen), endothelial function (von Willebrand factor [vWf]), platelet activation (soluble P-selectin) and thrombogenesis (plasminogen activator inhibitor [PAI-1], and fibrin D-dimer) in stroke and the effects of concurrent hypertension. In total, 86 consecutive patients (58 male, 28 female) aged < 75 years with acute stroke (ictus < 12 h) were studied. Baseline blood tests on admission were compared with 46 'hospital controls' (patients with uncomplicated essential hypertension) and 24 healthy normotensive controls. Further comparisons were made between stroke patients with hypertension (systolic BP > 160 mm Hg and/or diastolic BP > 90 mm Hg) on admission and those without hypertension. We also investigated whether these changes are affected by stroke subtype, and the presence of high BP levels on admission (as assessed by ambulatory BP monitoring).

While the results showed that there were clear abnormalities of haemorheology, endothelial dysfunction and thrombogenesis in acute stroke, these levels did not appear to be affected by stroke subtype (ischaemic/thrombotic, haemorrhagic or TIA) or the height of the BP. This was despite the postulated hypercoagulable state conferred by hypertension and the relationship of haemostatic abnormalities to vascular complications. However, the possibility arises that, despite their raised BP levels, some of these patients may not actually have had chronic hypertension, but rather transiently elevated BPs due to a 'white coat' effect or acute hypertensive reaction as a consequence of hospital admission or of having a stroke. Furthermore, this study was limited by its cross-sectional nature and small numbers within the stroke pathological subtypes and therefore could not imply causality whether the changes in the measured indices were the cause or the effect of the stroke. This could only be answered in a prospective longitudinal study.

Why are strokes related to hypertension? Classic studies and hypotheses revisited.

Dickinson CJ. *J Hypertens* 2001; **19**(9): 1515–21.

B A C K G R O U N D . Although it seems obvious that excessive intravascular pressure is the cause of spontaneous intracerebral haemorrhage, the available evidence instead suggests that haemorrhage arises from previous ischaemic damage to the walls of small blood vessels.

I N T E R P R E T A T I O N . This interpretation unifies the aetiology of cerebral infarction and intracerebral haemorrhage. It is supported by much pathological evidence and also fits with observations on spontaneous stroke-prone hypertensive rats, which have smaller cerebral arteries than Wistar-Kyoto rats. Ischaemic damage to the brain probably occurs during spontaneous dips in aortic pressure in the presence of atheromatous arterial lesions and arteriolar narrowing by lipohyaline deposits. It may also follow long-lasting arterial spasm provoked by sudden pressure elevations. Local factors, especially unevenness of cerebral perfusion, probably determine the site of an infarct and whether it becomes haemorrhagic or not. In the long-term, hypotensive drugs will lessen atheroma deposition. In the short term, they may act by reducing or preventing damaging arteriolar spasm.

Comment

As previously discussed, the main complications of hypertension (stroke and myocardial infarction) are paradoxically thrombotic rather than haemorrhagic. This review, however, looked into the 'Birmingham paradox' from a different dimension, such that spontaneous intracerebral haemorrhage and/or the 'paradox', may not be related to abnormal haemorheology, endothelial function or thrombogenesis, but rather, could arise from previous ischaemic damage to the walls of small blood vessels. The author raised four interesting questions: 1) Why does hypertension predispose to intracerebral haemorrhage? 2) Why is cerebral infarction closely related to cerebral haemorrhage? 3) Why does lowering BP protect against strokes? and 4) Is the stroke-prone spontaneously hypertensive rat relevant to the study of strokes in man?

Stress-induced blood pressure reactivity and incident stroke in middle-aged men.

Everson SA, Lynch JW, Kaplan GA, Lakka TA, Sivenius J, Salonen JT. *Stroke* June 2001; **32**(6): 1263–70.

BACKGROUND. Exaggerated BP reactivity to stress is associated with atherosclerosis and hypertension, which are known stroke risk factors, but its relationship to stroke is unknown. Previous work also indicates that the association between reactivity and cardiovascular diseases (CVDs) may be influenced by socioeconomic status.

INTERPRETATION. Excessive sympathetic reactivity to stress may be etiologically important in stroke, especially ischaemic strokes, and low socioeconomic status confers added risk.

Comment

The present study investigated the relationship between stress-induced BP reactivity (in anticipation of an exercise tolerance test [ETT]) and subsequent 11-year risk of stroke in a population sample of >2300 middle-aged men from the Kuopio

Ischaemic Heart Disease (KIHD) risk factor study, an ongoing study of bio-psychosocial risk factors for CVD. To our knowledge, this is the first study to link reactivity to excess risk of stroke. Men with exaggerated systolic (but not diastolic) reactivity had 72% greater risk of any stroke and 87% greater risk of ischaemic stroke relative to less reactive men. Moreover, men who were high reactors and poorly educated were nearly three times more likely to suffer a stroke than better educated, less reactive men. Adjustment for stroke risk factors had little impact on these significant associations. The study provided clear evidence, considering their novelty, careful ascertainment of cases, and thorough assessment of possible covariates. However, it is unknown how the SBP rise in anticipation of ETT relates to more conventional measures of reactivity. In addition, though both socio-economic status and reactivity seem uniquely contributed to excess stroke risk, the interactive effects between CV reactivity and social economic status to stroke risk is not entirely clear. Furthermore, as pointed out by the authors, additional research is needed to corroborate these findings in other populations, particularly in those who are most vulnerable to stroke.

Target organ damage: non-dippers have higher risk

Introduction

Several factors are known to influence blood pressure-dependent target organ damage (TOD) in hypertension: duration and severity of hypertension load, diurnal variations of BP, and 24-h overall BP variability. The introduction of ambulatory blood pressure monitoring (ABPM) techniques has provided unique information about the diurnal variation of BP. These variations are of interest because they may be related to hypertensive TOD or to poor CV prognosis. The mechanism of such phenomenon is complex and poorly understood though the non-dipping pattern has been described in many different conditions including renal disease, diabetes, sleep apnoea syndrome and secondary hypertension associated with altered autonomic CV regulation. In several cross-sectional studies and one longitudinal survey, non-dippers have been reported to have more clinical and subclinical TOD in the heart (e.g. left ventricular hypertrophy), brain (e.g. cerebral ischaemia), and kidneys (e.g. microalbuminuria) than do dippers, hence, such marked changes in diurnal haemodynamic variation may predict CV events such as stroke. However, others have reported no substantial differences between the extent of target organ damage in hypertensive dippers and non-dippers though their 24-h average BP values were similar. It should be emphasized however that the reproducibility of the diurnal variation in BP over time and such arbitrary subdivision of hypertensive subjects into dippers and non-dippers are both arguable. Nevertheless, many such studies have been reported with the advent of 24-h ABPM device. The articles below are only examples.

Target organ damage and non-dipping pattern defined by two sessions of ambulatory blood pressure monitoring in recently diagnosed essential hypertensive patients.

Cuspidi C, Macca G, Sampieri L, *et al. J Hypertens* 2001; **19**(9): 1539–45.

BACKGROUND. **The clinical manifestations of high BP-dependent TOD in untreated essential hypertension patients are related to several factors, such as duration and severity of hypertension, diurnal variations of BP and 24-h overall BP variability.**

INTERPRETATION. This study suggests that a blunted reduction in nocturnal BP, persisting over time, may play a pivotal role in the development of some expressions of TOD, such as LVH and intima media (IM) thickening, during the early phase of essential hypertension, despite similar clinic BP, 24-h and 48-h BP levels being observed in non-dippers and dippers.

Comment

The mechanisms of dipping are complex and not well understood. The non-dipping status is thought to be of clinical and prognostic relevance. Several cross-sectional and one longitudinal study have reported an increase in TOD and a greater risk of CV morbidity in non-dippers as compared to dippers.

This study investigated the potential impact of a reduced nocturnal fall in BP on cardiac and extracardiac TOD (by assessing microalbuminuria, carotid ultra-sonography and amydriatic photography of ocular fundi) in 141 never-treated recently diagnosed hypertensive patients in whom the definition of dipper and non-dipper status was made by two concordant ABPM recordings. The results showed that echo LVH was 2 to 4-fold higher in non-dippers, and this was associated with greater carotid intimal thickness. There were no differences between the two groups in the prevalence of retinal changes and microalbuminuria. In addition, the two groups did not differ in office, average 24-h and 48-h BP level, suggesting that the greater extent of CV alterations seen in non-dippers may not be secondary to higher overall BP load.

The interesting feature of this study was that the dipping status was based on two concordant ABPMs, which according to the authors is the more accurate way with better reproducibility in patients' classifications into dippers and non-dippers. Clearly, different definitions will make comparisons between studies difficult. However, the main question remains: would treatment be different between the two groups? At first glance, it would seem that non-dippers are higher risk group, therefore need closer attention. However, until we understand the fundamental mechanism that drives the risk in non-dippers, we have no basis for treatment.

Stroke prognosis and abnormal nocturnal blood pressure falls in older hypertensives.

Kario K, Pickering TG, Matsuo T, *et al. Hypertension* 2001; **38**: 852–7.

BACKGROUND. It remains uncertain whether abnormal dipping patterns of nocturnal BP influence the prognosis for stroke.

INTERPRETATION. In older Japanese hypertensive patients, extreme dipping of nocturnal BP may be related to silent and clinical cerebral ischaemia through hypoperfusion during sleep or an exaggerated morning rise of BP, whereas reverse dipping may pose a risk for intracranial haemorrhage.

Comment

Briefly, a variety of abnormal BP diurnal variation patterns have been described in which the nocturnal fall of BP may be > 20% (extreme-dippers), < 10% (non-dippers), or even reversed (reverse-dippers). These variations may be related to hypertensive target organ damage. Elderly hypertensive patients who were extreme dippers may have an increased risk of silent cerebral infarcts (SCI) and may be

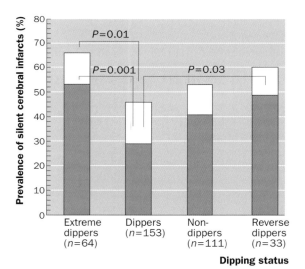

Fig. 3.1 Prevalence of SCIs: white area indicates 1 SCI detected by brain MRI per person; solid area, multiple SCIs (defined as ≥ 2 SCIs per person). Overall, χ^2 values for 4-group comparisons are 7.53 for any SCI ($P = 0.057$) and 12.8 for multiple SCIs ($P = 0.005$). Source: Kario *et al.* (2001).

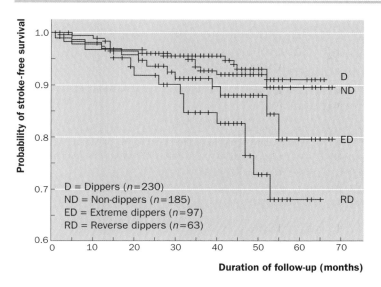

Fig. 3.2 Stroke-free survival curves. Overall log rank statistic for 4-group comparison is 14.5 (P = 0.002). Log-rank statistic is 3.12 (P = 0.08, extreme-dippers *vs* dippers), 12.5 (P = 0.0004, reverse-dippers *vs* dippers), and 8.7 (P = 0.003, reverse-dippers *vs* non-dippers). Source: Kario *et al.* (2001).

more prone to develop a stroke secondary to cerebral hypoperfusion when treated with antihypertensive therapy.

This study is based on stroke events in 575 elderly patients with sustained hypertension. Patients were subclassified into different patterns of diurnal BP variation (according to ambulatory systolic BP monitoring). Baseline brain magnetic resonance imaging (MRI) identified those extreme-dippers had the highest percentages of multiple silent cerebral infarcts (53%) followed by reverse-dippers (49%), non-dippers (41%) and dippers (29%). There was a J-shaped relationship between dipping status and stroke incidence (extreme-dippers, 12%; dippers, 6.1%; non-dippers, 7.6%; and reverse-dippers, 22%), and this remained significant after controlling for confounding variables. Intracranial haemorrhage was more common in reverse-dippers, whereas in the extreme-dippers, 27% of strokes were ischaemic strokes that occurred during sleep (*versus* 8.6% of strokes in the other three subgroups). Results remained unchanged even when diastolic BP was used to classify dipping status.

However, despite the relatively large size of this prospective study, the number of stroke events is relatively small, especially when trying to draw comparisons among the four groups. Nonetheless, what this data set clearly shows is that the two

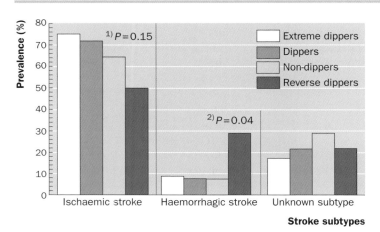

Fig. 3.3 Prevalence of stroke subtypes, by nocturnal dipping status. [1]P value for correlation (γ-coefficient) of dipping status (observed categories) and prevalence of ischaemic stroke. [2]P value for χ^2 test contrasting reverse dippers with the three other groups. Source: Kario *et al.* (2001).

extreme patterns of nocturnal dipping (extreme-dipping and reverse-dipping) are collectively associated with a more than doubling in the risk of stroke.

The association of blunted nocturnal blood pressure dip and stroke in a multiethnic population.

Phillips RA, Sheinart KF, Godbold JH, Mahboob R, Tuhrim S. *Am J Hypertens* 2000; **13**(12): 1250–5.

BACKGROUND. **Non-dipping has been defined as a reduction in the mean systolic (SBP) and diastolic BP (DBP) of <10% from awake to sleep. The hypothesis was made that non-dipping might be associated with stroke in minority populations.**

INTERPRETATION. The strength of the contribution of non-dipping to stroke risk was similar in all ethnic groups. Non-dipping was associated with stroke in both men and women. Given the previous reports that non-dipping contributes to stroke risk in European and Asian populations, these data suggest that non-dipping may be universally associated with risk for stroke.

Comment

The case-control study of a multiethnic population by Phillips *et al.* again showed that non-dippers are at greater risk for CV events, in this case, cerebrovascular events than dippers, even after being adjusted for traditional stroke risk factors. They monitored BP over a 24-h period with an ambulatory device in 166 cases from a multiethnic population of stroke survivors (63 blacks, 61 non-Hispanic whites, and 42 Caribbean Hispanics, aged 69.5 ± 11 years) and 217 community control subjects (73 blacks, 107 non-Hispanic whites, and 67 Caribbean Hispanics, aged 69 ± 9 years). Prevalence of non-dipping was significantly greater among cases than among control subjects (64% *vs* 37%, $P < 0.001$). In a multiple logistic regression model adjusted for traditional risk factors for stroke, non-dipping conferred an increased risk for stroke. The probability of stroke associated with non-dipping (odds ratio [OR] 2.5, confidence interval [CI] 1.6 to 4.0) was equal to that of traditional risk factors. The risk of stroke for non-dippers was seen in both non-Hispanic whites (OR 4.2, $P < 0.001$) as well as in the minority blacks/Caribbean Hispanics (OR 1.9, $P = 0.03$). In addition, they also found that non-dipping was associated with age in stroke survivors but not in control subjects. Thus, non-dipping seems to be a more powerful risk factor for stroke in an elderly population than in younger subjects.

It is of note that several studies in a variety of populations of European and Asian descent have also demonstrated a relationship between non-dipping and risk for CV events, including stroke. However, a causal relationship cannot be established in a case-control study. Hence, more prospective data are needed to determine the role that non-dipping contributes to causation of stroke and to recurrent stroke rate.

No impact of blood pressure variability on microalbuminuria and left ventricular geometry: analysis of daytime variation, diurnal variation and 'white coat' effect.

Kristensen KS, Hoegholm A, Bang LE, Gustavsen PH, Poulsen CB. *Blood Press Monit* 2001; **6**(3): 125–31.

B ACKGROUND . **To investigate the influence of blood pressure variability on target organ involvement.**

I NTERPRETATION . BP variability data obtained by non-invasive ABPM does not seem to improve the information inherent in the BP level.

Comment

Unlike the previous two studies described above, this cross-sectional study reported by Kristensen *et al.* failed to demonstrate a link between BP variability and increase level of target organ damage (as assessed by echocardiography determination of left ventricular mass index and relative wall thickness and early morning urine albumin/creatinine ratio) in 420 patients with newly diagnosed untreated essential hypertension recruited from a hypertension clinic at a district general hospital. The study demonstrated that hypertensive patients with high variability exhibited no more significant target organ damage than patients with low variability, but patients with established hypertension had significantly more target organ damage than the 'white coat' hypertensives. However, the 'white coat' effect as such was not associated with increased target organ involvement. On the other hand, non-dippers had significantly more cardiac target organ damage than dippers, but the difference disappeared after correction for different 24-h BP level.

Ambulatory blood pressure monitoring: dippers compared with non-dippers.
White WB. *Blood Press Monit* 2000; **5**(Suppl 1): S17–23.

BACKGROUND. Epidemiologic studies have demonstrated that the peak incidence of most types of CVD follows a circadian (24 h) pattern. Ambulatory monitoring studies have documented a reproducible 24-h rhythm for BP, characterized by a period of low values during sleep, an early-morning increase in pressures, and a plateau period while the individual is awake and active. Hypertensive patients who display the typical nocturnal decrease in BP are termed 'dippers', whereas patients in whom the nocturnal decrease in BP is absent or blunted are termed 'non-dippers'. The circadian rhythm may be influenced by demographic, neurohormonal and pathophysiological factors.

INTERPRETATION. The non-dipper profile appears to be of prognostic significance because it is associated with increased target-organ damage and a worsened cardiovascular outcome. Chronotherapy is a new pharmacologic concept whereby medication is delivered at a time and in a concentration that varies according to physiologic need during the dosing period.

Comment

It is known that the risk for myocardial infarction and stroke is at its highest during the early morning or on awakening. One reason for such phenomena may be related to an activation of the sympathetic nervous system and the renin–angiotensin–aldosterone system leading an early-morning BP surge and thus greatest risk for CV events. Several studies have demonstrated that hypertensive patients who are also a dipper are at lesser risk for CV events when compared to non-dippers during the early morning hours. The mechanism for such observational facts is not known. However, this has implication as to the timing of therapy i.e. chronotherapy for those at risk. In the near future, the benefits of a chrono-therapeutic approach to the management of hypertension should be elucidated by large-scale outcome studies.

Stroke: left ventricular hypertrophy and treatment

Introduction

Left ventricular (LV) geometric abnormalities such as LVH, both on electro- and echocardiography have been shown to be a potent predictor of increased CV morbidity and mortality in subjects with or without known CVD, independent of BP. The predictive risk is especially high in those with CV risk factors such as hypertension or diabetes mellitus. The increased risk of stroke or transient ischaemic attacks associated with LVH is complex and multifactorial.

Although the mechanisms by which LVH develops are also incompletely understood, the renin–angiotensin system may play an important role. Indeed, recent evidence from Heart Outcome Prevention Evaluation (HOPE) study has provided us with the first evidence that LVH regression by ramipril, an angiotensin converting enzyme inhibitor (ACEI), reduced the risk of death, myocardial infarction, congestive heart failure as well as stroke, independent of blood pressure lowering. Similarly, the recently published Losartan Intervention For End-point reduction (LIFE) study has provided further evidence that reversal of LVH can reduce the risk of fatal or non-fatal stroke, also independent of its reduction on BP, and thus extends the results of the placebo-controlled HOPE trial.

Left ventricular hypertrophy as an independent predictor of acute cerebrovascular events in essential hypertension.
Verdecchia P, Porcellati C, Reboldi G, *et al. Circulation* 2001; **104**: 2039–44.

BACKGROUND. It is uncertain whether LVH confers an increased risk for cerebrovascular disease in apparently healthy patients with essential hypertension.

INTERPRETATION. In apparently healthy patients with essential hypertension, LVH diagnosed by electrocardiography (ECG) or echocardiography confers an excess risk for stroke and transient ischaemic attack independently of BP and other individual risk factors.

Comment

Cerebrovascular events are well-recognised consequences of elevated BP which in turn may lead to LVH. It may be difficult to differentiate the relative role of elevated BP from a direct contribution of LVH to the increased risk of developing stroke. As pointed out by Devereux |**1**|, long-term prognostic studies of stroke in populations with baseline measurements of both left ventricular mass (LVM) and ambulatory BP are needed to resolve this uncertainty. The present study, consisting of 2363 initially untreated hypertensive patients (mean age 51 ± 12 years, 47% women)

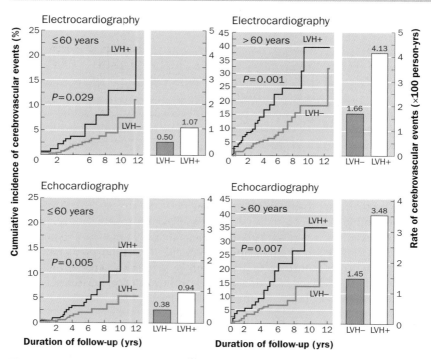

Fig. 3.4 Cumulative incidence and crude rate of cerebrovascular events in hypertensive subjects < 60 (left) and > 60 (right) years old with and without LVH determined by electrocardiography (ECG) (top) and echocardiography (bottom). Source: Verdecchia *et al.* (2001).

free of previous CVD and followed up for up to 14 years (mean 5 years), has clearly answered the question above. By contrast, however, it is still unclear whether LVH regression will lead to reduction of stroke risk.

Treatment of hypertension to prevent stroke

Treatment of hypertension to prevent stroke: translating evidence into clinical practice.
Kaplan RC. *J Clin Hypertens* 2001; **3**(3): 153–6.

B A C K G R O U N D . **Although programmes such as the National High Blood Pressure Education Project emphasize that all patients with hypertension should be treated, it** is perhaps natural for physicians to question the usefulness of aggressively treating those patients who have modestly elevated BP levels but are otherwise healthy, asymptomatic individuals.

INTERPRETATION. The evidence suggests that treating patients with non-severe hypertension would prevent a larger proportion of the population-wide burden of stroke than treating only those with more severe hypertension. To determine the best population-wide strategy for preventing hypertension-associated morbidity and mortality, epidemiological data serve as an important complement to the clinical trial results. The evidence we need is available to us, and our present challenge is to translate this evidence into practice.

Comment

The prevention of stroke remains a formidable challenge in the treatment of hypertension. Using the example of stroke, this review summarizes the clinical trial data demonstrating the efficacy of antihypertensive therapy in patients with severe and non-severe forms of hypertension. The evidence suggests that treating patients with non-severe hypertension would prevent a larger proportion of the population-wide burden of stroke than treating only those with more severe hypertension. It is shown how such measures as relative risk reduction (RRR), number needed to treat

Table 3.1 Impact of antihypertensive drug treatment of the occurrence of stroke among patients with hypertension

	Will the patient's stroke risk decrease?	How many patients of this type need to be treated to prevent one stroke?		How much of the populationwide burden of strokes would be prevented by successful treatment?	
Untreated blood pressure level	Relative risk reduction (RRR) associated with treatment	5-year stroke incidence, if untreated	Number needed to treat (NNT) to prevent one stroke*	Population frequency	Population attributable fraction (PAF)
90–110 mmHG DBP	39%	2.2%	118	6.9%	8.6%
Up to 115 mmHG DBP	30%	6.5%	52	0.5%	1.5%
Above 115 mmHg DBP	43%	8.2%	29	0.5%	2.7%

This table is based on data from Hennekens and Braunwald |2| and summarizes the results of 17 randomized clinical trials. For computation of PAF, these data were used to eliminate the 5-year stroke incidence among hypertensive individuals treated with placebo, and a background incidence of 0.5% among non-hypertensive individuals was assumed. Data from the Third National Health and Nutrition Examination Survey (NHANES-III) 24 were used to estimate population frequency.
*Over 5 years of treatment.

Source: Hennekens et al. (2001) |2|.

(NNT) and population-attributable fraction (PAF) can be applied in the management of hypertensive patient populations.

However, the common theme that is shared by all consensus treatment guidelines for hypertension is: best practice based on best available evidence. Physicians treating patients with hypertension should follow these guidelines. While emphasizing the importance of primary prevention in the long-term, patients who have the highest absolute risk for events would gain the most benefit from treatment and hence, be the most cost-effective in the short-term.

Antihypertensive drug therapies and the risk of ischaemic stroke.

Klungel OH, Heckbert SR, Longstreth WT Jr, *et al. Arch Intern Med* 2001; **161**: 37–43.

BACKGROUND. The relative effectiveness of various antihypertensive drugs with regard to the reduction of stroke incidence remains uncertain. This study assesses the association between first ischaemic stroke and use of antihypertensive drugs.

INTERPRETATION. In this study of pharmacologically treated hypertensive patients, antihypertensive drug regimens that did not include a thiazide diuretic were associated with an increased risk of ischaemic stroke compared with regimens that did include a thiazide. These results support the use of thiazide diuretics as first-line antihypertensive agents.

Comment

This is a population-based case-control study among pharmacologically treated hypertensive patients. Klungel *et al.* used medical records and telephone interviews to gather drug information on 380 hypertensive patients who had had a fatal or non-fatal ischaemic stroke. They found that patients taking a beta-blocker, calcium channel blocker (CCB), or ACEI in combination with a thiazide diuretic seemed to have the same risk of stroke as patients taking a diuretic alone. In contrast, patients taking two of the drugs listed above other than a diuretic appeared to have a 2.48-fold increase in the risk of stroke, when compared to the use of a diuretic only. However, the association with risk of stroke was slightly less pronounced in patients with known CVD.

Hence, this study adds to the growing body of evidence that the choice of drug used to lower BP in hypertensives really does matter for specific end-organ protection. Again, ongoing large-scale clinical trials should help clarify this issue. In the absence of additional clinical trial evidence, the results of this study support the use of thiazide diuretics as first-line antihypertensive agents.

Stroke: more HOPE than PROGRESS

Randomized trial of a perindopril-based blood-pressure-lowering regimen among 6105 individuals with previous stroke or transient ischaemic attack.

PROGRESS Collaborative Group. *Lancet* 2001; **358**: 1033–41.

BACKGROUND. BP is a determinant of the risk of stroke among both hypertensive and non-hypertensive individuals with cerebrovascular disease. However, there is uncertainty about the efficacy and safety of blood-pressure-lowering treatments for many such patients. The perindopril protection against recurrent stroke study (PROGRESS) was designed to determine the effects of a blood-pressure-lowering regimen in hypertensive and non-hypertensive patients with a history of stroke or transient ischaemic attack.

INTERPRETATION. This BP-lowering regimen reduced the risk of stroke among both hypertensive and non-hypertensive individuals with a history of stroke or transient ischaemic attack (TIA). Combination therapy with perindopril and indapamide produced larger BP reductions and larger risk reductions than did single drug therapy with perindopril alone. Treatment with these two agents should now be considered routinely for patients with a history of stroke or transient ischaemic attack, irrespective of their BP.

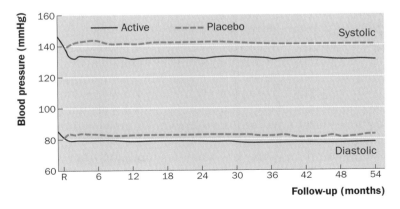

Fig. 3.5 Changes in systolic and diastolic BP among participants assigned active treatment and those assigned placebo. Source: PROGRESS Collaborative Group (2001).

Comment

This study was published as a fast-track paper as according to the authors the results were overwhelming and showed for the first time that antihypertensive therapy with a combination of the ACEI (perindopril) and the diuretic (indapamide) prevents the recurrence of stroke even in patients with normal BP. However, this claim was not supported by the accompanying editorial commentary.

PROGRESS included 6105 hypertensive and non-hypertensive patients who had had stroke (haemorrhagic or ischemic) or TIA with no major disability within the previous 5 years, were randomized to a flexible regimen of active treatment (perindopril 4mg once daily, with indapamide 2.5mg once daily added at the discretion of the treating physician) or matched placebo. There was no entry BP criteria, i.e. they could be either normotensive or hypertensive, but around half the patients did have raised BP. The primary outcome was total fatal or non-fatal stroke. After 4 years of follow-up, active treatment (60% received both drugs, and 40% received perindopril alone) reduced BP by 9/4 mmHg and stroke recurrence by 28% compared with placebo and that of major CV complications by 26%. Both hypertensive and non-hypertensive patients had similar reductions in their risk of stroke. The results also showed significant reductions in stroke recurrence in patients who had previously suffered either an ischaemic or haemorrhagic stroke.

Nevertheless, one or two odd findings are worth highlighting. In the subgroup of active treatment patients who received both perindopril and indapamide, BP was

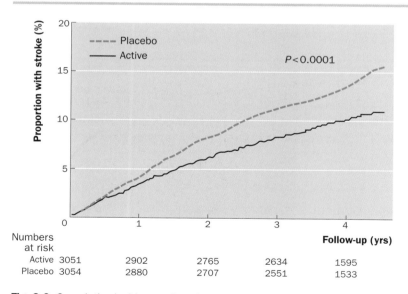

Fig. 3.6 Cumulative incidence of stroke among participants assigned active treatment and those assigned placebo. Source: PROGRESS Collaborative Group, (2001).

reduced by 12/5 mmHg, and the risk of stroke was cut by 43%. Single-drug therapy with perindopril alone reduced BP by 5/3 mmHg, but produced no reduction in the risk of stroke. As 5 mmHg reduction in systolic BP should translate into an approximate 20% reduction in stroke risk, the fact that the study showed no benefit in the perindopril-only group was rather surprising. It is not only out of line within

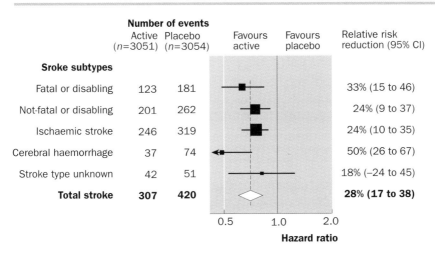

Fig. 3.7 Effects of study treatment on stroke subtypes. Source: PROGRESS Collaborative Group, (2001).

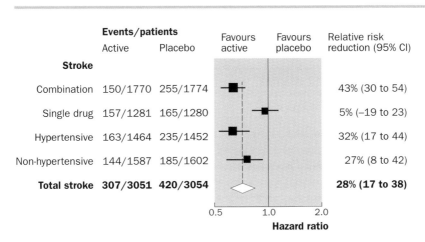

Fig. 3.8 Effects of study treatment on stroke in subgroups of patients. Source: PROGRESS Collaborative Group, (2001).

the context of PROGRESS itself but also with the evidence on the primary preven-tion of stroke in many previous outcome studies. However, the authors explained that such findings might be the result of chance. In addition, there are some who cannot accept at all that ACEI may have special ancillary effects beyond its efficacy in BP lowering properties. It should also be remembered that in previous trials, such as the CAPtopril Prevention Project (CAPPP), fatal or non-fatal stroke were 1.25 times more common in patients randomized to captopril (an ACEI) than in those assigned conventional therapy with diuretics, beta-blockers, or both. On the other hand, in the Post-stroke Antihypertensive Treatment Study (PATS), 2.5 mg of indapamide daily decreased BP by 5/2 mmHg and reduced the recurrence of fatal and non-fatal stroke by 29%.

Thus, it is probably correct to say a '… pril for every cardio or reno … ill', but the current evidence of a '… pril for cerebro … ill' is certainly less convincing until the results of on-going megatrials such as ASCOT or ALLHAT become available.

HOPE substudy confirms ramipril prevents stroke, reduces stroke severity, regardless of BP lowering.
Probstfield J, HOPE Collaborative Investigators. American Stroke Association 27th International Stroke Conference, 2002.

BACKGROUND. **HOPE has previously noted that control of hypertension in diabetics and treatment of high-risk diabetic patients with the ACE inhibitor ramipril prevent stroke.**

INTERPRETATION. HOPE substudy confirms ramipril prevents stroke, reduces stroke severity, regardless of BP lowering and diabetes status.

Comment

New data from the HOPE study subanalysis confirm the benefit of treatment with the ACEI ramipril over placebo in preventing strokes, both total stroke and all stroke subtypes. Moreover, patients who had a stroke while on ramipril also tended to have less severe motor and cognitive deficits compared to those on placebo.

The data seem to be more widely applicable than that published in the diabetic group as data now has shown similar benefit in stroke prevention regardless of their

Table 3.2 HOPE: Total stroke and subtypes

Stroke type	Ramipril	Placebo	RR (95% CI)
Total stroke	3.4%	4.9%	0.68 (0.56–0.84)
Ischaemic stroke	2.2%	3.4%	0.64 (0.50–0.82)
Non-ischaemic stroke	1.4%	1.7%	0.80 (0.57–1.12)

Source: Probstfield *et al.* (2002).

diabetic status. In HOPE, the overall reduction in total stroke was 32%, and 31% among diabetics. This subanalysis showed that non-fatal stroke was reduced by 24%, and fatal stroke by 61%. Recurrent strokes were also reduced by about 33%. Ischaemic and haemorrhagic strokes were both reduced, by 36% and 26% respectively. Strokes not documented by computed tomography, magnetic resonance imaging or autopsy evidence were classified as 'uncertain'. Haemorrhagic strokes and strokes of uncertain type are combined as 'non-ischaemic' strokes in the table below.

Again, as in the overall study, the estimates of treatment benefit were consistent across all subgroups examined: those with and without hypertension, with and without prior coronary heart disease, with and without prior peripheral vascular disease and with and without diabetes. Further characterization of cognitive and motor changes after a stroke while on assigned therapy showed that patients taking ramipril had less severe deficits than those on placebo. Changes such as those in cognition or consciousness, ocular or visual symptoms, face or limb weakness, dysarthria or dysphasia, or frank dysphagia, were significantly less frequent among those on treatment.

However, the controversy continues as to whether or not the BP reduction in HOPE accounts for the reduction in stroke and myocardial infarction.

References

1. Devereux RB. Therapeutic options in minimizing left ventricular hypertrophy. *Am Heart J* 2000; **139**(1 Pt 2): S9-14.

2. Hennekens CH, Braunwald E. Clinical Trials in Cardiovascular Disease: *A Companion to Braunwald's Heart Disease*. Philadelphia, PA: W.B. Saunders; 1999.

4

Pregnancy and hypertension

Hypertension in pregnancy

Introduction

Hypertension is a common complication of pregnancy occurring in about 10% of pregnancies. Hypertension in pregnancy is nevertheless due to a number of different and distinct aetiologies and pathophysiological mechanisms, many of which are poorly understood. It is therefore not surprising that the classification of the hypertensive disorders of pregnancy has been difficult and controversial and thus limits the ability to prevent and treat this disorder. It is likely that the cause of pregnancy-induced hypertension is multifactorial and involves both genetic and other factors.

There have been several attempts to classify the hypertensive syndromes in pregnancy but none is entirely satisfactory. Nevertheless, it is important to attempt to ascertain which syndrome is present in individual patients so that appropriate treatment can be instituted.

Pregnancy-induced hypertension can simply be divided into pre-eclampsia and gestational hypertension. Unlike gestational hypertension, pre-eclampsia is a systemic disease characterized not only by hypertension but also by increased vascular resistance, diffuse endothelial dysfunction, proteinuria and coagulopathy. However, both conditions may represent different manifestations of one disease process. Indeed, it may be difficult to differentiate pre-eclampsia from gestational hypertension in the absence of severe disease manifestations.

In addition, essential hypertension can sometimes be misdiagnosed as pregnancy-induced hypertension when a woman's first blood pressure (BP) determination is in the second trimester of pregnancy, a time when BP has normally fallen from pre-pregnancy values. The subsequent return to usual BP in the third trimester may be mistaken for new-onset hypertension in pregnancy.

The close relationship between essential hypertension and insulin resistance and hyperinsulinaemia is well established. However, the possible role of insulin resistance in the pathogenesis of pregnancy-induced hypertension has only recently been reported. Such observations may have implications for treatment or preventive strategies before and during pregnancy. Whether links to insulin resistance for both pre-eclampsia and gestational hypertension suggest a common pathophysiology still remains to be determined.

Pathogenesis and genetics of pre-eclampsia.
Roberts JM, Cooper DW. *Lancet* 2001; **357**: 53–6.

BACKGROUND. **After more than a century of intensive research, pre-eclampsia and eclampsia remain an enigmatic set of conditions. Aberration of the interaction between placental and maternal tissue is probably the primary cause, but the exact nature of the differences from normal pregnancy remain elusive. In this review, attempts to understand the sequence of physiological changes have concentrated on vascular endothelium and oxidative stress issues.**

INTERPRETATION. There are genetic components to susceptibility, but the relative contributions of maternal and fetal genotypes are still unclear. Whole-genome mapping could ultimately define the causative genes.

Comment

The definitions of hypertension in pregnancy (according to the National High Blood Pressure Education Working Group Report on High Blood Pressure in Pregnancy) are shown in Table 4.1. The most severe presentations of hypertension in pregnancy are gestational proteinuric hypertension (pre-eclampsia) and eclampsia. Pre-eclampsia complicates about 10% of hypertensive pregnancies (see definition) and remains a major cause of maternal and neonatal morbidity and mortality. As discussed in the review by Roberts and Cooper, the exact pathophysiology of pre-eclampsia remains poorly understood and hence pre-eclampsia has been referred to as the 'disease of theories'.

Pre-eclampsia only occurs in the presence of a placenta and its resolution begins with the removal of the placenta. The pathophysiology of pre-eclampsia is much

Table 4.1 Classification of hypertension in pregnancy

Preeclampsia
   Hypertension developing after 20 weeks' gestation with proteinuria and/or oedema

Gestational hypertension (also termed transient hypertension of pregnancy)
   Hypertension developing after 20 weeks' gestation without other signs of pre-eclampsia

Chronic hypertension
   Hypertension before 20 weeks' gestation in the absence of neoplastic trophoblastic disease

Pre-eclampsia superimposed on chronic hypertension
   Pre-eclampsia developing in a woman with pre-existing hypertension

Hypertension is defined as systolic blood pressure ≥140 mmHg or diastolic blood pressure ≥ 90 mmHg; or systolic blood pressure increase of ≥30 mmHg or diastolic blood pressure of ≥15 mmHg over first trimester of prepregnancy values. Proteinuria refers to 24-hour urine protein ≥300 mg or dipstick protein ≥1 g/L.
Source: Solomon *et al.* (2001).

Table 4.2 Risk factors for pre-eclampsia

Preconceptional and/or chronic risk factors

Partner-related risk factors:
Nulliparity/primipaternity
Limited sperm exposure, teenage pregnancy, donor insemination
Partner who fathered a pre-eclamptic pregnancy in another woman

Maternal-specific risk factors:
History of previous pre-eclampsia
Increasing maternal age, interval between pregnancies
Family history
Patient requiring occyte donation

Presence of specific underlying disorders:
Chronic hypertension and renal disease
Obesity, insulin resistance, low maternal birthweight
Gestational diabetes, type-1 diabetes mellitus
Activated protein C resistance (factor V Leiden), protein S deficiency
Antiphospholipid antibodies
Hyperhomocysteinaemia

Exogenous factors:
Smoking (risk decrease)
Stress, work-related psychosocial strain

Pregnancy-associated risk factors
Multiple pregnancy
Urinary tract infection
Structural congenital anomalies
Hydrops fetalis
Chromosomal anomalies (trisomy 13, triploidy)
Hydatidiform moles

Source: Dekker *et al.* (2001).

more than the increased BP and altered renal function – clinical features that facilitate diagnosis. Perfusion is decreased to virtually all organs, secondary to intense vasospasm due to an increased sensitivity of the vasculature to any pressor agent. This low perfusion in many cases is secondary to abnormal placentation. Whereas pregnancy is associated with striking modifications of the spiral arteries that provide the blood supply to the placenta, these changes do not take place normally in pre-eclampsia. In normal pregnancy, the luminal diameter of the spiral arteries is very enlarged and the walls are remodelled such that they contain very little smooth muscle.

Perfusion is further compromised by activation of the coagulation cascade, especially platelets, with attendant microthrombi formation. Additionally, plasma volume is decreased by loss of fluid from the intravascular space, further compromising organ blood flow. Increased platelet activation and markers of endothelial activation antedate clinically evident pre-eclampsia by weeks to months in groups of women destined to develop the disorder.

These changes extend into the vessels to the inner third of the myometrium to provide a large bore, flaccid, low-resistance circuit for perfusion of the intervillous space. These modifications are associated with endovascular invasion of fetal trophoblast into these maternal vessels. Endovascular invasion and spiral artery remodelling occur either very superficially or not at all in pre-eclampsia.

The maternal fetal tolerance that allows the intimate interaction of genotypically disparate cells in the intervillous space does not happen normally in pre-eclampsia, compromising appropriate endovascular invasion. Other conditions can also decrease placental blood supply and increase pre-eclampsia risk. Pre-existing maternal conditions that are associated with microvascular disease, such as hypertension or diabetes, or that are thrombophilic (e.g. anticardiolipin antibody syndrome), increase the risk of pre-eclampsia. In addition, obstetric conditions that increase placental mass, such as hydatidiform moles or multiple gestations increase the risk of pre-eclampsia, apparently by a decrease of placental blood flow.

Elevated levels of S-nitrosoalbumin in pre-eclampsia plasma.

Tyurin VA, Liu SX, Tyurina YY, *et al. Circ Res* 2001; **88**(11): 1210–5.

BACKGROUND. The availability of nitric oxide (NO), which is required for the normal regulation of vascular tone, may be decreased in pre-eclampsia, thus contributing to the vascular pathogenesis of this pregnancy disorder. Because ascorbate is essential for the decomposition of S-nitrothiols and the release of NO, we speculated that the ascorbate deficiency typical of pre-eclampsia plasma might result in decreased rates of decomposition of S-nitrosothiols.

INTERPRETATION. S-nitrosoalbumin and total S-nitrosothiol concentrations are significantly increased in pre-eclampsia plasma and may reflect insufficient release of NO groups in this condition.

Comment

Pre-eclampsia, a life-threatening complication of pregnancy that accounts for about 75 000 maternal deaths each year worldwide, could be caused by decreased availability of NO. Although specific pathways through which a shortage of ascorbate translates into functional endothelial deficiency are not completely understood, ascorbate has been shown to reverse NO-dependent endothelial dysfunction in atherosclerosis, hypertension, hypercholesterolaemia and diabetes. Oxidative stress is usually accompanied by a pronounced depletion of ascorbate which is thought to contribute to the endothelial dysfunction of pre-eclampsia.

A decreased availability of the NO required for the normal regulation of vascular tone, which may contribute to the pathogenesis of pre-eclampsia, could be due to suppressed NO production by endothelium and/or improper storage and delivery to its targets. NO, which is one of the major mediators of blood vessel relaxation, is either used immediately after production, or is bound to albumin, forming S-nitrosoalbumin.

Tyurin *et al.* report a study of plasma samples from 21 pregnant women with pre-eclampsia who were compared with samples taken from 21 women at the same gestational stage of a normal pregnancy. The women with pre-eclampsia had significantly higher levels of S-nitrosalbumin in their blood, consistent with the hypothesis that nitric oxide is being stored in the blood and is not being released in large enough quantities to maintain a healthy blood flow, leading to profound vasoconstriction throughout the woman's body.

Plasma from women who had pre-eclampsia contained 11.1 ± 2·9 nmol/ml of total S-nitrosothiols whereas plasma from women with no symptoms of the disorder contained 9·4 ± 1.5 nmol/ml. Increased levels of S-nitrosothiols were almost completely accounted for by the increased concentrations of S-nitrosoalbumin. Low levels of vitamin C may lead to decreased availability of NO in the general circulation and this might cause the vasoconstriction and vasospasm that are associated with the typical symptoms of pre-eclampsia–hypertension, proteinuria, and oedema.

Brief review: hypertension in pregnancy: a manifestation of the insulin resistance syndrome?

Solomon CG, Seely EW. *Hypertension* 2001; **37**: 232–9.

BACKGROUND. Pregnancy-induced hypertension (PIH), which includes both gestational hypertension and pre-eclampsia, is a common and morbid pregnancy complication for which the pathogenesis remains unclear. Emerging evidence suggests that insulin resistance, which has been linked to essential hypertension, may play a role in PIH.

INTERPRETATION. Conditions associated with increased insulin resistance, including gestational diabetes, polycystic ovary syndrome and obesity, may predispose to hypertensive pregnancy. Furthermore, metabolic abnormalities linked to the insulin resistance syndrome are also observed in women with PIH to a greater degree than in normotensive pregnant women. These include glucose intolerance, hyperinsulinaemia, hyperlipidaemia, and high levels of plasminogen activator inhibitor-1, leptin, and tumour necrosis factor-alpha. These observations suggest the possibility that insulin resistance may be involved in the pathogenesis of PIH and that approaches that improve insulin sensitivity might have benefit in the prevention or treatment of this syndrome, although this requires further study.

Table 4.3 Correlates of insulin resistance associated with pregnancy-induced hypertension

Conditions	Biomarkers
Gestational diabetes mellitus	Hyperglycaemia
Polycystic ovary syndrome	Hyperinsulinaemia
Obesity/excessive weight gain	Hyperlipidaemia
	Increased TNF-α
	High PAI-1 Levels
	Hyperleptinaemia

Source: Solomon *et al.* (2001).

Comment

Despite the significant morbidity associated with new-onset hypertension in pregnancy, the pathogenesis remains unclear. Although it is likely that the cause of PIH is multifactorial, insulin resistance may be an important contributor.

This overview by Solomon and Seely discusses the association of essential hypertension with insulin resistance and hyperinsulinaemia. Indeed, it was not until recent years that more widespread interest developed in the possible role of insulin resistance in the pathogenesis of PIH. Postulated mechanisms through which insulin resistance might increase blood pressure in pregnancy, as in essential hypertensives, include sympathetic nervous system activation, renal sodium retention, increased cation transport, and associated endothelial dysfunction. Conditions associated with increased insulin resistance, including gestational diabetes, polycystic ovary syndrome and obesity, also predispose to hypertensive pregnancy. Furthermore, metabolic abnormalities such as glucose intolerance, hyperinsulinaemia, hyperlipidaemia, and high levels of plasminogen activator inhibitor-1, leptin and tumor necrosis factor-alpha, can be found. Such observations may have implications for treatment or preventive strategies before and during pregnancy.

Sympathetic neural mechanisms in normal and hypertensive pregnancy in humans.

Greenwood JP, Scott EM, Stoker JB, Walker JJ, Mary DA. *Circulation* 2001; **104**(18): 2200–4.

B ACKGROUND. Direct recordings from peripheral sympathetic nerves have shown an increased sympathetic drive in PIH and pre-eclampsia. It is unknown whether sympathetic drive is altered in normal pregnancy when arterial BP can be normal or relatively low. The aim of this study was to measure and compare peripheral sympathetic discharge, its vasoconstrictor effect and its baroreceptor control, during

pregnancy and postpartum in women with normal pregnancy (NP) and PIH and in normotensive non-pregnant (NN) women.

INTERPRETATION. Central sympathetic output was increased in women with normal pregnancy and was even greater in the hypertensive pregnant group. The findings suggest that the moderate sympathetic hyperactivity during the latter months of normal pregnancy may help to return the arterial pressure to non-pregnant levels, although when the increase in activity is excessive, hypertension may ensue.

Comment

Very little is known about the activity of the peripheral sympathetic system in normal pregnancy compared with the non-pregnant state. During the third trimester of normal pregnancy, arterial BP tends to rise toward normal non-pregnant levels but it is unknown whether central sympathetic drive is involved in this process. The use of indirect measures of sympathetic output, such as changes in haemodynamic variables and circulating catecholamines, has yielded conflicting results in both normal and hypertensive pregnancy.

The paper by Greenwood *et al.* aims to measure and compare peripheral sympathetic discharge, its vasoconstrictor effect and its baroreceptor control, during pregnancy and postpartum in 21 women with NP and 18 PIH and in 21 NN women. They found that central sympathetic output was increased in women with normal pregnancy and was even greater in the hypertensive pregnant group, suggesting that the moderate sympathetic hyperactivity during the latter months of normal pregnancy may help to return the arterial pressure to non-pregnant levels. Nevertheless, when the increase in activity is excessive, hypertension may ensue.

Evaluation

Introduction

Accurate BP measurement in pregnancy is critical because even small elevations of pressure radically affect the patient's care. In pregnancy, the main sources of variation are the methods for measuring the diastolic pressure (DBP) and the posture of the patients. For many years, both obstetricians and physicians have tended to take the DBP at the phase of muffling of diastolic sounds rather than the phase of disappearance of sounds. The debate still continues and this has led to considerable confusion in reporting pregnancy-related BP in the literature. However, analysis of the techniques reported in the international obstetric literature shows an increasing trend to adopt phase 5 as the indicator for DBP.

With the advent of ambulatory blood pressure monitoring (ABPM) devices, predictable patterns of BP variation along gestation have been identified for both clinically healthy and hypertensive pregnant women. Indeed, the use of a reliable and accurate automated device for ABPM has been suggested as the logical approach to overcoming many of the problems associated with office BP measurement. However, it should be borne in mind that posture effect, especially during the late pregnancy stage where the gravid uterus may cause some vena caval compression, can lead to a fall in cardiac output and thus BP. This may significantly affect the validity of the 24-h BP measurement using the ABPM device, especially when the subject is resting on her back at night. Furthermore, it should be noted that most automatic and semiautomatic BP monitoring systems have not been validated in pregnancy.

Evaluation of the blood pressure load in the diagnosis of hypertension in pregnancy.

Hermida RC, Ayala DE. *Hypertension* 2001; **38**: 723–9.

BACKGROUND. The use of a set of new end-points obtained from ABPM, in addition to the BP values themselves, has been advocated to improve sensitivity and specificity in the diagnosis of hypertension and the evaluation of a patient's response to treatment. Among these parameters is the use of BP load, the percentage of values above a given constant reference limit or computed by reference to daytime and night-time limits.

INTERPRETATION. The optimum reference limits for calculating the BP load, markedly < 140/90 mmHg, must be defined as a function of gestational age, in keeping with the predictable trends in BP along pregnancy previously documented.

Comment

See below

Influence of parity and age on ambulatory monitored blood pressure during pregnancy.

Ayala DE, Hermida RC. *Hypertension* 2001; **38**(3 Pt 2): 753–8.

BACKGROUND. Studies based on casual BP measurements concluded that both age and parity have significant effects on BP during pregnancy. These results were tested on clinically healthy normotensive women who were systematically studied by ambulatory BP monitoring during their pregnancies.

INTERPRETATION. Reference thresholds for BP to be used in the early identification of hypertensive complications in pregnancy could thus be developed as a function of the rest-activity cycle and gestational age, independent of parity or maternal age.

Comment

See below

Differences between office and 24-hour ambulatory blood pressure measurement during pregnancy.

Churchill D, Beevers DG. *Obstet Gynecol* 1996; **88**(3): 455–61.

BACKGROUND. To compare BP measurements in ambulatory pregnant women with well-taken office readings.

INTERPRETATION. There are important differences between ambulatory and office BPs measured throughout pregnancy, findings that could not be explained by activity or present knowledge of cardiovascular haemodynamics in pregnancy. Ambulatory BP readings must be considered different entities than office BP readings. Care should be taken in predicting obstetric outcome from the results of ambulatory BP recordings.

Comment

Generally, isolated BP measurements in detecting hypertensive complications in pregnancy are unreliable and the use of ABPM has been advocated. Indeed, there is a trend of decreasing BP up to the middle of gestation followed by increasing BP up to the day of delivery in normal pregnancies – but this is not found in pregnancies complicated with gestational hypertension or pre-eclampsia.

Moreover, differences between healthy and complicated pregnancies in the circadian pattern of BP can be observed by ABPM as early as in the first trimester of pregnancy, before the actual clinical diagnosis of gestational hypertension or pre-eclampsia. A cautious approach is advocated by Churchill and Beevers, suggesting that there are important differences between ambulatory and office BPs measured throughout pregnancy. Thus, ambulatory BP readings – whilst useful – must be considered different entities than office BP readings, and care should be taken in predicting obstetric outcome from the results of ambulatory BP recordings.

The paper by Hermida *et al.* analysed data from 205 normotensive pregnant women and 123 women who developed gestational hypertension or pre-eclampsia. In their paper, they suggest optimum reference limits for calculating the BP 'load', which must be defined as a function of gestational age.

The subsequent paper from the same researchers, again based on systematic ambulatory monitoring in normotensive pregnant women, indicates the lack of differences in BP according to parity (Figure 4.1). They suggest that reference thresholds for BP, to be used in the early identification of hypertensive complications in pregnancy, could thus be developed as a function of rest-activity cycle and gestational age, independent of parity or maternal age.

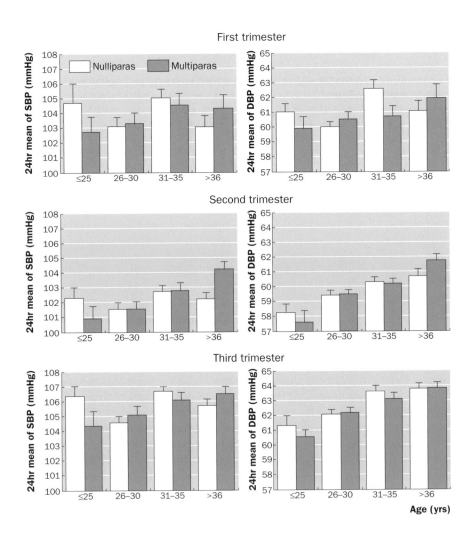

Fig. 4.1 Influence of parity and age in the 24-h mean of SBP (left) and DBP (right) of clinically healthy pregnant women sampled by 48-h ABPM in different trimesters of their gestation. Source: Lip *et al.* (2001).

Blood pressure monitoring during pregnancy.

Feldman DM. *Blood Press Monit* 2001; **6**: 1–7.

BACKGROUND. Conventional (office, mercury column or aneroid manometry) BP measurement is the most common screening test performed during prenatal visits. During the past several years, investigators have focused on the use of 24-h ambulatory and automated self (or home) BP monitoring during pregnancy.

INTERPRETATION. Since the 1980s, the importance of ambulatory and home BP monitoring in diagnosing and managing hypertensive patients has been well established. In pregnancy, there is a growing interest in these forms of out-of-office BP assessment as evidenced by numerous publications in the obstetric and hypertension literature. However, further research is needed in order to better define the role of ambulatory and home BP monitoring in both routine and high-risk obstetric practice.

Comment

The use of ambulatory and home BP monitoring in pregnancy is a relatively new and promising method of managing patients with hypertension in pregnancy. This review discusses the benefits of out-of-office BP monitoring compared to conventional BP assessment and provides a summary of the available literature on both home and ABPM in pregnancy and how they relate to various clinical aspects of hypertension in pregnancy.

Table 4.4 Haemodynamic alterations during pregnancy

Parameter	Early pregnancy*	Late pregnancy**
Mean arterial pressure	decreased	maintained or increased
Plasma volume	increased	maintained
Red cell volume	increased	increased
Heart rate	increased	increased
Cardiac output	increased	decreased
Stroke volume	increased	decreased
Systemic vascular resistance	increased	maintained

* Less than 20 weeks' gestation. ** More than 30 weeks' gestation.

Source: Feldman (2001).

Management

Introduction

Hypertensive disorders occur in 8–10% of pregnancies and contribute significantly to still-births and neonatal morbidity and mortality. Hypertensive disorders are also the second leading cause of maternal mortality after embolism. Despite this, there are still no definitive guidelines as to when and how patients should be treated. However, it is important that those patients at highest risk are stratified early with appropriate treatment and close monitoring. Due to numerous and differing classification systems in the past, hypertension in pregnancy can be a difficult condition to diagnose and treat. However, management considerations should be made between chronic hypertension that is present before pregnancy and those occurring as part of the pregnancy-specific condition pre-eclampsia, as well as management considerations in women with comorbid conditions that may cause hypertension and influence the choice of antihypertensive therapy. Unfortunately, there have been very few randomized controlled trials assessing its management.

Pre-eclampsia occurs in about 5% of first pregnancies and in about 15% of women with chronic hypertension. It is a serious syndrome associated with intra-uterine growth retardation or death as well as maternal morbidity and mortality, and thus requires careful assessment and management. It can be seen in the early stages of pregnancy occasionally with normal blood pressures and proteinuria alone. Patients generally have no symptoms and can only be detected by routine screening. Prevention of pre-eclampsia is a big step forward in prenatal care. There can be three distinctive stages in the prevention of pre-eclampsia: primary, secondary or tertiary. Primary prevention means avoiding occurrence of a disease. Secondary prevention in the context of pre-eclampsia implies breaking off the disease process before emergence of clinically recognisable disease. Tertiary prevention means prevention of complications caused by the disease process and is thus more or less synonymous with treatment.

What's in a name? Problems with the classification of hypertension in pregnancy.
Brown MA, Buddle ML. *J Hypertens* 1997; **15**: 1049–54.

Comment

Hypertension is an important cause of both maternal and fetal morbidity and mortality. The classification system proposed by Brown and Buddle (1997), which accounts for the multisystem involvement which can occur in pre-eclampsia and eclampsia, divides hypertension in pregnancy into three main groups: pre-eclampsia, gestational hypertension and chronic hypertension (Table 4.5).

Table 4.5 Hypertension in pregnancy

1. Pre-eclampsia: *De novo* hypertension arising after 20 weeks gestation returning to normal within 3 months postpartum and one or more of:
- Proteinuria ≥300 mg/day or dipstix result persistently ≥1g/l
- Renal insufficiency
- Liver disease: AST>40IU/l or severe right upper quadrant or epigastric pain or both
- Neurological problems: convulsions (eclampsia), hyper-reflexia with clonus or severe headache with hyper-reflexia
- Haematological disturbances: thrombocytopenia or haemolysis or both
- Retardation of fetal growth

2. Gestational hypertension: *De novo* hypertension after 20 weeks gestation without any features of pre-eclampsia returning to normal within 3 months post partum. This diagnosis can clearly only be made in retrospect.

3. Chronic hypertension:
- **Essential hypertension:** Blood pressure ≥140mmHg systolic or ≥90mmHg diastolic, or both, before conception or during the first half of pregnancy without an apparent secondary cause or evidence of white-coat hypertension
- **Secondary hypertension:** Usually this is due to underlying renal disease, but occasionally coarctation of the aorta or phaeochromocytoma are encountered.

Source: Brown *et al.* (1997)

Table 4.6 Dosages of recommended agents

Drug	Indication	Doses
Methyldopa	Mild/moderate chronic and gestational hypertension	250 mg 2–3 times/day; increase at 2 day intervals as need to maximum dose of 3 g/day
Labetalol	Mild/moderate chronic and gestational hypertension	400–800 mg/day in divided doses
	Severe hypertension/pre-eclampsia	200 mg orally or 40 mg bolus IV; then 200 mg orally 2 times/day in addition to hydralazine/nifedipine
Nifedipine	Moderate chronic and gestational hypertension	Nifedipine LA 30–60 mg once/day; nifedipine 10 mg 2–3 times/day
	Severe hypertension/pre-eclampsia	Nifedipine 10–20 mg orally followed by same dose every 8 hours
Hydralazine	Severe hypertension/pre-eclampsia	Initial IV bolus 5 mg; repeat every 15 minutes as required to achieve BP control; maintenance infusion of 60–300 µg/kg/hr
Magnesium sulphate	Prophylaxis in pre-eclampsia and prevention of further fits in eclampsia	4 g IV loading bolus; maintenance infusion of 1–2 g/hour for at least 24 hours after the last fit

Source: Brown *et al.* (2001).

Little benefit to the fetus has been shown from treating gestational and chronic hypertension, but studies in this area have been small in size and would not have the power to show a difference in outcome between treated and untreated groups. However, the reduction in morbidity and mortality in the treatment of pre-eclampsia is significant. It should not be forgotten that the definitive treatment for severe hypertension is delivery of the fetus despite risks to fetal morbidity and mortality. This will reduce BP, but hypertension *per se* may still persist postpartum requiring short-term therapy.

Primary, secondary and tertiary prevention of pre-eclampsia.
Dekker G, Sibai B. *Lancet* 2001; **357**: 209–15.

BACKGROUND. Pre-eclampsia remains one of the major obstetrical problems in less-developed countries. The causes of this condition are still unknown, thus effective primary prevention is not possible at this stage. Research in the past decade has identified some major risk factors for pre-eclampsia, and manipulation of these factors may result in a decrease in its frequency.

INTERPRETATION. In the early 1990s, aspirin was thought to be the wonder drug in secondary prevention of pre-eclampsia. Results of large trials have shown that this is not the case: if there is an indication for using aspirin it is for the patient with very high risk of developing severe early-onset disease. The calcium story followed a more or less similar pattern, with the difference being that existing evidence shows that women with a low dietary calcium intake are likely to benefit from calcium supplementation. Proper antenatal care and timed delivery are of utmost importance in tertiary prevention of pre-eclampsia. There is evidence to suggest that the intrinsic direct effect of moderate degrees of maternal hypertension is beneficial to the fetus. Severe hypertension needs treatment. If antihypertensive treatment is indicated, there is no clear choice of a drug. Hydralazine should no longer be thought of as the primary drug; most studies show a preference for calcium channel blockers.

Comment

There is a paucity of good randomized clinical trials of sufficient size or power to provide firm clinical guidelines for the treatment of hypertension in pregnancy.

Recommendations regarding the level of BP that warrants treatment during pregnancy are controversial, especially since BP normally falls to a nadir in the mid-trimester of pregnancy. A general policy is to treat chronic hypertension if BP is consistently >140/90 mmHg after the first trimester, or if BP rises by >30 mmHg systolic or >15 mmHg diastolic, above the values prior to pregnancy or during the first trimester. This view can be challenged now that it is known that the treatment of mild hypertension confers no benefit to the mother or the fetus. It is therefore the policy only to treat diastolic pressures of 100 mmHg or more on repeated

Table 4.7 Laboratory tests in hypertension in pregnancy

Test	Rationale
Full blood count	• Haemoconcentration is found in pre-eclampsia and is an indicator of severity.
	• Decreased platelet count suggests severe pre-eclampsia.
Blood film	• Signs of microangiopathic haemolytic anaemia favour the diagnosis of pre-eclampsia.
Urinalysis	• If dipstix proteinuria of ≥1g/l, a quantitative measurement of 24-h protein excretion is required.
	• Hypertensive pregnant women with proteinuria should be considered to have pre-eclampsia until proven otherwise.
Biochemistry, including serum creatinine, urate, liver function tests	• Abnormal or rising levels suggest pre-eclampsia and are an indicator of disease severity.
Lactate dehydrogenase	• Elevated levels are associated with haemolysis and hepaticin involvement, suggesting severe pre-eclampsia.
Serum albumin	• Levels may be decreased even with mild proteinuria, perhaps due to capillary leak or hepatic involvement in pre-eclampsia.

Source: adapted from recommendations of the National High Blood Pressure Education Program Working Group Report on High Blood Pressure in Pregnancy. *Am J Obstet Gynecol* 1990; **163**: 1689–1712.

measurements. In the absence of any information on the value of reducing systolic pressures, the policy is to withhold drugs unless the systolic pressure exceeds 160 mmHg.

This excellent review by Gus Dekker and Baha Sibai provides an authoritative overview on best practice for the management of pre-eclampsia.

5

Diabetes

Hypertension, diabetes and renal disease: the high-risk patients

Introduction

Few will deny the importance of blood pressure (BP) control in diabetic patients with hypertension. Most patients with both disorders have a markedly worsened risk for premature microvascular and macrovascular complications. Over the past few years, many randomized, controlled trials, in particular the UK Prospective Diabetes Study (UKPDS), have provided data supporting more aggressive BP lowering in this high-risk group. Most treatment guidelines now recommend lower goal BP level (< 130/80 mmHg) using multiple antihypertensive drugs if necessary in order to reduce or slow the onset of renal disease and cardiovascular (CV) events.

The UKPDS has shown that aggressive management of high BP is more important in reducing CV events and slowing renal disease progression than is intensive control of blood glucose levels. However, despite numerous randomized trials, there is still controversy over which particular class of agent is best for patients with hypertension and diabetes mellitus (DM). Nevertheless, few will argue the importance of interrupting the renin–angiotensin system (RAS) in these patients. On the basis of their apparent superiority in slowing diabetic nephropathy, angiotensin-converting enzyme inhibitors (ACEIs) should probably be the first choice. Studies have shown that use of ACEIs can prevent the progression of microalbuminuria to overt proteinuria, reduce proteinuria in patients with overt diabetic nephropathy, slow the deterioration of the glomerular filtration rate, delay progression to end-stage renal disease (ESRD), and lower BP. It is of note, however, that most of this evidence was mainly derived from trials on patients with type 1 DM. Although in UKPDS the overall events may be similar to beta-blocker/diuretic treatment compared with an ACE/diuretic regimen, there appears to be an advantage to the latter regimen in type 2 diabetic persons. However, several major clinical trials have indicated that most patients require an average of more than three different antihypertensive agents to reach the BP goal of < 130/80 mmHg.

Until very recently, the therapeutic benefit of ACEIs in patients with type 2 DM and overt nephropathy was less clear. Meta-analyses of several small trials that have included type 2 diabetic patients and non-diabetic hypertensive patients suggest that there is a renoprotective benefit of ACEIs in both patient populations; this benefit is linked in part to BP reduction, but a component may be independent of the antihypertensive effect of this class of drugs. Three recently completed randomized blinded trials address the previously unanswered questions of whether angiotensin receptor blockers (ARBs) delay the progression of nephropathy (Reduction of Endpoints in NIDDM [non-insulin-dependent diabetes mellitus] with the Angiotensin II Antagonist Losartan [RENAAL], Irbesartan Diabetic Nephropathy Trial [IDNT], see below) or reduce proteinuria (IRbesartan MicroAlbuminuria [IRMA] II) in patients with type 2 DM. These trials have provided exciting data and based on these novel results, there is little doubt that ARBs are beneficial for diabetic patients with or at risk for renal disease, and that the renal benefit may supercede the BP effect. Taken together with the results from Micro-HOPE (Heart Outcomes Prevention Evaluation), it is unarguable that patients with type 2 DM will certainly benefit tremendously from agents that interrupt the RAS system. It is unclear, however, whether ARBs will produce similar benefits in patients with type 1 DM. Until more evidence for harder end-points from on-going trials is available, one should be prepared to shift to more flexible pharmacological treatment strategies given the knowledge that both types of DM share similar pathophysiology with high risk of CV disease, and both ACEIs and ARBs block the RAS system.

The importance of ethnic differences in our therapeutic approaches in any disease has long been realized but little attention has been paid to the ethnic minorities when designing therapeutic clinical trials. For a variety of reasons, including genetic predisposition for CV diseases, the ethnic minorities have been found to have higher prevalence and poorer prognosis. The African American Study of Kidney Disease and Hypertension (AASK) trial is innovative; it is the largest trial to focus on only one ethnic group, African American, designed to evaluate the impact on progression of hypertensive kidney disease. The results were novel and will be discussed below.

Indeed, the results of on-going randomized hypertension trials with large subpopulations of patients with DM, such as the Antihypertensive and Lipid Lowering treatment to prevent Heart Attack Trial (ALLHAT) and the ASCOT, may provide additional useful information about the treatment of this vulnerable group of patients.

A practical approach to achieving recommended blood pressure goals in diabetic patients.
Bakris GL. *Arch Intern Med* 2001; **161**: 2661–7.

BACKGROUND. Approximately 11 million Americans have both hypertension and DM. This double diagnosis places such patients at high risk for renal damage, especially ESRD. Recent data suggest that an even lower diastolic BP (DBP) goal (i.e. < 80 mmHg) may be necessary.

INTERPRETATION. All diabetic patients with BP greater than 130/80 mmHg should begin ACEI treatment and be titrated to moderate or high doses until the BP goal is

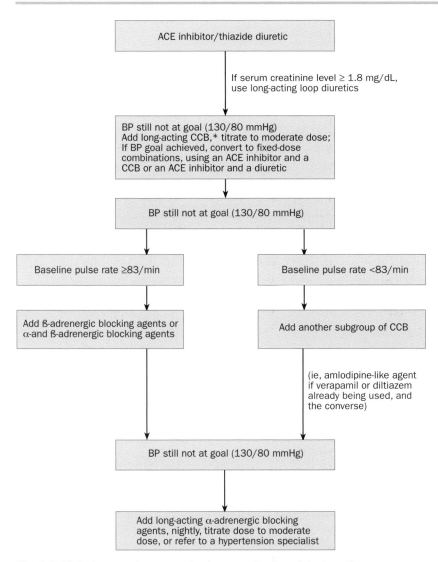

Fig. 5.1 Clinical approach to managing hypertension in a diabetic patient.

Everyone with DM, renal insufficiency, or both should be instructed on lifestyle modifications as per the Sixth report of the Joint National Committee on Prevention, Detection, Evaluation, and Treatment of High Blood Pressure (JNC VI). Everyone, however, should initiate therapy if BP is greater than 130/85 mmHg. If BP is less than 15/10 mmHg above goal (i.e. 130/80 mmHg), then ACEIs can be used alone. Asterisk indicates that calcium channel blockers (CCBs) (e.g. verapamil and diltiazem) have been shown to reduce CV mortality rates and progression of diabetic nephropathy independent of ACEI use. To convert serum creatinine levels to micromoles per litre, multiply milligrams per decilitre by 88.4. Source: modified with permission from Bakris (2001).

achieved. Multiple antihypertensive agents are often necessary to reach target BP, and may offer more renoprotection than one agent used singly.

Comment

The review article by a highly respected expert in the field excellently outlined an evidence-based practical approach in the management of hypertensive diabetics. A

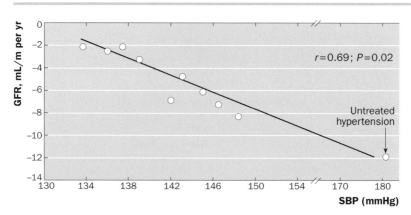

Fig. 5.2 Rates of decline in glomerular filtration rate (GFR) *vs* the systolic BP (SBP) in studies extending for 3 years or more in patients with type II DM nephropathy. Source: adapted from Bakris (2001).

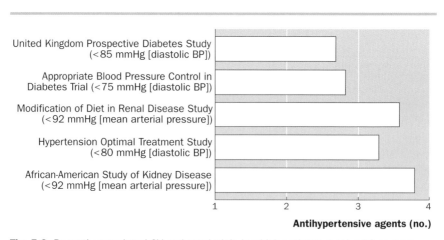

Fig. 5.3 Recently completed CV and renal trials in which patients received 2 or more antihypertensive agents for intensive BP control. BP indicates blood pressure. Source: Bakris (2001).

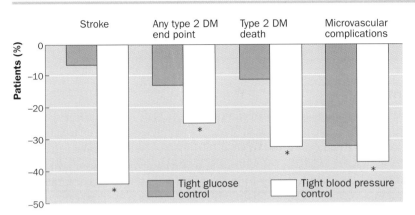

Fig. 5.4 Comparative effects of tight glucose control *vs* tight BP control in the United Kingdom Prospective Diabetes Study. Asterisk indicates *P* < 0.05 compared with glucose control; DM, diabetes mellitus. Source: Bakris (2001).

treatment algorithm was included to simplify the choice of antihypertensive agent(s) which depend only on three readily available clinical indices: BP, serum creatinine and heart rate. A case study that applies these evidence-based concepts in outpatient practice is also included. Clearly, ACEI is the first choice. Not only do they lower BP, they can also prevent the progression of microalbuminuria to overt proteinuria, reduce proteinuria in patients with overt diabetic nephropathy, slow the deterioration of the glomerular filtration rate and delay progression to ESRD as well as death.

It should be emphasized that in patients with type 2 DM and uncontrolled BP despite antihypertensive monotherapy, combination therapy is more effective for obtaining a further BP reduction than increasing the dose of the monotherapy or switching to another monotherapy belonging to another drug class. In addition, these patients also exhibit more frequently several CV risk factors on top of their hypertension. An intensified multifactorial intervention is known to delay the progression to nephropathy as well as the severity of retinopathy in patients with type 2 DM and microalbuminuria.

Effect of type 2 diabetes mellitus on left ventricular geometry and systolic function in hypertensive subjects.
Palmieri V, Bella JN, Arnett DK, *et al. Circulation* 2001; **103**: 102–7.

BACKGROUND. Type 2 diabetes is a CV risk factor. It remains to be elucidated in a large, population-based sample whether diabetes is associated with changes in left ventricular (LV) structure and systolic function independent of obesity and SBP.

INTERPRETATION. In a relatively healthy, population-based sample of hypertensive adults, type 2 diabetes was associated with higher LV mass, more concentric LV geometry, and lower myocardial function, independent of age, sex, body size and arterial BP.

Comment

The present report compared the diabetic and non-diabetic among 1950 hypertensive participants in the Hypertension Genetic Epidemiology Network (HyperGEN) Study without overt coronary heart disease (CHD). The results showed a diabetes-associated increase in LV mass, concentric LV geometry and relative wall thickness, independent of covariates e.g. BP, body mass index (BMI), age, sex, duration of hypertension or insulin resistance. Diabetic hypertensives had significantly lower stress-corrected midwall shortening despite similar endocardial ejection fractions independent of covariates. Such findings may contribute in part to high rates of overt CHD and heart failure to which diabetic individuals are predisposed.

 Separate and joint effects of systemic hypertension and diabetes mellitus on left ventricular structure and function in American Indians (the Strong Heart Study).
Bella JN, Devereux RB, Roman MJ, *et al. Am J Cardiol* 2001; **87**(11): 1260–5.

BACKGROUND. Although the association of systemic hypertension (SH) with DM is well established, the cardiac features and haemodynamic profile of patients with SH and DM diagnosed by American Diabetes Association criteria have not been elucidated.

INTERPRETATION. DM and SH each have adverse effects on LV geometry and function, and the combination of SH and DM results in the greatest degree of LV hypertrophy (LVH), myocardial dysfunction and arterial stiffness.

Comment

The Strong Heart Study is a population-based prospective cohort survey of CV risk factors, and prevalence and incidence of CV disease in American Indians. It is of note that American Indians have higher prevalence of DM, thus current results may not be generalizable to other groups. Nevertheless, this study has clearly shown that DM and SH are associated with independent and additive increases in the prevalence and degree of abnormalities of LV structure and function. Moreover, it would be even more interesting to see if the corresponding CV events over the 2 years follow-up would also be highest in the DM and SH combined group and whether the medications used had any influence.

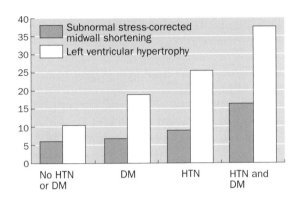

Fig. 5.5 Prevalence of LVH and subnormal stress-corrected midwall shortening in participants with neither DM nor systemic hypertension, DM alone, systemic hypertension alone, or both conditions. Source: Bella *et al.* (2001).

The impact of diabetes on left ventricular filling pattern in normotensive and hypertensive adults: the Strong Heart Study.

Liu JE, Palmieri V, Roman MJ, *et al. J Am Coll Cardiol* 2001; **37**(7): 1943–9.

B A C K G R O U N D . Diastolic abnormalities have been extensively described in hypertension but are less well characterized in DM, which frequently coexists with hypertension.

I N T E R P R E T A T I O N . Diabetes mellitus, especially with worse glycaemic control, is independently associated with abnormal LV relaxation. The severity of abnormal LV relaxation is similar to the well-known impaired relaxation associated with hypertension. The combination of DM and hypertension has more severe abnormal LV relaxation than groups with either condition alone. In addition, abnormal relaxation (AbnREL) in DM is associated with worse glycaemic control.

Comment

This study sought to determine the effect of DM on LV filling pattern in normotensive (NT) and hypertensive individuals. By analysing the transmitral inflow velocity profile at the mitral annulus in four groups from the Strong Heart Study, NT-non-DM ($n = 730$), hypertensive-non-DM ($n = 394$), NT-DM ($n = 616$) and hypertensive-DM ($n = 671$) (the DM subjects were further divided into those with normal filling pattern [$n = 107$} and those with AbnREL [$n = 447$]), Liu *et al.*

found that the peak E velocity was lowest in hypertensive-DM, intermediate in NT-DM and hypertensive-non-DM and highest in the NT-non-DM group ($P < 0.001$), with a reverse trend seen for peak A velocity ($P < 0.001$). In multivariate analysis, E/A ratio was lowest in hypertensive-DM and highest in NT-non-DM, with no difference between NT-DM and hypertensive-non DM ($P < 0.001$). Likewise, mean atrial filling fraction and deceleration time were highest in hypertensive-DM, followed by hypertensive-non-DM or NT-DM and lowest in NT-non-DM (both $P < 0.05$). Among DM subjects, those with AbnREL had higher fasting glucose ($P = 0.03$) and haemoglobin A1C ($P = 0.04$).

Lipid and blood pressure treatment goals for type 1 diabetes. Ten-year incidence data from the Pittsburgh Epidemiology of Diabetes Complications Study.

Orchard TJ, Forrest KY, Kuller LH, *et al. Diabetes Care* 2001; **24**: 1053–9.

BACKGROUND. Subjects with type 1 diabetes are at high risk for many long-term complications, including early mortality and coronary artery disease (CAD). Few data are available on which to base goal levels for two major risk factors, namely BP and lipid/lipoproteins. The objective of this study was to determine at which levels of low-density lipoprotein (LDL) and high-density lipoprotein (HDL) cholesterol, triglycerides and BP, the relative risks of type 1 diabetic complications increase significantly.

INTERPRETATION. Although observational in nature, these data strongly support the case for vigorous control of lipid levels and BP in patients with type 1 diabetes.

Comment

Little data are available on the predictive power of baseline lipid and BP measurements in people with type 1 DM. Most of the existing recommendations are extrapolated from type 2 diabetics who are typically older with different microvascular complications. However, according to the authors of this study, aggressive lipid- and BP-lowering goals in people with type 1 diabetes are both essential and attainable. Their study is timely, appearing in print within weeks of the National Cholesterol Education Programs Adult Treatment Panel III report (NCEP III) in which diabetics, for the first time, are to be considered at a risk level for subsequent CV events on a par with people who already have heart disease.

Based on 10-year prospective observations of young adults with type 1 DM, Orchard *et al.* propose re-thinking traditional 'cut-off' measurements for lipids and BP in these patients, with the aim of preventing diabetes complications. The 'cut-off' levels were identified by linking baseline measurements of BP and lipid fractions in 589 patients with childhood-onset (< 17 years) type 1 DM to incidence of six diabetes complications especially on total mortality, CAD and overt nephropathy. Like the LDL guidelines specified in the recent NCEP report, as well as in the American Diabetes Association (ADA) 2001 clinical practice guidelines in the ADA's position statement, *Management of Dyslipidemia in Adults with Diabetes*, Orchard *et al.* suggest that diabetics should aim to keep their LDL levels below 100 mg/dl (2.6 mmol/l). They also concur with ADA recommendations for HDL target levels of >45 mg/dl (1.1 mmol/l). (The NCEP guidelines make no specific recommendations for HDL.) Where Orchard *et al.* claim their observations depart from the ADA recommendations is for triglycerides, pointing to target levels of less than 150 mg/dl (1.7 mmol/l), 25% lower than that stipulated in the ADA guidelines at 200 mg/dl. BP cut-offs extrapolated from their data are also lower than that set by the JNC VI, which set targets for diabetics at 130/85 mmHg. By contrast, the data from this observational study suggest that a systolic BP of < 120 mmHg and a diastolic BP of < 80 mmHg might be more appropriate goals for reducing risk. In addition, age, sex and glycaemic control had little influence on these goals.

It should be noted that their recommendations are based solely on observational analysis and therefore do not necessarily stand on their own. Although definitive clinical trial results would be 'desirable', it is unlikely that this will be conducted in type 1 diabetics given the current evidence of the benefits of lowering lipid levels and BP in type 2 diabetics and general populations.

Diabetes, hypertension, and cardiovascular disease: an update.

Sowers JR, Epstein M, Frohlich ED. *Hypertension* 2001; **37**: 1053–9.

BACKGROUND. Hypertension is approximately twice as frequent in patients with diabetes compared with patients without the disease. Conversely, recent data suggest that hypertensive persons are more predisposed to the development of diabetes than are normotensive persons. Furthermore, up to 75% of CV diseases (CVD) in diabetes may be attributable to hypertension, leading to recommendations for more aggressive treatment (i.e. reducing BP to < 130/85 mmHg) in persons with coexistent diabetes and hypertension.

INTERPRETATION. This update reviews the current knowledge regarding the CVD risk factors and their treatment, with special emphasis on the cardiometabolic syndrome, hypertension, microalbuminuria, and diabetic cardiomyopathy. This update also examines the role of the RAS in the increased risk for CVD in diabetic patients and the impact of interrupting this system on the development of clinical diabetes as well as CVD.

Comment

The authors are to be congratulated for writing such a thorough review on the recent advances from the three main multicentre clinical trials (UKPDS, CAPPP and

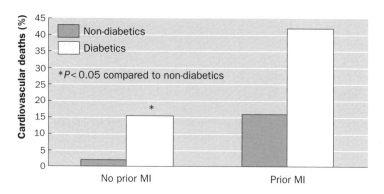

Fig. 5.6 Incidence of death from CV causes in diabetic and non-diabetic individuals after a 7-year follow-up. MI indicates myocardial infarction. Source: Sowers *et al.* (2001).

HOPE) on the diabetic hypertensive patients, as well as on the newer fundamental findings that add importantly to our overall knowledge of the CV complications of DM. There was special emphasis on the impact of ACEIs in altering the course of disease progress in these high-risk patients, including details on the possible mechanisms at the cellular level. The therapeutic implications were also briefly discussed.

Reduced cardiovascular morbidity and mortality in hypertensive diabetic patients on first-line therapy with an ACE inhibitor compared with a diuretic/β-blocker-based treatment regimen: a subanalysis of the Captopril Prevention Project.

Niskanen L, Hedner T, Hansson L, *et al. Diabetes Care* 2001; **24**: 2091–6.

BACKGROUND. The Captopril Prevention Project (CAPPP) evaluated the effects of an ACEI-based therapeutic regimen on CV mortality and morbidity in hypertension. One planned subanalysis of the CAPPP was to evaluate the outcome in the diabetic patient group.

INTERPRETATION. Captopril is superior to a diuretic/beta-blocker antihypertensive treatment regimen in preventing CV events in hypertensive diabetic patients, especially in those with metabolic decompensation.

Comment

In this subanalysis of the CAPPP, 572 (4.9% of 10 985 hypertensive patients) diabetic patients were evaluated. The primary end-point, fatal and non-fatal myocardial infarction and stroke as well as other CV deaths, was markedly lower in the captopril than in the conventional therapy group (RR = 0.48; P = 0.084). However, such an impressive result should be interpreted with caution, as this is a subgroup analysis. Nevertheless, as in many other studies, hypertensive diabetics with impaired metabolic control have consistently benefited the most from ACEI–based therapy compared to other therapy. The results also seem to support those from the HOPE study that the choice of antihypertensive drug regimen may be of importance when there are multiple risk factors and when the protective effect is well beyond that obtained by BP reduction *per se.*

Effects of losartan on renal and cardiovascular outcomes in patients with type 2 diabetes and nephropathy: RENAAL (Reduction of Endpoints in NIDDM with the Angiotensin II Antagonist Losartan) Study.
Brenner BM, Cooper ME, Zeeuw DD, *et al. N Engl J Med* 2001;
345: 861–869.

BACKGROUND. Diabetic nephropathy is the leading cause of ESRD. Interruption of the RAS slows the progression of renal disease in patients with type 1 diabetes, but similar data are not available for patients with type 2, the most common form of diabetes. The role of the angiotensin-II-receptor antagonist losartan in patients with type 2 diabetes and nephropathy was assessed.

INTERPRETATION. Losartan conferred significant renal benefits in patients with type 2 diabetes and nephropathy, and it was generally well tolerated.

Comment

Two trials (RENAAL and IDNT) performed with ARBs have examined the potential of these drugs in slowing the progression of diabetic nephropathy and protecting against CV morbidity and mortality. In RENAAL, a total of 1513 patients were enrolled in this randomized, double-blind study comparing losartan (50–100 mg once daily) with placebo, both taken in addition to conventional antihypertensive treatment (except ACEIs). All had type 2 diabetes, proteinuria and elevated serum creatinine. The primary outcome was a composite of time to first occurrence of either a doubling of serum creatinine, ESRD or death. Secondary end-points included a composite of morbidity and mortality from CV causes, proteinuria, and the rate of progression of renal disease. After 3.4 years of follow-up, the primary end-point was significantly reduced with losartan therapy, as well as two of the three measures making up the composite. The benefit exceeded that attributable to changes in BP. The secondary end-point was similar in the two groups, but the rate of first hospitalization for heart failure and level of proteinuria was 32% and 35% lower with losartan, respectively.

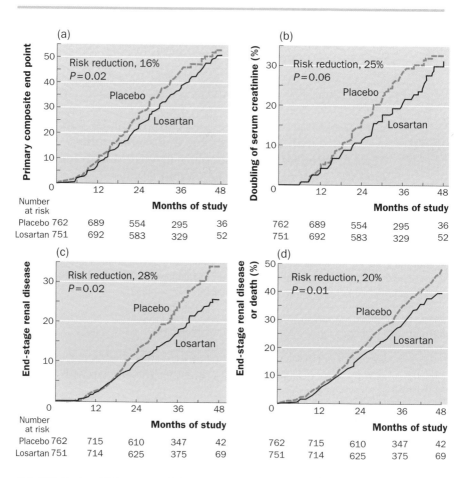

Fig. 5.7 Kaplan–Meier curves of the percentage of patients with the primary composite end point (panel a) and its individual components, a doubling of the serum creatinine concentration (panel b), ESRD (panel c), and the combined end-point of ESRD or death (panel d). The mean follow-up time was 3.4 years (42 months). Source: Brenner *et al.* (2001).

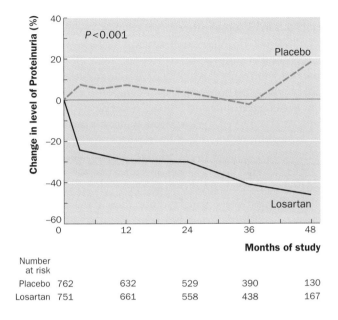

Number at risk

Placebo	762	632	529	390	130
Losartan	751	661	558	438	167

Fig. 5.8 Median changes from baseline in the level of proteinuria. Proteinuria was measured as the urinary albumin-to-creatinine ratio in a first morning specimen. The mean follow-up time was 3.4 years. Source: Brenner *et al.* (2001).

Renoprotective effect of the angiotensin-receptor antagonist irbesartan in patients with nephropathy due to type 2 diabetes.

Lewis EJ, Hunsicker LG, Clarke WR, *et al.* *N Engl J Med* 2001; **345**: 851–60.

BACKGROUND. **It is unknown whether either the angiotensin-II-receptor blocker irbesartan or the calcium-channel blocker amlodipine slows the progression of nephropathy in patients with type 2 diabetes independently of its capacity to lower the systemic BP.**

INTERPRETATION. The angiotensin-II-receptor blocker irbesartan is effective in protecting against the progression of nephropathy due to type 2 diabetes. This protection is independent of the reduction in BP it causes.

Comment

In this trial, Lewis and colleagues randomized 1715 men and women with hypertension and type 2 diabetes with frank kidney disease (proteinuria > 900 mg/day), to treatment with irbesartan (75–300 mg once daily), amlodipine (2.5–10 mg once daily), or placebo on a background of antihypertensive therapy (excluding ACEIs). Irbesartan and amlodipine doses were given as a forced titration to the maximum tolerated dose. The primary end-point was timed to a composite end-point of death, doubling of baseline serum creatinine and ESRD. The target BP was 135/85 mmHg or less in all groups. After a mean 2.6 years of follow-up, the incidence of a primary end-point event was significantly reduced by irbesartan therapy, by 20% compared to placebo, and by 23% compared to amlodipine. The risk of a doubling of the serum creatinine concentration was 33% and 37% lower in the irbesartan group than in the placebo and amlodipine group, respectively. These results were highly statistically and clinically significant. Furthermore, these differences were not explained by differences in the BPs that were achieved. There were no significant differences in the rates of death from any cause or in the CV composite end-

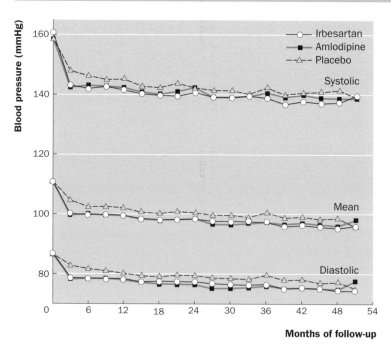

Fig. 5.9 Average systolic, mean arterial, and DBPs at randomization (0 months) and during follow-up, according to treatment group. The mean arterial blood pressure (MAP) during follow-up was, on average, 3.3 mmHg lower in the irbesartan and amlodipine groups than in the placebo group. Source: Lewis *et al.* (2001).

point. However, when secondary composite outcome broke down separately, patients on amlodipine experienced significantly more congestive heart failure.

Taken together with the RENAAL trial, these intervention studies show very similar results. Both point to a protection of the kidneys afforded by angiotensin II receptor blockade that cannot be accounted for exclusively by the BP reduction *per se.*

The date of onset of ESRD could not be determined for one patient in the placebo group and two patients in the amlodipine group. These three patients were excluded from the analyses shown in Panels A and C.

The association between microalbuminuria and the progression of diabetic nephropathy has been clearly established in patients with type 1 DM. However, recent studies from several laboratories have established that microalbuminuria is a marker of CV morbidity in non-diabetic patients with essential hypertension as well as in patients with type 2 DM.

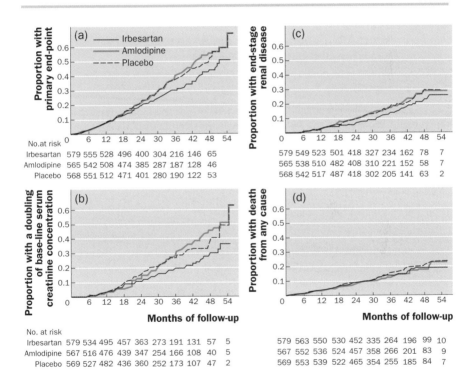

Fig. 5.10 Cumulative proportions of patients with the primary composite end-point (panel a) and its components, a doubling of the base-line serum creatinine concentration (panel b), ESRD (panel c), and death from any cause (panel d). Source: Lewis *et al.* (2001).

Microalbuminuria is associated with insulin resistance, atherogenic dyslipi-daemia and central obesity, and is a part of the metabolic CV syndrome associated with hypertension. Persistent albuminuria is the most important surrogate end-point in clinical trials aimed at the prevention of diabetic nephropathy. Urinary albumin measurements are used to determine both the diagnosis of diabetic nephropathy and its progression to ESRD. Furthermore, increased urinary albu-min excretion may contribute to the pathogenesis of glomerular lesions. Sustained reduction in albuminuria during antihypertensive treatment is associated with a diminished rate of decline in the glomerular filtration rate and an improved prog-nosis. IRMA II has reaffirmed that antihypertensive treatment enhances renopro-tection in patients with type 2 DM and microalbuminuria. Beyond BP control, irbesartan directly reduces the rate of clinical albuminuria and diabetic nephropathy.

Effect of irbesartan on the development of diabetic nephropathy in patients with type 2 diabetes. IRbesartan MicroAlbuminuria type 2 diabetes mellitus in hypertensive patients (IRMA II).

Parving HH, Lehnert H, Brochner-Mortensen J, *et al. N Engl J Med* 2001; **345**(12): 870–8.

BACKGROUND. Microalbuminuria and hypertension are risk factors for diabetic nephropathy. Blockade of the RAS slows the progression to diabetic nephropathy in patients with type 1 diabetes, but similar data are lacking for hypertensive patients with type 2 diabetes.

INTERPRETATION. Irbesartan is renoprotective independently of its blood-pressure-lowering effect in patients with type 2 diabetes and microalbuminuria.

Comment

This trial randomized 590 patients with hypertension, type 2 diabetes, micro-albuminuria (urinary albumin excretion rate [UAER] 20–200 μg/min) and normal kidney function to two doses of irbesartan (150 and 300 mg once daily) or placebo on a background of antihypertensive therapy (excluding ACEIs, ARBs, or dihydropyridine-CCBs). The primary end-point was timed to the onset of diabetic nephropathy (clinical proteinuria), defined as UAER > 200 μg/min, and an increase of > 30% from baseline. After two years, the number of patients progress-ing from microalbuminuria to clinical proteinuria was significantly reduced by 70% with the highest dose of irbesartan therapy. Clinical CV end-points were also reduced by irbesartan treatment over placebo, from 8.7% in the control group, to 4.5% in the 300 mg irbesartan group. The percentage of patients with a reduction of microalbuminuria to normal levels was significantly increased with any irbesartan therapy. The trial results clearly demonstrated that irbesartan could significantly benefit this patient population.

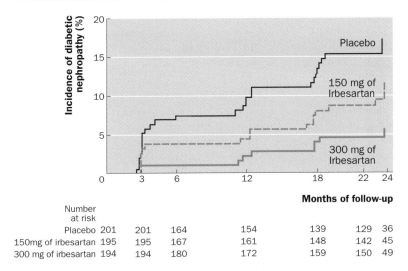

Fig. 5.11 Incidence of progression to diabetic nephropathy during treatment with 150 mg of irbesartan daily, 300 mg of irbesartan daily, or placebo in hypertensive patients with type 2 diabetes and persistent microalbuminuria. Source: Parving *et al.* (2001).

The difference between the placebo group and the 150 mg group was not significant ($P = 0.08$ by the log-rank test), but the difference between the placebo group and the 300 mg group was significant ($P < 0.001$ by the log-rank test).

The average urinary albumin excretion rate (geometric mean) was significantly reduced in both irbesartan groups ($P < 0.001$). There were no significant differences among the three groups in the initial or the sustained (3–24-month) rate of decline in creatinine clearance. The average trough MAP during the study was 103 mmHg in the placebo group, 103 mmHg in the 150 mg group, and 102 mmHg in the 300 mg group ($P = 0.005$ for the comparison between the 300 mg group and the placebo group).

The calcium channel blocker controversy in patients with diabetic nephropathy: is there an issue?
Ruilope LM, Campo C, Segura J. *Curr Hypertens Rep* 2001; **3**(5): 419–21.

BACKGROUND. Chronic renal failure, proteinuria and arterial hypertension run in parallel in the presence of diabetic nephropathy. New goal BP levels have been established in diabetic patients: 130/85 mmHg and 125/75 mmHg depending on the level of proteinuria being below or above 1 g/day. New and lower threshold BP

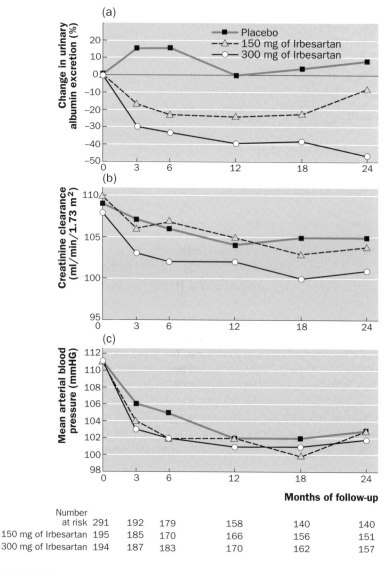

Fig. 5.12 Geometric mean rate of urinary albumin excretion (panel a), estimated mean creatinine clearance (panel b), and trough MAP (panel c) in hypertensive patients with type 2 diabetes and persistent microalbuminuria, according to treatment group. Source: Parving *et al.* (2001).

(> 130/85 mmHg) to initiate pharmacological therapy is required in the presence of DM in order to facilitate the strict BP control that is required. It must be considered that both renal and CV protection are obtained with strict BP control, which otherwise seems to require blockade of angiotensin II effects when proteinuria above 1 g/day is present.

INTERPRETATION. While awaiting the publication of long-term follow-up studies looking at renal and CV outcome in diabetic and other nephropathies in which calcium channel blockers are compared with other antihypertensive drugs, calcium channel blockers will remain the drugs needed to attain the expected goal BP in diabetics, both alone (in the absence of microalbuminuria or macroalbuminuria) or in combination, particularly with ACEIs.

Comment

See below

Effect of ramipril *vs* amlodipine on renal outcomes in hypertensive nephrosclerosis. The African American Study of Kidney Disease and Hypertension (AASK).

Agodoa LY, Appel L, Bakris GL, *et al. JAMA* 2001; **285**(21): 2719–28.

BACKGROUND. Incidence of ESRD due to hypertension has increased in recent decades but the optimal strategy for treatment of hypertension to prevent renal failure is unknown, especially among African Americans. This study compared the effects of an ACEI (ramipril), a dihydropyridine CCB (amlodipine), and a beta-blocker (metoprolol) on hypertensive renal disease progression.

INTERPRETATION. Ramipril, compared with amlodipine, retards renal disease progression in patients with hypertensive renal disease and proteinuria and may offer benefit to patients without proteinuria.

Comment

AASK was a 3 × 2 factorial double-blind designed study of 1094 hypertensive African Americans (non-diabetic) with mild to moderate renal insufficiency, randomized to receive 1 of 3 drugs/classes, ramipril, metoprolol, or amlodipine, with other agents added to achieve one of two BP targets, either an aggressive goal of 125/75 mmHg, or the standard target of 140/90 mmHg. The primary end-point of the trial was the change in GFR slope, including both the total and chronic slopes. The secondary end-point of the study - regarded as potentially more clinically relevant - was a composite of a 50% decrease in the GFR, an absolute decrease in GFR of 25 ml/min/1.73m², ESRD or death. The present paper is an interim analysis and compares only the amlodipine and ramipril arms following suspension of the amlodipine arm in October 2000 after the trial's data and safety monitoring board (the National Institutes of Health) noted that amlodipine was significantly less effective than ramipril or metoprolol in slowing progression of renal disease especially in patients with baseline evidence of kidney damage (urine protein–creatinine ratio [UP/Cr] >0.22 or proteinuria of approximately 300 mg/day). Participants with protein excretion above this level showed the greatest benefit of ramipril compared with those receiving amlodipine in all outcome parameters. Indeed, in the first 6 months, ramipril treatment appeared to decrease proteinuria by 20%, whereas protein excretion in patients treated with amlodipine increased by almost 60%. Moreover, in the entire patient cohort, ramipril reduced the combined end-point of ESRD and death by 41%, and the combined end-point of GFR, ESRD, and death by 38%. Such findings were highly contentious and of great clinical relevance for a number of reasons: 1) the risk of hypertensive ESRD for African-Americans is 20-fold greater than in whites; 2) African-Americans have traditionally been thought to be less responsive to ACEIs; 3) CCBs are currently one of the most commonly prescribed drugs for hypertension in African Americans. Dihydropyridine-calcium channel blockers increase proteinuria and may not slow the progression of established renal disease despite substantial reductions in BP. In terms of reno/cardioprotection, ACEI once again proved to be superior to CCBs. A recent meta-analysis by Furberg *et al.* (*see page 198*) has shown detrimental effects of CCBs: CCBs were associated with 25% higher rates of both acute myocardial infarction and heart failure.

AASK is a landmark study that has shown for the first time the benefit of ACE inhibition in African-Americans, an understudied group that is at greatly increased risk of serious, costly and fatal disease. Indeed, the full trial results have been presented at the American Heart Association Scientific Sessions November 2001 and confirmed the interim results of this paper. In addition, amlodipine appeared to

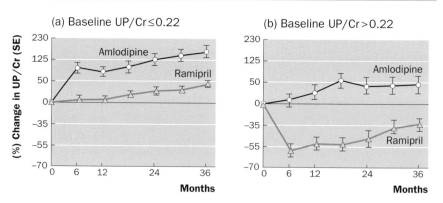

Fig. 5.13 Percent changes in proteinuria from baseline. UP/Cr indicates urinary protein to creatinine ratio. Shown are the estimated percentage changes from baseline in the geometric mean UP/Cr. Baseline UP/Cr of 0.22 corresponds approximately to proteinuria of 300 mg/d. Error bars represent SE. Source: Agodoa *et al.* (2001).

have minimal or no detrimental effect on renal function in people with no protein-uria. The relative benefit of the two BP targets has also been announced. Unlike diabetics with hypertension in other trials, non-diabetic patients in AASK showed no difference in benefit between the two BP targets.

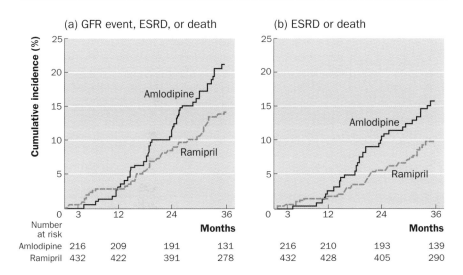

Fig. 5.14 Cumulative incidence of renal events and death. GFR indicates glomerular filtration rate; ESRD, end-stage renal disease. The adjusted risk reduction for ramipril *vs* amlodipine for the GFR event, ESRD, or death composite outcome was 38% (95% confidence interval [CI], 13%–56%; *P* = 0.005) (a) and for ESRD or death was 41% (95% CI, 14%–60%; *P* = 0.007) (b). The risk reductions are adjusted for baseline levels of log transformed UP/Cr, history of heart disease, MAP, sex, and age. Source: Agodoa *et al.* (2001).

Blood pressure and angiotensin converting enzyme inhibitor use in hypertensive patients with chronic renal insufficiency.

Hsu CY, Bates DW, Kuperman GJ, Curhan GC. *Am J Hypertens* 2001; **14**(12): 1219–25.

BACKGROUND. Hypertension treatment is important in managing chronic renal insufficiency (CRI). Little is known, however, about the BP control achieved or the pattern of antihypertensive drug prescription among CRI patients.

INTERPRETATION. The BP control achieved among hypertensive CRI subjects, although no worse than that among those without CRI, was found to be suboptimal.

Patients with creatinine clearance (CrCl) 21 to 40 ml/min were less likely to be prescribed ACEIs than were those with CrCl >60 mL/min. Improvement is needed in the clinical management of these factors that can influence the progression of CRI.

Comment

Disappointingly, but not surprisingly, the BP control is still suboptimal whether or not there is concurrent CRI. Perhaps there is slight consolation that the BP control in patients with CRI is not worse than other hypertensives with preserved renal function. However, patients with a CrCl 21 to 40 ml/min—a population that should be targeted for ACEI treatment—were actually less likely to be prescribed ACEI. The study would be more interesting if one could compare treatment of hypertension by nephrologists versus non-nephrologists. Nevertheless, this study identified areas in which the care of patients with CRI can be improved. Education concerning the importance of aggressive BP lowering and appropriate ACEIs use, as well as earlier referral to nephrologists for co-management of CRI patients, may improve the care of the large number of ambulatory patients with reduced renal function.

Study rationale and design of ADVANCE: action in diabetes and vascular disease – preterax and diamicron MR controlled evaluation.

The ADVANCE Investigators. *Diabetologia* 2001; **44**(9): 1118–20.

BACKGROUND. **Patients with Type 2 NIDDM are at increased risk of macrovascular and microvascular disease, both of which are reduced by controlling raised BP in hypertensive patients. Intensive glycaemic control has also been shown to reduce microvascular disease but the effects on macrovascular disease remain uncertain.**

INTERPRETATION. ADVANCE is designed to provide reliable evidence on the balance of benefits and risks conferred by BP lowering therapy and intensive glucose control therapy in high-risk diabetic patients, regardless of initial BP or glucose concentrations. Primary outcomes are, first, the composite of non-fatal stroke, non-fatal myocardial infarction or CV death and, secondly, the composite of new or worsening nephropathy or diabetic eye disease. The scheduled average duration of treatment and follow-up is 4.5 years.

Comment

The objective of ADVANCE is to determine the effects on macrovascular and microvascular disease of first, lowering BP using a very low dose ACEI–diuretic combination (perindopril–indapamide) compared with placebo; and secondly, intensive glucose control with modified-release gliclazide-based glucose control regimen targeting a glycated haemoglobin A1c concentration of 6.5% or less compared with usual glucose control, in 10 000 high-risk hypertensive adults and non-hypertensive individuals with type 2 diabetes. The study is a 2 × 2 factorial randomized, controlled trial with a scheduled period of treatment and follow-up of 4.5 years. The primary outcomes are, first, the composite of non-fatal stroke, non-fatal myocardial infarction or CV death and, secondly, the composite of new or worsening nephropathy or diabetic eye disease. Secondary outcomes include cause-specific CV end-points in addition to dementia and all-cause mortality.

Renal function: the Cinderella of cardiovascular risk profile.

Ruilope LM, van Veldhuisen DJ, Ritz E, Luscher TF. *J Am Coll Cardiol* 2001; **38**(7): 1782–7.

BACKGROUND. The presence of an altered renal function in essential hypertension, advanced heart failure (HF) and after an MI is associated with higher CV morbidity and mortality. Indices of altered renal function (e.g. microalbuminuria, increased serum creatinine concentrations, decrease in estimated creatinine clearance or overt proteinuria) are independent predictors of CV morbidity and mortality in any of the three clinical situations. These parameters should then be routinely evaluated in clinical practice. These facts have several therapeutic implications.

INTERPRETATION. First, although there is no evidence-based information on the level of BP that confers optimal renal protection, levels substantially lower than past recommendations are advisable. Second, hypertensive kidney damage should be prevented by early treatment of hypertensive patients, particularly those with microalbuminuria. Finally, to avoid further aggravation of high CV risk, antihypertensive agents devoid of unwanted metabolic side effects should be used for the treatment of hypertensive vascular damage. In HF, the combination of an ACEI and a beta-blocker seem to be the most renoprotective. Renal outcome is also improved by ACE inhibition after an MI. Finally, renal and CV outcome seem to run in parallel in all these situations.

Comment

See below

Renal function and intensive lowering of blood pressure in hypertensive participants of the hypertension optimal treatment (HOT) study.

Ruilope LM, Salvetti A, Jamerson K, *et al. J Am Soc Nephrol* 2001; **12**(2): 218–25.

BACKGROUND. This article reports further analyses of the Hypertension Optimal Treatment (HOT) Study data with the aim of describing 1) the value of baseline serum creatinine and its clearance (estimated by Cockroft and Gault formula) as predictors of CV events; 2) the effects of intensive lowering of BP on CV events and renal function in patients with reduced renal function; and 3) the effects on CV events of adding acetylsalicylic acid to antihypertensive therapy in patients with reduced renal function.

INTERPRETATION. The results show that 1) baseline elevation in serum creatinine and a reduction in estimated creatinine clearance are powerful predictors of CV events and death; 2) reduced renal function at baseline did not preclude the desired control of BP; 3) the results of this reanalysis of the HOT Study suggest, though do not prove, that the association of acetylsalicylic acid with intensive antihypertensive therapy offers additional benefit in hypertensive patients with reduced renal function.

Comment

Data from the above reanalysis of the HOT study have demonstrated that serum creatinine values above the cut-off point for mild renal insufficiency predict an elevated CV risk even when BP control is excellent. Indeed, in this study, serum creatinine values were the most powerful predictors of mortality, stronger than any of the known accompanying risk factors. The investigators also assessed the prognostic value of a diminished creatinine clearance, as estimated by the Cockcroft and Gault formula. Values < 60 ml/min were associated with a significantly higher cardiovascular risk. Similarly, in the Hypertension Detection and Follow-up Program trial, the presence of elevated serum creatinine values (> 1.7 mg/dl) at baseline was found to be a very potent predictor for five- and eight-year all-cause mortality. Furthermore, in the Cardiovascular Health Study, baseline serum creatinine values > 1.7 mg/dl were associated with a 70% increase in risk for all-cause mortality in elderly men and women followed for five years. The risk conferred was similar to that associated with the presence of congestive heart failure at baseline.

It is of note that in the general population, the presence of an elevated serum creatinine concentration is also associated with a high prevalence of CVD, as in the case of essential hypertension. Such increased risk has been attributed to the fact that elevated serum creatinine concentrations coexist with several other CV risk factors.

Does treatment of non-malignant hypertension reduce the incidence of renal dysfunction? A meta-analysis of ten randomized, controlled trials.
Hsu CY. *J Hum Hypertens* 2001; **15**(2): 99–106.

BACKGROUND. It remains controversial whether non-malignant 'benign' hypertension causes renal dysfunction. The effect of lowering BP on the incidence of renal dysfunction among patients with non-malignant hypertension is not clear. This meta-analysis was conducted to determine whether antihypertensive drug therapy reduces the incidence of renal dysfunction in patients with non-malignant hypertension.

INTERPRETATION. Among patients with non-malignant hypertension enrolled in randomized trials, treated patients did not have a lower risk of renal dysfunction. The 95% CI suggests that a 25% or more true protective effect of antihypertensive drugs is unlikely.

Comment

While it is well established that malignant hypertension damages the kidneys, it remains unclear whether treating patients with non-malignant 'benign' hypertension would prevent renal dysfunction in the long-term. This meta-analysis included ten randomized controlled trials of antihypertensive drug therapy, involving a total of 26 521 individuals with non-malignant hypertension (equivalent to 114 000 person-years) but with normal baseline renal function. As expected, treated patients had lower BP and fewer CV events. However, patients randomized to antihypertensive therapy (or more intensive therapy) did not have a significant reduction in their risk of developing renal dysfunction (relative risk = 0.97; 95% CI 0.78–1.21; $P = 0.77$). While the majority of us agree that lowering BP in patients with hypertension would lead to reduction of both cardiac and cerebrovascular events, many of us would also expect a reduction in the risk of renal dysfunction. The conclusion of this study that BP lowering had no evident renoprotective effect in the studied population is certainly a surprise to many of us at first glance. As usual, the interpretation of any conclusion generated from meta-analyses should be made with caution as patients' inclusion/exclusion criteria could be significantly different. Furthermore, it is of note that the trials included in the analysis had no renal end-points as primary outcome, such as doubling of serum creatinine or time to dialysis, thus lowering the power to detect any renal events. Quite rightly, however, the author recognized the importance of treating BP in these patients as there are clear 'non-renal benefits' with BP lowering.

Part III

Therapy

6

Current drugs

Angiotensin-converting enzyme inhibitors and angiotensin receptor antagonists in hypertension

Introduction

It has been more than twenty years since the introduction of the angiotensin converting enzyme inhibitors (ACEIs); 'the…pril'. The indications and expectations regarding their use has widened considerably, and much of this has been the result of great interest in research of the renin–angiotensin system (RAS) which plays a critical role in the pathogenesis of various vascular diseases. It is now well recognized that many of the adverse effects of the RAS are mediated by angiotensin II (Ang II) and the angiotensin-1 (AT-1) receptor, and thus the creation of angiotensin receptor blockers (ARBs); 'the …sartan'.

ACEIs are now considered among the most successful therapies for hypertension, congestive heart failure, post-myocardial infarction and diabetic microvascular complications as well as preventing stroke. Theoretically, the ARBs may exceed the promise of the ACEIs in the prevention of end-organ damage by reaping the benefits of unopposed angiotensin type 2 (AT_2) receptors while simultaneously blocking the untoward effects of AT_1 receptors and also cause less of a cough. Indeed, more clinical studies have reported what seem to be equivalent cardiovascular (CV) protections as seen in those studies afforded by ACEIs. We will discuss these recently published studies below. Large scale comparative clinical trials of ACEIs *vs* ARBs would probably not be carried out as most of the '…pril' drugs are coming to the end of their patent rights and obviously, such studies are not profitably attractive. Nevertheless, smaller scale comparative studies would still be worthwhile in order to explore further the many questions surrounding the RAS.

It has been accepted by many clinicians that tolerability of ACEIs is a potential stumbling block to their use. Most notably is the ACEI-induced cough which may be the result of the agents' ability to slow the metabolism of bradykinin. Many now have regarded ARB as an 'ACEI without a cough'. It is commonly assumed that all drugs of a class share their mechanisms of action and, thus, are clinically interchangeable. But, the question is: are ACEIs interchangeable with ARBs? We will discuss this further below.

ACEIs: a 'pril' for every ill

Reduction of cardiovascular risk by regression of electrocardiographic markers of left ventricular hypertrophy by the angiotensin-converting enzyme inhibitor ramipril.

Mathew J, Sleight P, Lonn E, *et al. Circulation* 2001; **104**(14): 1615–21.

BACKGROUND. **Electrocardiographic (ECG) markers of left ventricular hypertrophy (LVH) predict poor prognosis. It was determined whether the ACEI, ramipril, prevents the development and causes regression of ECG LVH and whether these changes are associated with improved prognosis independent of blood pressure (BP) reduction.**

INTERPRETATION. The ACEI ramipril decreases the development and causes regression of ECG-LVH independent of BP reduction, and these changes are associated with reduced risk of death, myocardial infarction (MI), stroke, and congestive heart failure (CHF).

Comment

In this substudy of the Heart Outcomes Prevention Evaluation (HOPE) trial, the ACEI ramipril reduced the development of LVH and resulted in LVH regression by ECG. This effect was seen not only in persons with high BP, but also in those with normal or controlled BP. Importantly, this decrease in ECG-LVH translates into a reduced risk of CV death, MI, stroke and CHF. This represents one of the first trials that convincingly shows that LVH regression really does matter, even in patients without hypertension.

The substudy compared baseline and end-of-study ECGs from 8281 patients at high CV risk who were randomized to ramipril or placebo and followed for 4.5 years in the main HOPE trial. Ramipril prevented LVH, or caused a gradual regression of LVH, in 91.9% of patients, irrespective of their BP reduction. Interestingly, however, 90.2% of patients assigned to placebo also had regression or prevention of LVH. Patients who experienced regression or prevention of LVH had a reduced risk of the predefined primary outcome and of CHF.

The regression of LVH seen in patients assigned to placebo could be related to multiple risk factor modification in patients who participate in clinical trials, as well as the use of concomitant medications, including beta-blockers and other BP-lowering drugs. It also raises the recurrent question of how typical is the population entered into trials, where motivated patients and research staff with regular, careful follow-up get a good package of care that includes education, advice on non-pharmacological measures to reduce CV risk, etc.

However, unanswered questions remain. Afro-Caribbean patients are at particular risk of developing LVH, but whether LVH regression in this group would be beneficial is still unknown. Recent evidence from other trials suggests that black patients with left ventricular dysfunction do not respond well to ACE inhibitors, especially if they have a past history of hypertension.

Randomized trial of a perindopril-based blood-pressure-lowering regimen among 6105 individuals with previous stroke or transient ischaemic attack.

PROGRESS Collaborative Group. *Lancet* 2001; **358**(9287): 1033–41.

BACKGROUND. Blood pressure is a determinant of the risk of stroke among both hypertensive and non-hypertensive individuals with cerebrovascular disease. However, there is uncertainty about the efficacy and safety of BP-lowering treatments for many such patients. The Perindopril pROtection aGainst REcurrent Stroke Study (PROGRESS) was designed to determine the effects of a BP-lowering regimen in hypertensive and non-hypertensive patients with a history of stroke or transient ischaemic attack (TIA).

INTERPRETATION. This BP-lowering regimen reduced the risk of stroke among both hypertensive and non-hypertensive individuals with a history of stroke or TIA. Combination therapy with perindopril and indapamide produced larger BP reductions and larger risk reductions than did single drug therapy with perindopril alone. Treatment with these two agents should now be considered routinely for patients with a history of stroke or TIA, irrespective of their BP.

Comment

It is estimated that five million people die from stroke each year and at least 15 million others suffer non-fatal strokes that are frequently disabling. About 1 in 5 survivors will suffer another stroke or heart attack within 5 years. The HOPE study suggests the value of an ACEI in patients with vascular disease, in the reduction of CV end-points. Few clinical trials have addressed the value of ACEIs in cerebrovascular disease, or more generally the effects of BP lowering in patients post-stroke. Indeed, it has generally been thought that antihypertensive drugs were only useful for stroke patients with high BP.

The publication of PROGRESS was therefore timely, with addition data on the value of ACEI-based therapy in stroke patients. In this trial, antihypertensive therapy with a combination of perindopril and indapamide has been shown for the first time to prevent the recurrence of stroke even in 6100 patients who had had stroke (haemorrhagic or ischaemic) or TIA within the past 5 years but did not have major disability.

Patients were randomized to either antihypertensive drug therapy or placebo. Those randomized to drug therapy received either the ACEI perindopril (4 mg daily) with or without indapamide (2.5 mg daily). Among those patients with hypertension on entry, BP was reduced by an average of 10 mmHg in the treated group. In the normotensive group, BP was reduced by an average of 8 mmHg in the treated group.

After 4 years of follow-up, active treatment reduced BP by 9/4 mmHg and stroke recurrence by 28% compared to placebo. Both hypertensive and non-hypertensive patients had similar reductions in their risk of stroke. In the portion of active treatment patients who received both perindopril and indapamide, BP was reduced by 12/5 mmHg, and the risk of stroke was cut by 43%. Single-drug therapy with perindopril alone reduced BP by 5/3 mmHg, but produced no reduction in the risk of stroke. This observation has generated some controversy, as a 5 mmHg reduction in systolic BP (SBP) should translate into an approximate 20% reduction in stroke risk. Indeed, in the CAPtopril Prevention Project (CAPPP), fatal or non-fatal stroke were 1.25 times more common in patients randomized to captopril than in those assigned conventional therapy with diuretics, beta-blockers, or both. Conversely, in the Post-stroke Antihypertensive Treatment Study (PATS), indapamide 2.5 mg daily decreased BP by 5/2 mmHg and reduced the recurrence of fatal and non-fatal stroke by 29%.

In addition to reducing strokes, antihypertensive therapy also showed a significant 38% reduction in non-fatal MI. The benefits seen in this trial occurred despite the fact that 80% of patients entered were already on antihypertensive therapy of some type, and this medication was continued. Half the patients were already on antihypertensives to lower their BP, and another third were taking them for some other reason such as angina. In addition, most patients were taking aspirin.

ACEIs and progression of renal disease in non-diabetics

Angiotensin-converting enzyme inhibitors and progression of non-diabetic renal disease: a meta-analysis of patient-level data.
Jafar TH, Schmid CH, Landa M, *et al. Ann Intern Med* 2001; **135**(2): 73–87.

BACKGROUND. ACEIs are highly effective in slowing the progression of renal disease due to type 1 diabetes, and evidence of their efficacy in type 2 diabetes is growing. However, although 14 randomized, controlled trials have been completed; no consensus exists on the use of ACEIs in non-diabetic renal disease.

INTERPRETATION. Antihypertensive regimens that include ACEIs are more effective than regimens without ACEIs in slowing the progression of non-diabetic renal disease. The beneficial effect of ACEIs is mediated by factors in addition to decreasing BP and urinary protein excretion and is greater in patients with proteinuria. Angiotensin-converting inhibitors are indicated for treatment of non-diabetic patients with chronic renal disease and proteinuria and, possibly, those without proteinuria.

Comment

This meta-analysis of trials addressing the impact of ACEIs on renal disease suggests that antihypertensive regimens that include an ACEI can slow progression of kidney failure, even in non-diabetics and in those with a greater degree of kidney damage at baseline. The primary outcomes for the meta-analysis were end-stage renal disease (ESRD), and the combined outcome of ESRD or a two-fold increase in serum creatinine, a well-accepted surrogate outcome for worsening renal disease over the short-term.

In a previous meta-analysis of 11 ACEI trials, ACE Inhibition in the Progressive Renal Disease Study Group showed that ACE inhibition was associated with decreased progression of renal disease in the entire grouped population.

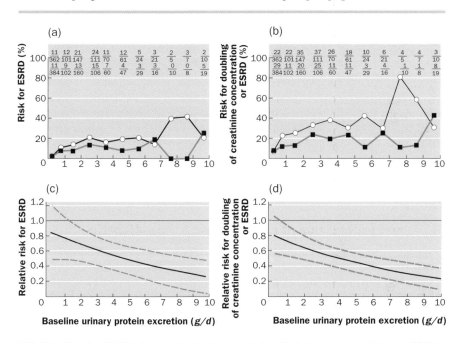

Fig. 6.1 Risk for ESRD (a), combined outcome of doubling of serum creatinine or ESRD (b), or relative risk for these outcomes (c and d) in patients taking ACEIs (squares) and controls (circles), according to baseline urinary protein excretion. The values above the graphs in panels (a) and (b) are the fraction of patients with events in the control group (upper row) and ACEI group (lower row). Relative risks were calculated from multivariable models controlling for significant baseline patient and study characteristics. The solid horizontal line at a relative risk of 1.0 in panels (c) and (d) indicates no difference between the ACEI and control groups; the solid and dotted curved lines represent point estimates and 95% confidence intervals (CIs) for the relative risks. P values for tests for interaction between baseline urinary protein excretion and treatment were 0.03 and 0.001, respectively. Source: Jafar et al. (2001).

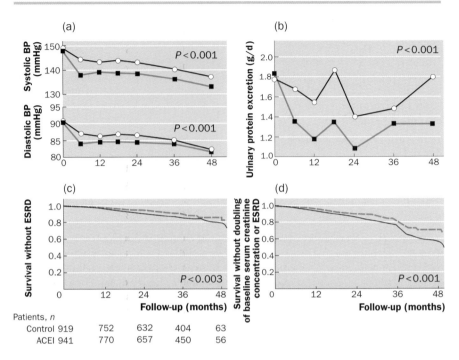

Fig. 6.2 Blood pressure (a), urinary protein excretion (b), survival without ESRD (c), or the combined outcome of doubling of baseline serum creatinine concentration or ESRD (d) during follow-up among patients taking ACEIs (dotted line) and controls (solid line). Follow-up measurements were reported more often during the first 2 years and less often thereafter. Mean BP and mean urinary protein excretion during follow-up were defined as the mean of all available follow-up values for each patient. Change during follow-up was defined as the baseline value minus the mean follow-up value for each patient. The number of patients with follow-up data available for analysis of survival without ESRD is shown below the x-axis of panel (c). Slightly fewer patients had follow-up measurements of BP and urinary protein excretion than for ascertainment of ESRD.
Source: Jafar *et al.* (2001).

Out of the total of 1860 non-diabetic patients enrolled in the 11 studies and with data available for analysis by Jafar *et al.*, 919 were assigned to the 'control' group (having been randomized to either placebo or a drug other than an ACEI), and 941 were assigned to the ACEI group. Enalapril was the ACEI studied in 7 of the 11 studies, while captopril, benazepril, cilazapril and ramipril were evaluated in one study each.

After a mean of 2.2 years, patients in the ACEI group had a greater mean decrease in systolic and diastolic BP (DBP) and urinary protein excretion. After adjustment, the relative risk for ESRD was 0.69, and 0.70 for the combined outcome of ESRD and doubling of serum creatinine in the ACEI group. Those with higher urinary protein excretion at baseline appeared to benefit most from ACE inhibition in terms of both ESRD alone ($P = 0.03$) and ESRD/serum creatinine doubling ($P = 0.001$). At urinary protein excretion values lower than 0.5g/day, the effect was not statistically significant.

ACEIs and diabetic hypoglycaemia

Activity of angiotensin-converting enzyme and risk of severe hypoglycaemia in type 1 diabetes mellitus.

Pedersen-Bjergaard U, Agerholm-Larsen B, Pramming S, Hougaard P, Thorsteinsson B. *Lancet* 2001; **357**(9264): 1248–53.

BACKGROUND. The insertion (I) allele of the angiotensin-converting-enzyme (ACE) gene occurs at increased frequency in endurance athletes. This association suggests that low ACE activity is favourable for performance in conditions with limited substrate availability. Such conditions occur in endurance athletes during competition and in diabetic patients during insulin-induced hypoglycaemia. Patients rely on preserved functional capacity to recognise hypoglycaemic episodes and avoid progression by self-treatment.

INTERPRETATION. ACE activity is a clinically significant marker of the risk of severe hypoglycaemia in patients with type 1 diabetes, especially in those with impaired defence against hypoglycaemia. These findings need to be confirmed in prospective studies.

Comment

See below

Diabetes, hypertension, and cardiovascular disease: an update.

Sowers JR, Epstein M, Frohlich ED. *Hypertension*. 2001; **37**: 1053–9.

BACKGROUND. Hypertension is approximately twice as frequent in patients with diabetes compared with patients without the disease. Conversely, recent data suggest that hypertensive persons are more predisposed to the development of diabetes than are normotensive persons. Furthermore, up to 75% of CV diseases (CVD) in diabetes may be attributable to hypertension, leading to recommendations for more aggressive treatment (i.e., reducing BP to < 130/85 mmHg) in persons with coexistent diabetes and hypertension.

INTERPRETATION. This update reviews the current knowledge regarding the CVD risk factors and their treatment, with special emphasis on the cardiometabolic syndrome, hypertension, microalbuminuria, and diabetic cardiomyopathy. This update also examines the role of the renin-angiotensin system in the increased risk for CVD in diabetic patients and the impact of interrupting this system on the development of clinical diabetes as well as CVD.

Comment

Cardiovascular disease accounts for up to 80% of deaths in people with type 2 diabetes, and is 7.5 times more likely to occur among type 2 diabetics than in people without diabetes. Moreover, hypertension is twice as frequent in diabetics, and up to 75% of CV deaths in people with diabetes may be attributable to hypertension. The recent MICRO-HOPE analysis demonstrates the clear beneficial effect of the ACEI ramipril in reducing CV events in this high-risk patient group.

ACEIs may also have a role in the prevention of severe hypoglycaemia in diabetics. Indeed, ACE activity in patients with type 1 diabetes is a strong independent marker of the risk of severe hypoglycaemia. The ACE gene can be present as an I allele or a D allele. The I allele confers low tissue and blood activity of ACE, as it produces an ACE protein that has only one of the putative two active sites.

Pedersen-Bjergaard *et al.* investigated ACE activity as a potential marker by conducting a study in which 207 consecutive adult outpatients with type 1 diabetes, untreated with ACEIs or angiotensin-II-receptor antagonists, reported their experience of mild and severe hypoglycaemia during the previous two years. The patients were then tested for serum ACE concentrations and ACE genotype. The patients with the DD genotype were 3 times more likely to have had severe hypoglycaemia in the previous 2 years than those who had the II genotype (relative risk [RR] 3.2 95% CI 1.4–7.4). ACE activity was also related to the risk of severe hypoglycaemia, with those in the highest quartile having a 3.5 times higher risk than those in the lowest quartile.

What are the clinical implications? First, measurement of ACE activity might enable stratification of diabetic patients at the time of diagnosis according to their long-term risk of severe hypoglycaemia. In patients with high ACE activity, awareness of hypoglycaemia and residual-cell function could be assessed regularly during the course of diabetes by simple means for further risk stratification.

Secondly, drugs that modulate the activity of the angiotensin system or the bradykinin pathway might be valuable in the prevention of severe hypoglycaemia. Thus, trials are warranted on the protective effect of ACEIs against severe hypoglycaemia in high-risk patients with high ACE activity, who may constitute as much as 10–20% of unselected patients with type 1 diabetes.

Effect of ramipril *vs* amlodipine on renal outcomes in hypertensive nephrosclerosis: a randomized controlled trial. African American Study of Kidney Disease and Hypertension (AASK) Study Group.
Agodoa LY, Appel L, Bakris GL, *et al. JAMA* 2001; **285**(21): 2719–28.

BACKGROUND. Incidence of ESRD due to hypertension has increased in recent decades, but the optimal strategy for treatment of hypertension to prevent renal failure is unknown, especially among African Americans. To compare the effects of an ACEI (ramipril), a dihydropyridine calcium channel blocker (CCB) (amlodipine), and a beta-blocker (metoprolol) on hypertensive renal disease progression.

INTERPRETATION. Ramipril, compared with amlodipine, retards renal disease progression in patients with hypertensive renal disease and proteinuria and may offer benefit to patients without proteinuria.

Comment

Current guidelines recommend CCBs as first-line therapy for treatment of hypertension in African-American patients, as it has been believed, for various reasons, that ACEIs are not effective in this population.

The African-American Study of Kidney Disease and Hypertension (AASK) study shows that ACEIs are effective in preventing progression to renal failure in African Americans with hypertensive renal disease, and are more effective than CCBs, the currently recommended treatment for this population.

In this study (terminated early) which enrolled 1094 African-American patients from 21 centres, patients were randomized to receive 1 of 3 drugs: ramipril, the beta-blocker metoprolol or amlodipine. Patients were also randomized to 1 of 2 BP targets, either an aggressive goal of 125/75 mmHg, or the more usual target of 140/90 mmHg.

Table 6.1 Comparison of antihypertensive agents in reducing GFR, ESRD, or death

Drugs compared	RR	P value
Ramipril *vs* metoprolol	22%	0.042
Ramipril *vs* amlodipine	38%	0.005
Metoprolol *vs* amlodipine	19%	0.19
Ramipril *vs* amlodipine in patients with minimal renal dysfunction*	46%	0.004
Metoprolol *vs* amlodipine in patients with minimal renal dysfunction*	37%	0.003

*Patients with baseline urine protein–creatinine ratio of > 0.22 or ~300 mg protein/day

Source: Agodoa *et al.* (2001).

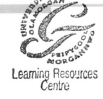

Learning Resources
Centre

Table 6.2   Mortality rates for patients receiving ACEIs *vs* patients not receiving ACEIs

End-points	ACE inhibitors	No ACE inhibitors
CAD mortality	18%	26%
CVA mortality	11%	10%
CVD mortality	29%	36
Other mortality	2%	1%
All deaths	31%	37%

Source: Agodoa *et al.* (2001).

Those treated with ramipril were significantly less likely to progress to more severe renal dysfunction, dialysis, or death than those treated with amlodipine, a CCB. The interim analysis of the AASK at 3 years revealed a renoprotective effect of ramipril as compared to amlodipine in patients with mild to moderate renal insufficiency. This differential effect was independent of the BP levels reached and was evident in proteinuric patients and suggestive in patients with baseline proteinuria < 300 mg/d, but was not conclusive. Furthermore, aggressive BP lowering beyond usual levels was not associated with additional slowing of renal disease progression.

Over a period of approximately 10 years, 74 patients (31%) in the ACEI group and 212 (37%) in the non-ACEI group died. After correcting for baseline differences, patients not receiving ACEIs had 80% higher mortality compared to those not taking them (relative risk of 1.8 [CI 1.3–2.6]), indicating a strong protective effect of ACEIs in African American men with coronary heart disease. The benefit was seen regardless of which ACEI was used.

If not ACEIs –Angiotensin II receptor blockers?

The Ang II antagonists are an important new class of CV drugs that block the RAS. Certainly, the evidence so far indicates Ang II antagonists are safe and well tolerated drugs, with benefits in many CV conditions, including hypertension and heart failure. It seems likely that Ang II antagonists will have their own unique benefits and should not be simply regarded as 'new'ACEIs without the cough.

Yes, for the prevention of renal disease progression in type 2 diabetes.

Effects of losartan on renal and cardiovascular outcomes in patients with type 2 diabetes and nephropathy.
Brenner BM, Cooper ME, de Zeeuw D, *et al. N Engl J Med* 2001; **345**(12): 861–9.

B A C K G R O U N D . Diabetic nephropathy is the leading cause of ESRD. Interruption of the RAS slows the progression of renal disease in patients with type 1 diabetes, but similar data are not available for patients with type 2, the most common form of diabetes. We assessed the role of the angiotensin-II-receptor antagonist losartan in patients with type 2 diabetes and nephropathy.

INTERPRETATION. Losartan conferred significant renal benefits in patients with type 2 diabetes and nephropathy, and it was generally well tolerated.

Comment

See below

Irbesartan in patients with type 2 diabetes and microalbuminuria study group. The effect of irbesartan on the development of diabetic nephropathy in patients with type 2 diabetes.

Parving HH, Lehnert H, Brochner-Mortensen J, Gomis R, Andersen S, Arner P. *N Engl J Med* 2001; **345**(12): 870–8.

BACKGROUND. Microalbuminuria and hypertension are risk factors for diabetic nephropathy. Blockade of the RAS slows the progression to diabetic nephropathy in patients with type 1 diabetes, but similar data are lacking for hypertensive patients with type 2 diabetes.

INTERPRETATION. Irbesartan is renoprotective independently of its BP-lowering effect in patients with type 2 diabetes and microalbuminuria.

Comment

The beneficial effects of ACEIs in diabetic renal disease are well established, but some patients do not tolerate ACEIs due to cough and other side effects. Thus, a viable alternative treatment is with Ang II receptor (AT1R) antagonists, which have also been shown to slow the progression of renal disease in patients with type 2 diabetes, hypertension and proteinuria, a marker of kidney disease.

Three recent trials confirm the benefits of the angiotensin receptor antagonists in type II diabetes. The RENAAL study with losartan and the Irbesartan Diabetic Nephropathy Trial (IDNT) study using irbesartan showed these drugs provided a renoprotective effect, reducing morbidity independent of BP lowering.

In the Reduction of Endpoints in NIDDM (non-insulin dependent diabetes mellitus) with the Angiotensin II Antagonist Losartan (RENAAL) study, 1513 patients from centres in 29 countries were randomized to treatment with losartan (50–100 mg/qd) or placebo. All had type 2 diabetes, proteinuria and elevated serum creatinine. Most (94%) had hypertension, and were treated with antihypertensive medications, but could not be treated with either an Ang II antagonist or an ACEI to be included in this trial.

The primary end-point was a composite of time to first occurrence of either a doubling of serum creatinine, ESRD or death. The researchers reported that, after 3.4 years of follow-up, the primary end-point was significantly reduced with losartan therapy, as well as two of the three measures making up the composite.

A composite end-point of MI, stroke, revascularization, hospitalization for unstable angina, hospitalization for heart failure and CV death was not significantly different between the groups, nor were the components of this end-point different, with the exception of hospitalization for heart failure, which was significantly reduced by 32% ($P = 0.005$) with losartan treatment.

The drug was well tolerated: discontinuation of therapy occurred in 17% of treated patients, 22% of placebo patients. The most common reasons for withdrawal included heart failure, ESRD, MI, stroke and worsening renal insufficiency. The researchers also presented an economic analysis, suggesting that over the 3.5-year study period, losartan treatment plus conventional BP therapy reduced the number of days with ESRD by about 32%, a reduction estimated to produce a net $3000 savings for Medicare per treated diabetic patient, after factoring in the cost of the drug.

The two trials investigating the effects of irbesartan were part of the larger PRogram for Irbesartan Mortality and Morbidity Evaluations (PRIME), which aimed to look at the drug's effect in those with type 2 diabetes and hypertension, and microalbuminuria in the IRbesartan MicroAlbuminuria Type 2 Diabetes Mellitus in Hypertensive Patients (IRMA II) and in those with diabetes, hypertension, and proteinuria, a marker of nephropathy, in the IDNT trial. In the IDNT trial, 1715 men and women with hypertension and type 2 diabetes were randomized to treatment with irbesartan, in a dose of 75–300 mg once daily, the CCB amlodipine in a dose of 2.5–10 mg once daily, or placebo on a background of antihypertensive therapy. Patients in this trial already had frank kidney disease, with proteinuria > 900 mg/qd, and serum creatinine levels of 1.2–3.0 mg/dL in men, 1.0–3.0 mg/dL in women. The primary end-point was timed to a composite end-point of death, doubling of baseline serum creatinine and end-stage renal disease.

Table 6.3 Losartan *vs* placebo in RENAAL: Relative risk reduction in end-points

End-point	Losartan	Placebo	RR reduction	P value
Primary composite end-point	43.5%	47.1%	16%	0.024
ESRD	19.6%	25.5%	28%	0.002
2× serum creatinine	21.6%	26.0%	25%	0.006
Death	21.0%	20.3%	–	NS

Source: Parving *et al.* (2001).

Table 6.4 Comparison of UAER with valsartan *vs* amlodipine

End-point	Valsartan baseline	Valsartan 24 weeks	Amlodipine baseline	Amlodipine 24 weeks	*P* value
UAER (mcg/min)	57.97	32.3	55.4	50.7	P <0.001

More patients returned to normal albuminuric status after treatment with valsartan (29.9%) compared to amlodipine (14.5%), a statistically significant difference (*P* = 0.001). These differences were seen in conjunction with similar levels of blood pressure lowering.

Source: Parving *et al.* (2001).

After 2.5 years of follow-up, the incidence of a primary end-point event was significantly reduced by irbesartan therapy, by 33% compared to placebo, and by 37% compared to amlodipine.

In the IRMA II trial, 590 patients with hypertension, type 2 diabetes, microalbuminuria (urinary albumin excretion rate [UAER] 20–200 mcg/min), and normal kidney function were randomized to two doses of irbesartan (150 and 300 mg once daily) or placebo on a background of antihypertensive therapy, (excluding ACEIs, Ang II antagonists or dihydropyridine CCBs). The primary end-point was time to the occurrence of clinical proteinuria, defined as UAER greater than 200 mcg/min, and an increase of > 30% from baseline.

After two years, the number of patients progressing from microalbuminuria to clinical proteinuria was significantly reduced by 70% (*P* = 0.0004) with the highest dose of irbesartan therapy. Clinical CV end-points were also reduced by irbesartan treatment over placebo, from 8.7% in the control group, to 4.5% in the 300 mg irbesartan group.

In the Microalbuminuria Reduction with Valsartan (MARVAL) trial, 332 type 2 diabetes patients with microalbuminuria with and without hypertension were randomized to 80 mg/day of valsartan, or 5 mg/day of amlodipine, and followed for 24 weeks. A target BP of 135/85 mmHg was attempted for all patients, through dose doubling and the addition of an alpha blocker or thiazide diuretic. From baseline to the end of 24 weeks, the mean (lower and upper quartiles) in UAER was significantly reduced by valsartan compared to amlodipine.

More patients returned to normal albuminuric status after treatment with valsartan (29.9%) compared to amlodipine (14.5%), also a statistically significant difference (*P* = 0.001). These differences were seen in conjunction with similar levels of BP lowering.

Are all Ang II receptor antagonists the same?

A prospective, randomized, open-label trial comparing telmisartan 80 mg with valsartan 80 mg in patients with mild to moderate hypertension using ambulatory blood pressure monitoring.

Littlejohn T, Mroczek W, Marbury T, VanderMaelen CP, Dubiel RF.
Canadian Journal of Cardiology 2000; **16**(9): 1123–32.

BACKGROUND. To compare the antihypertensive efficacy and tolerability of
telmisartan 80 mg with valsartan 80 mg throughout a 24-h dosing interval in a
prospective, randomized, open-label, blinded end-point, parallel group study.

INTERPRETATION. Telmisartan 80 mg once daily was superior to valsartan 80 mg
once daily in reducing DBP during the last 6 h of the 24-h dosing interval. These results
may be due to telmisartan's longer plasma half-life or to a higher potency compared with
valsartan, such that a higher dose of valsartan may produce effects similar to those of
80 mg telmisartan. These data confirm the long duration of action of telmisartan with
consistent and sustained control of BP over 24 h and during the last 6 h of the dosing
interval. Both treatments were well tolerated; the adverse event data confirmed the
excellent tolerability profiles of telmisartan and valsartan that have been reported
previously.

Comment

See below

Comparative effects of candesartan cilexetil and losartan in patients with systemic hypertension. Candesartan *versus* Losartan Efficacy Comparison (CANDLE) Study Group.

Gradman AH, Lewin A, Bowling BT, *et al. Heart Dis* 1999; **1**(2): 52–7.

BACKGROUND. The antihypertensive efficacy and tolerability of the novel Ang-II
receptor blocker candesartan cilexetil and the prototype Ang-II receptor blocker,
losartan, were compared in an 8-week, multicentre, double-blind, randomized,
parallel-group, titration-to-effect study.

INTERPRETATION. The candesartan regimen was significantly more effective than the
losartan regimen in reducing trough sitting DBP at week 8 (11.0 mmHg *vs* 8.9 mmHg).
Candesartan also produced numerically greater reductions in secondary BP parameters,
including sitting SBP, trough standing DBP and SBP, and peak (6 ± 2.5 h after dose)
sitting and standing DBP and SBP. Responder rates (sitting DBP < 90 mmHg or
reduction in BP of ≥ 10 mmHg) and control rates (sitting DBP < 90 mmHg) were higher
with candesartan (64% *vs* 54% and 54% *vs* 43%, respectively). A total of 1.9% of the

patients taking candesartan and 6.5% of those taking losartan discontinued prematurely because of adverse events or lack of efficacy.

Comment
See below

Antihypertensive efficacy of candesartan in comparison to losartan: the CLAIM study.
Bakris G, Gradman A, Reif M, *et al. J Clin Hypertens* (Greenwich) 2001; **3**(1): 16–21.

BACKGROUND. An 8-week, multicentre, double-blind, randomized, parallel-group, forced-titration study was conducted to evaluate the antihypertensive efficacy of candesartan *vs* losartan in 654 hypertensive patients with a DBP between 95 and 114 mmHg from 72 sites throughout the US.

INTERPRETATION. This forced-titration study confirms that candesartan cilexetil is more effective than losartan in lowering BP when both are administered once daily at maximum doses. Both drugs were well tolerated.

Comment
See below

Effects of losartan and candesartan monotherapy and losartan/hydrochlorothiazide combination therapy in patients with mild to moderate hypertension.
Manolis AJ, Grossman E, Jelakovic B, *et al. Clin Ther* 2000; **22**(10): 1186–203.

BACKGROUND. The goal of this multicentre, double-blind, randomized, parallel-group study was to compare the effects of losartan potassium (hereafter referred to as losartan), candesartan cilexitil (hereafter referred to as candesartan), and losartan/hydrochlorothiazide (HCTZ) in patients with mild to moderate hypertension (sitting DBP [SiDBP] 95–115 mmHg).

INTERPRETATION. Losartan 50 mg/100 mg and candesartan 8 mg/16 mg were comparable treatments in terms of BP reduction. After titration, losartan 50 mg plus HCTZ 12.5 mg was superior to either candesartan 16 mg or losartan 100 mg in reducing hypertension. Losartan, but not candesartan, lowered serum uric acid levels and attenuated the expected increase in uric acid levels with HCTZ 12.5 mg.

Comment

The angiotensin receptor antagonists (sartans) are a relatively new class of drugs, with good efficacy and few side effects. Some of the early trials also reported that many patients treated with sartans had fewer adverse effects, compared to placebo. Recent data also suggests that sartans may improve sexual function!

With the increasing numbers of individual drugs within the sartans – in the UK, losartan, valsartan, candesartan, telmesartan and eprosartan are available, and jostling for market share – it is no surprise that many trials have attempted to compare one against the other, resulting in the so-called 'sartan wars'.

In this study by Littlejohn *et al.*, telmisartan 80 mg once daily was superior to valsartan 80 mg once daily in reducing DBP during the last 6 h of the 24 h dosing interval. These results may be due to telmisartan's longer plasma half-life or to a higher potency compared with valsartan, such that a higher dose of valsartan may produce effects similar to those of 80 mg telmisartan.

Gradman *et al.* and Bakris *et al.* similarly report a comparison between losartan and candesartan. Manolis *et al.* suggest a neutral comparison between losartan 50/100 mg and candesartan 8/16 mg in a multinational study, but advocate the uricosuric effects of losartan. Being the market leader at the time of writing, with many large outcome trials ongoing or reported, it comes as no surprise that losartan is the target comparator of many sartan comparisons. A well-proven safety and efficacy track record in clinical outcomes trials may yet win the day, but the counter-argument that 'it's all a class effect' is also heard from cynical clinical pharmacologists.

Combination of ACEIs and ARBs

Beyond the usual strategies for blood pressure reduction: therapeutic considerations and combination therapies.
Giles TD, Sander GE. *J Clin Hypertens* 2001; **3**(6): 346–53.

BACKGROUND. Rapidly accumulating clinical data have repeatedly demonstrated not only the critical importance of even small increases in BP as a pathophysiologic factor in the development of CVD, particularly in individuals with diabetes mellitus, but also the therapeutic necessity of more aggressive BP reduction and the achievement of progressively lower BP targets in reducing CV event rates.

INTERPRETATION. Achieving such target pressures is increasingly difficult, particularly in diabetic patients with chronic renal disease, who require complex multidrug antihypertensive regimens. This review attempts to provide some suggestions for constructing such antihypertensive regimens and provides considerations for the appropriate use of diuretics and the most effective drug combinations.

Comment

This review highlighted certain considerations and 'pearls' that may assist clinicians in designing pharmacologic regimens for their patients. The review also discussed certain pharmacologic properties of individual drugs that are often not considered because of the implications of such properties relative to multidrug regimens. The authors also suggested alternative combinations that may improve control of BP, as well as some combinations to be avoided. These suggestions are, of course, based on a desire to achieve lower BPs and have not been the subject of clinical outcome trials; they may be particularly appropriate for patients who have received drugs from four of the major classes – diuretics, beta-blockers, ACEIs/AT1R blockers and CCBs.

Coadministration of losartan and enalapril exerts additive antiproteinuric effect in IgA nephropathy.
Russo D, Minutolo R, Pisani A, *et al. Am J Kidney Dis* 2001; **38**(1): 18–25.

BACKGROUND. ACEI and AT1R antagonists (ARAs) are widely administered to reduce urinary protein loss and slow the progression of proteinuric nephropathy to end-stage renal failure. Our group recently observed that the combination of ACEIs and ARAs may have an additive antiproteinuric effect, which may occur because ACEIs do not completely reduce Ang II production. Ang II is also produced by chymase. Thus, combination therapy better antagonizes the effects of Ang II.

INTERPRETATION. This study shows that combination therapy with enalapril and losartan has an additive dose-dependent antiproteinuric effect that is likely induced by the drug-related reduction in systemic BP. In normotensive proteinuric patients, it is likely that even a small reduction in systemic BP may affect intraglomerular haemodynamics by a great extent because efferent arteriole regulation is hampered more completely by the coadministration of ACEIs and ARAs.

Comment

The purpose of this study is to ascertain whether the additive antiproteinuric effect of ACEIs plus ARAs is dose dependent and related to the drug-induced reduction in systemic BP.

Randomized controlled trial of dual blockade of renin–angiotensin system in patients with hypertension, microalbuminuria and non-insulin dependent diabetes: the candesartan and lisinopril microalbuminuria (CALM) study.

Mogensen CE, Neldam S, Tikkanen I, *et al. BMJ* 2000; **321**(7274): 1440–4.

BACKGROUND. The value of inhibiting the renin-angiotensin system (RAS) event microvascular complications in diabetes has been previously shown. However, it is also known that ACEIs often do not provide adequate control of BP in patients with diabetes. In addition, Ang II can be generated by pathways other than the ACE enzyme. An alternative approach is to block the receptors with an angiotensin II receptor blocking agent.

INTERPRETATION. Candesartan 16 mg once daily is as effective as lisinopril 20 mg once daily in reducing BP and microalbuminuria in hypertensive patients with type 2 diabetes. Combination treatment is well tolerated and more effective in reducing BP.

Comment

Blockade of the RAS at different sites using ACEIs or Ang II type 1 receptor antagonists is being widely used in the management of hypertension. This multicentre study was designed to evaluate the effect on BP and microalbuminuria of the combination of an ACEI, lisinopril (20 mg/day), and an Ang II blocker, candesartan (16 mg/day), compared with treatment with each drug singly in patients with microalbuminuria, hypertension and type 2 diabetes. The results clearly showed a beneficial effect of treatment with either drug on both systolic and DBP and on the albumin/creatinine ratio. The combination, however, gave an additional benefit with regard to both BP and microalbuminuria. For example, the mean reduction in DBP with candesartan was 10.4 mmHg, with lisinopril 10.7 mmHg, and with the combination 16.3 mmHg. The mean reductions in the urinary albumin/creatinine ratio were 24%, 39% and 50%, respectively. These treatment regimens were generally well tolerated, although 10% of patients reported cough or headache. There were no changes in haemoglobin A1c or in creatinine clearance. The study confirms that dual blockade of the RAS is more effective than monotherapy at reducing BP. It is already known that hypertension is a strong risk factor for microvascular disease in type 2 diabetes and that microalbuminuria adds to this risk. Combination therapy appears to reduce these two risk factors. Other studies such as the Val-HeFT, in addition to this one, have confirmed that this approach is safe. We shall await the results of the VALUE trial (see below).

Characteristics of 15 314 hypertensive patients at high coronary risk: the Valsartan Antihypertensive Long-term Use Evaluation (VALUE) trial.

Kjeldsen SE. Julius S. Brunner H, *et al. Blood Pressure* 2001; **10**(2): 83–91.

BACKGROUND. Valsartan is an orally active, selective antagonist of the Ang II-1 (AT1) receptor developed for the treatment of hypertension. The Valsartan Antihypertensive Long-term Use Evaluation (VALUE) Trial of Cardiovascular Events in Hypertension is a double-blind, randomized prospective, parallel group study designed to compare the effects of valsartan with those of the calcium-antagonist amlodipine on the reduction of cardiac morbidity and mortality.

INTERPRETATION. Patients with essential hypertension, aged 50 years and older, and at particularly high risk of coronary events were enrolled. 18 119 patients were screened and 15 314 patients in 31 countries were randomized mainly between January 1998 and December 1999. These hypertensives had a mean BP of 154.7/87.5 mmHg at the time of their randomization to blinded medication. The population comprises both genders (men 57.6%), Caucasians (89.1%), mean age 67.2 years, mean body mass index 28.6 kg/m^2, coronary heart disease (45.8%), high cholesterol (33.0%), type 2 diabetes mellitus (DM) (31.7%) and smokers (24.0%). More than 92% of the randomized participants had been treated for high BP for at least 6 months when screened for the study. The randomized population is now being treated (goal BP < 140/90 mmHg) in adherence with the protocol until at least 1450 patients experience primary cardiac end-point defined as clinically evident or aborted MI, hospitalization for heart failure or death caused by coronary heart disease.

Comment

Since ARBs inhibit the activation of the AT1 receptor by Ang II, while ACEIs increase the concentration of vasodilator peptides, such as bradykinin, the combination of both agents should provide a higher degree of blockade of the renin-angiotensin system than either agent alone, and thus represents an attractive possibility for therapy in patients requiring multiple drugs for BP control.

ACEI/ARB combination has been evaluated primarily in heart failure trials for determination of clinical outcome. However, in a small study of patients with chronic renal disease, Russo *et al.* report that the reductions in both systolic and DBP were greater with the combination than with an ARB alone. The combination did not cause further deterioration of renal function, and it may also have additive antiproteinuric effects.

The larger study by Mogensen *et al.* is in keeping with this, where candesartan 16 mg once daily was as effective as lisinopril 20 mg once daily in reducing BP and microalbuminuria in hypertensive patients with type 2 diabetes. At 24 weeks, the mean reduction in DBP with combination treatment (16.3 mmHg, $P < 0.001$)

was significantly greater than that with candesartan (10.4 mmHg, $P < 0.001$) or lisinopril (mean 10.7 mmHg, $P < 0.001$). Furthermore, the reduction in urinary albumin:creatinine ratio with combination treatment (50%, $P < 0.001$) was greater than with candesartan (24%, $P = 0.05$) and lisinopril (39%, $P < 0.001$). Thus, combination treatment was well tolerated and more effective in reducing BP.

ACEIs interchangeable to ARBs?

 Does the antihypertensive response to angiotensin-converting enzyme inhibition predict the antihypertensive response to angiotensin receptor antagonism?
Stergiou GS, Skeva II, Baibas NM, Kalkana CB, Roussias LG, Mountokalakis TD. *Am J Hypertens* 2001; **14**(7 Pt 1): 688–93.

BACKGROUND. Current guidelines recommend the use of AT1R antagonists in hypertensive patients in whom treatment with an ACEI is effective but poorly tolerated. This strategy is based on the assumption that because ACEIs and AT1R antagonists act on the same system there is little intra-individual variation in their antihypertensive response.

INTERPRETATION. In more than one third of hypertensive subjects, the BP response to ACE inhibition fails to predict the response to AT1R antagonism and *vice versa*. These data suggest that there are differences between these two drug classes that are not only of theoretical but also of practical significance.

Comment

The question addressed in this study was whether the antihypertensive response to ACE inhibition can predict the response to AT1R antagonism and *vice versa*. A crossover design in which all patients are exposed to all treatments is appropriate for addressing such a research question. Although the study was not blinded to the investigator, a selection bias was prevented by randomizing patients to the two treatment arms, and a placebo effect was minimised by using ambulatory BP monitoring (ABPM).

Thirty-three hypertensive patients were randomized to receive lisinopril (20 mg) or losartan (50 mg) for 5 weeks. Patients were then crossed-over to the alternative treatment for a second 5-week period. A 24-h ABPM was measured before randomization and on the final day of each period. The agreement in ABP response between the two drugs was assessed using the following approaches. Subjects were classified as responders and non-responders using as a threshold an arbitrary level of response (ABP fall ≥ 10 mmHg systolic or ≥ 5 mmHg diastolic) or the median ABP response achieved by each of the drugs. Disagreement between the two drugs in the responders–non-responders classification was expressed as the proportion of subjects whose ABP responded to one of the drugs only. The responders–

non-responders analysis showed that – irrespective of the criterion used for the definition of responders – in up to 40% of individuals, the antihypertensive response to ACE inhibition fails to predict the response to AT1R antagonism and *vice versa*. In other words, more than one third of individuals with poor response to treatment with one of these drug classes will respond well to the other, and *vice versa*.

It should be noted that, however, that the imperfect reproducibility of ABPM has probably affected, at least in part, the findings of this study. Furthermore, the differences in the pharmacological profile of the two drugs (antihypertensive efficacy and 24-h coverage) may have also affected the results. The better design might have been to study all patients on an ACEI and then to randomize them either to receive an AT1R antagonist or to continue the ACEI.

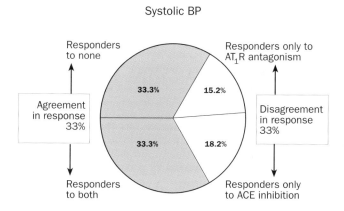

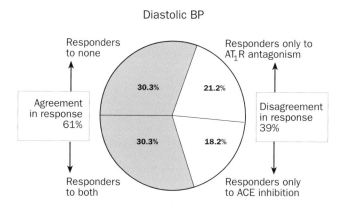

Fig. 6.3 Responders to ACE inhibition and/or to AT1R antagonism (24-h ambulatory BP). Source: Stergiou *et al.* (2001).

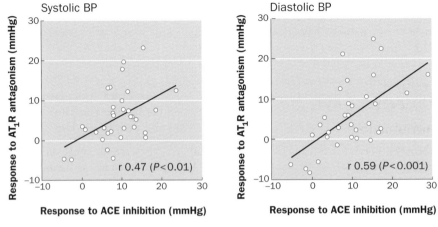

Fig. 6.4 Relationship between the antihypertensive responses to ACE inhibition and to AT$_1$R antagonism (24-h ambulatory BP; r = correlation coefficient).
Source: Stergiou *et al.* (2001).

Antihypertensive treatment in elderly patients aged 75 years or over: a 24-week study of the tolerability of candesartan cilexetil in relation to hydrochlorothiazide.
Neldam S. Forsen B. Multicentre Study Group. *Drugs & Aging* 2001; **18**(3): 225–32.

BACKGROUND. **To assess the safety and tolerability of the AT$_1$-receptor blocker candesartan cilexetil in relation to the diuretic HCTZ in elderly patients.**

INTERPRETATION. This study shows that antihypertensive treatment with candesartan cilexetil in elderly patients (aged ≥ 75 years) is well tolerated with a good safety profile and avoids the metabolic adverse effects of diuretic therapy.

Comment

This is a multicentre, double-blind, randomized, parallel group study principally recruited older hypertensive patients (*n* = 185, aged ≥ 75 years with mean sitting diastolic BP of 95 to 114 mmHg) to once daily treatment with candesartan cilexetil 8 mg or HCTZ 12.5 mg for 24 weeks. The results showed that once daily candesartan cilexetil 8 to 16 mg was very well tolerated with only few adverse effects reported which are comparable to HCTZ. The most common adverse events in both treatment groups were dizziness or vertigo and headache. However, hypokalaemia and hyperuricaemia were not found in patients treated with candesartan cilexetil but occurred in 8.1 and 6.5%, respectively, of patients treated with HCTZ. At week 24, the adjusted mean changes in sitting DBP (24 hours postdose) from baseline were similar between the two treatment arms: -12.0 mmHg [95% CI -1 0.4 to -13.6] in patients treated with candesartan cilexetil and -11.4 mmHg (95% CI -9.3 to -13.6) in patients treated with HCTZ.

Diuretics – new insights

Introduction

There are many reasons to believe that thiazide diuretics are the most successful antihypertensive drugs. Practically, they have been recommended as the first-line antihypertensive agent in every international treatment guidelines, not only because of lower cost, but, more importantly, they are effective, both as monotherapy and in combinations with other agents. Indeed, thiazide diuretics have been shown in many large clinical studies, particularly in the older patients, to be the best option for lowering BP as well as preventing CV events especially stroke and heart attacks, irrespective of race. It is of note that their use as first-line agents has constantly been recommended along with that of beta-blockers based on available evidence. However, despite abundant literature documenting their cost-effectiveness in the management of mild to moderate essential hypertension, the use of thiazides diuretics appear to be declining, as reported by one of the papers below. But, one thing is clear, a diuretic, based on a population-based study below and other outcome trials, should be included in most regimes to lower the risk of ischaemic stroke.

Antihypertensive drug therapies and the risk of ischemic stroke.

Klungel OH, Heckbert SR, Longstreth WT Jr, *et al. Arch Intern Med* 2001; **161**(1): 37–43.

BACKGROUND. The relative effectiveness of various antihypertensive drugs with regard to the reduction of stroke incidence remains uncertain.

INTERPRETATION. In this study of pharmacologically treated hypertensive patients, antihypertensive drug regimens that did not include a thiazide diuretic were associated with an increased risk of ischaemic stroke compared with regimens that did include a thiazide. These results support the use of thiazide diuretics as first-line antihypertensive agents.

Comment

Most clinical guidelines have advocated the use of thiazides as antihypertensive agents, which have proven efficacy in reducing MI and stroke, and are cheap and fairly well tolerated.

In this population-based case-controlled study, antihypertensive treatment that did not include a thiazide diuretic was associated with an 85% increased risk of ischaemic stroke when compared with the use of an antihypertensive drug regimen that included a thiazide. Patients taking a beta-blocker, CCB or ACEI in combination with a thiazide diuretic seemed to have the same risk of stroke as patients taking a diuretic alone. By contrast, patients taking drugs other than a diuretic appeared to have a 2.48-fold increase in the risk of stroke, when compared to the use of a diuretic only. In patients with known CVD, the association with risk of stroke was slightly less pronounced.

These data are also parallel the recent PROGRESS study, where a significant reduction in stroke was seen with a perindopril–indapamide combination whereas the stroke reduction with perindopril alone was not statistically significant.

Diuretics in isolated systolic hypertension

Risks of untreated and treated isolated systolic hypertension in the elderly: meta-analysis of outcome trials.

Staessen JA, Gasowski J, Wang JG, *et al. Lancet* 2000; **355**(9207): 865–72.

BACKGROUND. Previous meta-analysis of outcome trials in hypertension has not specifically focused on isolated systolic hypertension (ISH) or they have explained treatment benefit mainly as a function of the achieved DBP reduction. This study therefore undertook a quantitative overview of the trials to further evaluate the risks associated with SBP in treated and untreated older patients with ISH.

INTERPRETATION. Drug treatment is justified in older patients with ISH whose SBP is 160 mmHg or higher. Absolute benefit is larger in men, in patients aged 70 or more and in those with previous CV complications or wider pulse pressure. Treatment prevented stroke more effectively than coronary events. However, the absence of a relationship between coronary events and SBP in untreated patients suggests that the coronary protection may have been underestimated.

Comment

The prevalence of hypertension progressively increases with age. Meta-analyses of the randomized trials available to date have suggested that the absolute benefits of pharmacological treatment are even more pronounced among older adults. It is unsurprising to see the results of the above meta-analysis specifically focused on the treatment for isolated systolic hypertension in the elderly. Treatment of systolic hypertension is most effective in older patients who, because of additional risk factors or prevalent CVD, are at higher risk of developing a CV event. These patients are prime candidates for antihypertensive treatment. However, why antihypertensive treatment apparently provided less protection against coronary complications than against stroke remains unclear.

Effect of treating isolated systolic hypertension on the risk of developing various types and subtypes of stroke: the Systolic Hypertension in the Elderly Program (SHEP).
Perry HM Jr, Davis BR, Price TR, *et al. JAMA* 2000; **284**(4): 465–71.

BACKGROUND. The Systolic Hypertension in the Elderly Program (SHEP) demonstrated that treating isolated systolic hypertension in older patients decreased incidence of total stroke, but whether all types of stroke were reduced was not evaluated.

INTERPRETATION. In this study, antihypertensive drug treatment reduced the incidence of both haemorrhagic and ischaemic (including lacunar) strokes. Reduction in stroke incidence occurred when specific SBP goals were attained.

Comment
See below

Prevention of stroke by antihypertensive drug treatment in older persons with isolated systolic hypertension: final results of the Systolic Hypertension in the Elderly Program (SHEP).
SHEP Cooperative Research Group. *JAMA* 1991; **265**(24): 3255–64.

BACKGROUND. To assess the ability of antihypertensive drug treatment to reduce the risk of non-fatal and fatal (total) stroke in isolated systolic hypertension.

INTERPRETATION. In persons aged 60 years and over with isolated systolic hypertension, antihypertensive stepped-care drug treatment with low-dose chlorthalidone as step 1 medication reduced the incidence of total stroke by 36%, with 5-year absolute benefit of 30 events per 1000 participants. Major CV events were reduced, with 5-year absolute benefit of 55 events per 1000.

Comment
Older patients with ISH benefit from drug treatment, especially if they are men, over the age of 70, or have a history of CV complications or wider pulse pressure (PP). Antihypertensive drug therapy should be based on systolic, rather than diastolic, BP in this population.

In the paper by Staessen *et al.* a meta-analysis of ISH treatment in the elderly is presented, based on eight outcome trials in 15 693 patients > 60 years with ISH

Table 6.5 Active treatment resulted in reduction in both ischaemic and haemorrhagic events

Stroke type	Active treatment	Placebo	Adjusted RR (95% CI)
Ischaemic	85	132	0.63 (0.48–0.82)
Haemorrhagic	9	19	0.46 (0.21–1.02)
Unknown type	9	8	1.05 (0.40–2.73)

Among ischaemic strokes, four subtypes were observed, with reductions seen in particular among those with lacunar strokes and strokes of unknown type.

Source: SHEP Cooperative Research Group (2001).

Table 6.6 Ischaemic stroke subtype

Ischaemic stroke type	Active treatment	Placebo	Adjusted RR(95% CI)
Lacunar	23	43	0.53 (0.32–0.88)
Cardioembolic	9	16	0.56 (0.25–1.27)
Atherosclerotic	13	13	0.99 (0.46–2.15)
Unknown	40	60	0.64 (0.43–0.96)

Source: SHEP Cooperative Research Group (2001).

who were followed for 3–8 years. In all patients, BP at enrolment averaged 174/83 mmHg DBP. After treatment, the net reductions averaged 5.96% for systolic and 4.91% for DBPs. Drug therapy reduced total mortality by 13%, CV deaths by 18%, all CV complications by 26%, stroke by 30% and coronary events by 23%.

A 10 mmHg increase in SBP was significantly and independently correlated with increases by nearly 10% in the risk of all fatal and non-fatal complications, except for coronary events. Diastolic BP, on the other hand, was inversely correlated with total and CV mortality. At any given level of SBP, the risk of death rose with lower DBP and therefore with greater pulse pressure.

Recent analyses from the SHEP also showed that treatment of ISH resulted in reductions of both ischaemic and haemorrhagic stroke, particularly in patients reaching certain goal levels of SBP. Indeed, treatment of ISH (i.e. patients with SBP above 160 mmHg, but DBP – less than 90 mmHg) using a diuretic-based regime (chlorthalidone [12.5 mg per day] which could be doubled, then if goal was not reached, one of two drugs, atenolol or reserpine could be added) resulted in significant reduction of all strokes, fatal and non-fatal, by 36%. The treatment effect was seen within a year for the haemorrhagic strokes, but not until the second year of treatment for ischaemic strokes. Stroke mortality was similar between the groups. Along with this reduction in stroke was a 71% reduction in fatal and non-fatal MI, a reduction in all coronary heart disease of 27%, all CVD of 32% and total mortality of 13%. In addition, TIAs and episodes of CHF were also reduced.

Among ischaemic strokes, four subtypes were observed, with reductions seen in particular among those with lacunar strokes and strokes of unknown type.

Trends in antihypertensive drugs in the elderly: the decline of thiazides.

Onder G, Gambassi G, Landi F, Investigators of the GIFA Study (SIGG-ONLUS), *et al. J Hum Hypertens* 2001; **15**(5): 291–7.

BACKGROUND. **The last decade has seen the publication of different editions of guidelines for the pharmacological treatment of hypertension that were based on the results of large, randomized trials. Because of the wealth of data supporting the use of thiazide diuretics, this study focused on diuretic prescription to identify independent predictors of their utilisation.**

INTERPRETATION. Despite continued recommendations to use thiazide diuretics for the treatment of hypertension among older individuals, their use has been declining steadily between 1988 and 1997. A possible explanation is that the choice to prescribe a thiazide diuretic is influenced by age, functional status and comorbidity.

Comment

The international consensus for thiazide diuretics as the first-line antihypertensive agent has remained unchanged over the years though guidelines for treatment of hypertension have changed significantly in the last decade, especially regarding the role of ACEIs and CCBs as first-line agents. To investigate whether physicians adhere to treatment guidelines in the use of thiazide diuretics for hypertension treatment, Onder *et al.* analysed, between 1988 and 1997, the prescription pattern of antihypertensive agents for 5061 patients from among older hospitalised adults in Italy.

The results revealed the use of ACE-inhibitors has been rising steadily through the years, and they are the agents most commonly used since 1996. Calcium channel blockers also showed a similar trend and were the top prescribing drug until 1995; subsequently, the documentation of potentially severe side effects resulted in a nearly 20% reduction of their use. Surprisingly, beta-blockers have remained unpopular throughout the decade.

The prescription of diuretics as a class, however, showed a biphasic trend: an initial decrease with a prolonged steady state and a more recent rise. However, at a separate analysis, it was a evident that a progressive increase of the use of loop diuretics since 1988 has been paralleled by a nearly 50% reduction of thiazides prescriptions. The independent predictors of thiazide use were female gender, good functional status, preserved renal function, and absence of CV comorbidity.

So why are thiazide diuretics declining in popularity? The finding of a decline in the use of thiazide diuretics in Italy may also be similar elsewhere especially in the developed countries. There are many reasons why this could be the case: poor adherence to treatment guidelines, lack of marketing, physicians' preferences, other agents e.g. ACEIs, beta-blockers may be 'more cardioprotective' or for specific indications, metabolic adverse effects of thiazides especially at higher doses. It is of note that, however, though the use of thiazides as a first-line monotherapy is declining, most clinicians are actually quite happy to combine it with other agents

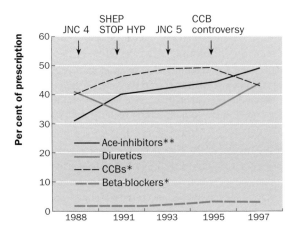

Fig. 6.5 Trends in the prescription of antihypertensive drugs among patients above 65 years of age. *$P <0.01$, **$P <0.001$ for trend. Source: Onder *et al.* (2001).

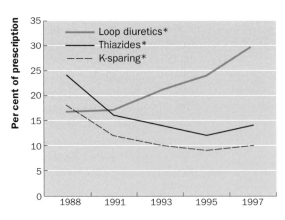

Fig 6.6 Trends in the prescription of diuretics by different classes. *$P <0.01$ for trend. Source: Onder *et al.* (2001).

i.e. as an add-on therapy! There is evidence that combination therapy with low dose thiazides can synergistically improve compliance and cost-effectiveness.

Calcium antagonists

Introduction

Calcium antagonists are widely used and effective antihypertensive drugs that reduce the risks for hypertensive complications compared with placebo. Indeed, calcium antagonists as a class are regarded as suitable first-line agent for the treatment of hypertension. In 1988 the Joint National Committee on Prevention, Detection, Evaluation, and Treatment of High Blood Pressure (JNC) IV recommended them as first-line agent, but subsequently JNC V withdrew this support. The current guidelines, JNC VI, have renewed emphasis on their use as first-line antihypertensive agents for treating isolated systolic hypertension in the older patients or hypertensive patients with angina or diabetes. However, for the past year, their use as a first-line agent has again been subjected to heavy debate. The recent meta-analysis by Pahor *et al.* *(see page 192)* has reported them to be less effective in preventing CV events (with the exception of stroke) especially the risk for acute MI compared to patients receiving other first-line antihypertensives. They concluded that calcium antagonists should be used as second-line agents for hypertension. However, such a claim has been heavily criticized by many hypertension experts, and hence many other similar meta-analyses have followed and been published. Analysis from the Blood Pressure Lowering Treatment (BPLT) Trialists' Collaboration concluded that there was strong evidence of benefit for calcium antagonists from placebo-controlled studies and that evidence of differences between calcium antagonist-based regimes and other therapies was weak.

It should be noted that calcium antagonists are a very heterogeneous group of drugs with properties differing significantly from one drug to another. Even different galenic formulations of the same molecule have significantly different effects on cardiovascular pathophysiology, besides lowering BP. Thus, the clinical effectiveness of every formulation must be evaluated separately in well-designed clinical studies. There is evidence that certain calcium antagonists may reduce the reinfarction rate and have the potential for decreasing atherogenesis. Calcium antagonists have also been shown to effectively reduce BP, left ventricular hypertrophy and more importantly, prevent stroke.

The data from the various meta-analyses in the use of calcium antagonists in preventing hard end-points was largely fragmented because of many possible sub-groupings across the class (e.g. Dihydropyridine *vs* non-dihydropyridine), patients (diabetics *vs* non-diabetics) and end-points (cardiovascular *vs* renal). Such meta-analyses have limited statistical power to really determine whether the small, but often significant, differences detected can be generalized to all calcium antagonists. Hence, it may be too early to deny a place for calcium antagonists as a whole in the long-term management of hypertension. Results from on-going large-scale trials such as the ALLHAT (Antihypertensive and Lipid-lowering Treatment to prevent Heart Attack Trial) study, capable of addressing the concerns, are eagerly awaited. We will discuss some of these issues in further detail below.

Effect of amlodipine on the progression of atherosclerosis and the occurrence of clinical events. PREVENT Investigators.

Pitt B, Byington RP, Furberg CD, *et al. Circulation* 2000; **102**(13): 1503–10.

B A C K G R O U N D . The results of angiographic studies have suggested that calcium channel-blocking agents may prevent new coronary lesion formation, the progression of minimal lesions, or both.

I N T E R P R E T A T I O N . Amlodipine has no demonstrable effect on angiographic progression of coronary atherosclerosis or the risk of major cardiovascular events but is associated with fewer hospitalizations for unstable angina and revascularization.

Comment

The Prospective Randomized Evaluation of the Vascular Effects of Norvasc Trial (PREVENT) was a multicentre, randomized, placebo-controlled, double-masked clinical trial designed to test whether amlodipine would slow the progression of early coronary atherosclerosis in 825 patients with angiographically documented coronary artery disease. The results showed no difference of the average 36-month reductions in the minimal diameter between placebo and amlodipine groups: 0.084 *vs* 0.095 mm, respectively ($P = 0.38$). In contrast, amlodipine had a significant effect in slowing the 36-month progression of carotid artery atherosclerosis: the placebo group experienced a 0.033 mm increase in intima-media thickness (IMT), whereas there was a 0.0126 mm decrease in the amlodipine group ($P = 0.007$). There was no treatment difference in the rates of all-cause mortality or major CV events, although amlodipine use was associated with fewer cases of unstable angina and coronary revascularization.

Relation between blood pressure variability and carotid artery damage in hypertension: baseline data from the European Lacidipine Study on Atherosclerosis (ELSA).

Mancia G, Parati G, Hennig M, *et al. J Hypertens* 2001; **19**(11): 1981–9.

B A C K G R O U N D . Baseline data from the ELSA have shown that carotid IMT is not related to DBP, but that it is related to clinic SBP or PP and more so to their 24-h average values. The aim of the present study was to determine whether IMT independently relates to additional information obtained through ambulatory BP, in particular to SBP or PP variability.

INTERPRETATION. This is the first demonstration from a large database that not only average 24-h PP and SBP values, but also 24-h BP fluctuations, are associated with, and possibly determinants of, the alterations of large artery structure in hypertension.

Comment

The CCB lacidipine has antiatherosclerotic effects in addition to its antihypertensive effect. ELSA is the largest prospective randomized double-blind trial to use carotid artery wall IMT as the primary end-point, and compared 2255 patients with mild-to-moderate hypertension from seven European countries, who were randomized to the beta-blocker atenolol or lacidipine and followed for 4 years. Among the 1519 patients who completed the 4-year treatment period, lacidipine had a significant treatment effect, reducing the yearly IMT progression rate by 40% compared with atenolol. Carotid IMT progression was 0.015 mm per year with atenolol compared with 0.006 mm per year with lacidipine ($P = 0.0073$). In ELSA, lacidipine-treated patients also showed 17% less plaque progression and 25% more plaque regression than those receiving atenolol ($P = 0.04$; intention-to-treat population).

Other studies have shown similar findings with other calcium blockers – the Verapamil in Hypertension and Atherosclerosis Study (VHAS) with verapamil and the PREVENT trial with amlodipine. The latter showed that amlodipine had a significant effect on a secondary measure – carotid atherosclerosis measured by ultrasound – although it was conducted in patients with angiographic evidence of coronary artery disease rather than a hypertensive population.

Cardiovascular protection and blood pressure reduction: a meta-analysis.
Staessen JA, Wang JG, Thijs L. *Lancet* 2001; **358**(9290): 1305–15.

BACKGROUND. Whether antihypertensive drugs offer CV protection beyond BP lowering has not been established. The aim was to investigate whether pharmacological properties of antihypertensive drugs or reduction of systolic pressure accounted for CV outcome in hypertensive or high-risk patients.

METHODS. In a meta-analysis, summary statistics from published reports were extracted, and pooled odds ratios for experimental *versus* reference treatment were calculated. A correlation was made across-trials odd ratios for differences in systolic pressure between groups.

FINDINGS. Nine randomized trials were analysed comparing treatments in 62 605 hypertensive patients. Compared with old drugs (diuretics and beta-blockers), CCBs and ACEIs offered similar overall CV protection, but CCBs provided more reduction in the risk of stroke (13.5%, 95% CI 1.3–24.2, $P = 0.03$) and less reduction in the risk MI (19.2%, 3.5–37.3, $P = 0.01$). Heterogeneity was significant between trials because of the high risk of CV events on doxazosin in one trial, and high risk of stroke on captopril in another; but systolic pressure differed between groups in these two trials by 2–3 mmHg. Similar systolic differences occurred in a trial of diltiazem *versus* old drugs, and in three trials of ACEI against placebo in high-risk patients. Meta-regression across 27 trials (136 124 patients) showed that odds ratios could be explained by achieved differences in systolic pressure. The findings emphasize that BP control is important. All antihypertensive drugs have similar long-term efficacy and safety. CCBs might be especially effective in stroke prevention. It was not found that ACEIs or alpha blockers affected CV prognosis beyond their antihypertensive effects.

Calcium channel blockers in hypertension: the saga goes on ...at least until ALLHAT/ASCOT

Calcium channel blockers in hypertension: the debate reawakens.
Lip GY, Beevers DG. *J Hum Hypertens* 2001; **15**(2): 85–7.

BACKGROUND. A series of pharmacosurveillance studies in the last decade implied an excess of mortality and MI, as well as cancer, bleeding and suicides attributable to use of calcium antagonists. No such excess is seen in randomized controlled trials using this class of drugs, but not to be outdone, the same campaigners against calcium antagonists have reported on a recent meta-analysis suggesting that the calcium antagonists are less effective than other antihypertensive agents, even causing a small excess in MI.

INTERPRETATION. All antihypertensive drugs lower BP and reduce end-points of stroke and MI.

Comment
See below

The INSIGHT and NORDIL trials: are calcium antagonists equivalent to established drug therapies for cardiovascular protection?
Ruddy MC. *Current Hypertension Reports* 2001; **3**(4): 289–96.

BACKGROUND. Calcium channel antagonists have come into worldwide use for treating hypertension and other circulatory disorders. In recent years, results of several observational studies have suggested that these drugs may not be as safe or effective as other available therapies, such as diuretics and beta-blockers, in the prevention of CV events.

INTERPRETATION. There is not yet sufficient evidence to prove whether cause-specific differences exist. Results of the NORDIL and INSIGHT studies support incorporating calcium antagonist-based therapy as an additional safe and effective approach for preventing BP-related illness and death.

Comment

One may extend the debate by speculating on the mechanisms whereby the calcium channel antagonists may differ from other antihypertensive agents, either beneficially or adversely. Indeed, calcium channel antagonists might be pro-arrhythmic, pro-haemorrhagic and may also cause coronary steal; they may also encourage apoptosis and activate the renin system. However, there are equal arguments in their favour, particularly as they may be antithrombotic. Perhaps the best response is to emphasize that the highest priority is to control the BP, and that there are subtle differences in outcome comparing the calcium channel antagonists with other agents, but these are very controversial and may be unproven.

The Nordic Diltiazem (NORDIL) study compared the effects of diltiazem with those of diuretics, beta-blockers, or both, on CV mortality and morbidity in hypertensive patients (aged 50–74 years, DBP $\geq$ 100 mmHg). After a mean follow-up of 4.5 years, SBP was significantly lower in both arms but was significantly greater in the diuretic and beta-blocker group (-23 mmHg) than in the diltiazem group (-20.3 mmHg, $P < 0.001$). However, there was no significant difference in the incidence of the primary end-point (composite of fatal and non-fatal stroke, MI and CV death) between the two groups. However, in the cause-specific end-points analysis, the occurrence of stroke (fatal or non-fatal) was significantly less in the diltiazem group compared with the diuretic and beta-blocker regime group.

Morbidity and mortality in patients randomized to double-blind treatment with a long-acting calcium-channel blocker or diuretic in the International Nifedipine GITS study: Intervention as a Goal in Hypertension Treatment (INSIGHT).

Brown MJ, Palmer CR, Castaigne A *et al. Lancet* 2000; **356**(9227): 366–72.

BACKGROUND. The efficacy of antihypertensive drugs newer than diuretics and beta-blockers has not been established. We compared the effects of the calcium-channel blocker nifedipine once daily with the diuretic combination co-amilozide on CV mortality and morbidity in high-risk patients with hypertension.

INTERPRETATION. Nifedipine once daily and co-amilozide were equally effective in preventing overall CV or cerebrovascular complications. The choice of drug can be decided by tolerability and blood-pressure response rather than long-term safety or efficacy.

Comment

INSIGHT is another large outcome study assessing the effect of calcium antagonist (nifedipine GITS, long acting formulation) *versus* a diuretic-based regime (co-amilozide: hydrocholorothiazide + amiloride) on morbidity and mortality in hypertensive patients (aged 55–88 years, with at least one additional CV risk factor such as diabetes) at high absolute risk of CV events. At the end of 36 months, BP was lowered effectively in both treatment groups. Again, as in the NORDIL trial, there was no significant difference of the primary end-points between the two treatment arms. However, a subgroup analysis has shown that the long-term protective effects of nifedipine GITS extended to hypertensive patients with DM. However, sub-studies of the INSIGHT have shown significantly less progression of carotid IMT and coronary calcifications in the nifedipine GITS group than the co-amilozide group. These observations were in agreement with that of the ELSA (with lacidipine) and PREVENT (with amlodipine) described above.

Health outcomes associated with calcium antagonists compared with other first-line antihypertensive therapies: a meta-analysis of randomized controlled trials.

Pahor M, Psaty BM, Alderman MH, *et al. Lancet* 2000; **356**: 1949–54.

B A C K G R O U N D . Several observational studies and individual randomized trials in hypertension have suggested that, compared with other drugs, calcium antagonists may be associated with a higher risk of coronary events, despite similar BP control. The aim of this meta-analysis was to compare the effects of calcium antagonists and other antihypertensive drugs on major CV events.

I N T E R P R E T A T I O N . In randomized controlled trials, the large available database suggests that calcium antagonists are inferior to other types of antihypertensive drugs as first-line agents in reducing the risks of several major complications of hypertension. On the basis of these data, the longer-acting calcium antagonists cannot be recommended as first-line therapy for hypertension.

Comment

With the calcium antagonists there appears to be a clear benefit on stroke reduction but less marked benefit on ischaemic heart disease, which is also partly dependant upon interpretation of the available data which has undergone various meta-analyses. Because meta-analyses look impressive, clinicians tend to believe them, but in fact they have many problems. Some of the trials included were designed to demonstrate drug equivalence, whilst others hoped to detect drug superiority. Some were open label studies with the risk of bias in randomization. There were also major differences in the methods of all trials included. Furthermore, the

Myocardial infarction

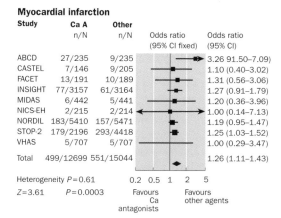

Study	Ca A n/N	Other n/N	Odds ratio (95% CI fixed)	Odds ratio (95% CI)
ABCD	27/235	9/235		3.26 91.50–7.09)
CASTEL	7/146	9/205		1.10 (0.40–3.02)
FACET	13/191	10/189		1.31 (0.56–3.06)
INSIGHT	77/3157	61/3164		1.27 (0.91–1.79)
MIDAS	6/442	5/441		1.20 (0.36–3.96)
NICS-EH	2/215	2/214		1.00 (0.14–7.13)
NORDIL	183/5410	157/5471		1.19 (0.95–1.47)
STOP-2	179/2196	293/4418		1.25 (1.03–1.52)
VHAS	5/707	5/707		1.00 (0.29–3.47)
Total	499/12699	551/15044		1.26 (1.11–1.43)

Heterogeneity P=0.61 0.2 0.5 1 2 5

Z=3.61 P=0.0003 Favours Ca antagonists Favours other agents

Stroke

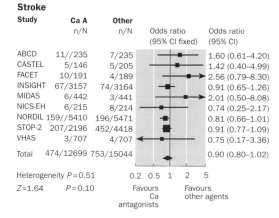

Study	Ca A n/N	Other n/N	Odds ratio (95% CI fixed)	Odds ratio (95% CI)
ABCD	11//235	7/235		1.60 (0.61–4.20)
CASTEL	5/146	5/205		1.42 (0.40–4.99)
FACET	10/191	4/189		2.56 (0.79–8.30)
INSIGHT	67/3157	74/3164		0.91 (0.65–1.26)
MIDAS	6/442	3/441		2.01 (0.50–8.08)
NICS-EH	6/215	8/214		0.74 (0.25–2.17)
NORDIL	159//5410	196/5471		0.81 (0.66–1.01)
STOP-2	207/2196	452/4418		0.91 (0.77–1.09)
VHAS	3/707	4/707		0.75 (0.17–3.36)
Total	474/12699	753/15044		0.90 (0.80–1.02)

Heterogeneity P=0.51 0.2 0.5 1 2 5

Z=1.64 P=0.10 Favours Ca antagonists Favours other agents

All-cause mortality

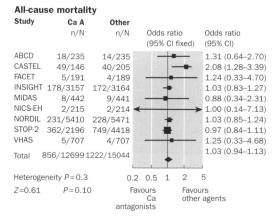

Study	Ca A n/N	Other n/N	Odds ratio (95% CI fixed)	Odds ratio (95% CI)
ABCD	18/235	14/235		1.31 (0.64–2.70)
CASTEL	49/146	40/205		2.08 (1.28–3.39)
FACET	5/191	4/189		1.24 (0.33–4.70)
INSIGHT	178/3157	172/3164		1.03 (0.83–1.27)
MIDAS	8/442	9/441		0.88 (0.34–2.31)
NICS-EH	2/215	2/214		1.00 (0.14–7.13)
NORDIL	231/5410	228/5471		1.03 (0.85–1.24)
STOP-2	362/2196	749/4418		0.97 (0.84–1.11)
VHAS	5/707	4/707		1.25 (0.33–4.68)
Total	856/12699	1222/15044		1.03 (0.94–1.13)

Heterogeneity P=0.3 0.2 0.5 1 2 5

Z=0.61 P=0.10 Favours Ca antagonists Favours other agents

Fig. 6.7 Numbers of events and odds ratios for comparison of calcium antagonists with other drugs. Source: Pahor *et al.* (2001).

meta-analyses themselves may be prone to bias as to which end-points are examined. There is also the problem that they rely heavily on the larger trials, some of which can be criticised for their design. Finally, the biggest problem is that meta-analyses do not take into account the possible influences of other drugs used as second-line agents. In reality, more than half of all hypertensive patients need an additional drug, and a third require three drugs or more, to bring about adequate control of BP. Large outcome trials such as ASCOT or ALLHAT may help allay the continuing debate.

Effects of ACE inhibitors, calcium antagonists, and other blood-pressure-lowering drugs: results of prospectively designed overviews of randomized trials.

Blood Pressure Lowering Treatment Trialists' Collaboration. *Lancet* 2000; **355**: 1955–64.

BACKGROUND. This programme of overviews of randomized trials was established to investigate the effects of ACEIs, calcium antagonists and other BP-lowering drugs on mortality and major CV morbidity in several populations of patients. Separate overviews of trials were carried out comparing active treatment regimens with placebo, comparing more intensive and less intensive blood-pressure-lowering strategies, and comparing treatment regimens based on different drug classes.

INTERPRETATION. Strong evidence of benefits of ACEIs and calcium antagonists is provided by the overviews of placebo-controlled trials. There is weaker evidence of differences between treatment regimens of differing intensities and of differences between treatment regimens based on different drug classes. Data from continuing trials of BP-lowering drugs will substantially increase the evidence available about any real differences that might exist between regimens.

Comment

These meta-analyses, armed with large numbers, seem to confirm the same trends of the three major trials, that there was no difference between calcium antagonists and other therapies on all cause mortality, but a trend, which reaches statistical significance, for an inferior effect on heart disease and a superior effect on stroke. It is clear that treating BP is beneficial, with strong evidence of benefits of ACEIs and calcium antagonists by the overviews of placebo-controlled trials. If the question is no longer 'do we treat hypertension?', but 'how to treat?' and 'who to treat?', some uncertainties arise. The meta-analyses suggest that there is weaker evidence of differences between treatment regimens of differing intensities and of differences between treatment regimens based on different drug classes.

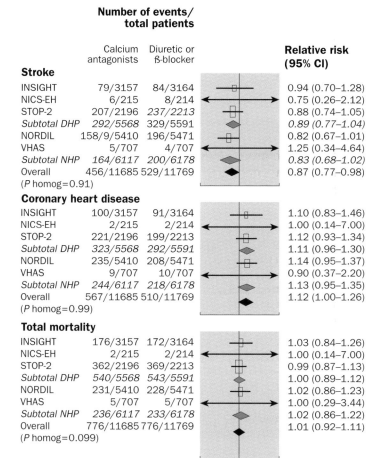

Number of events/ total patients

	Calcium antagonists	Diuretic or ß-blocker		Relative risk (95% CI)
Stroke				
INSIGHT	79/3157	84/3164		0.94 (0.70–1.28)
NICS-EH	6/215	8/214		0.75 (0.26–2.12)
STOP-2	207/2196	237/2213		0.88 (0.74–1.05)
Subtotal DHP	*292/5568*	*329/5591*		*0.89 (0.77–1.04)*
NORDIL	158/9/5410	196/5471		0.82 (0.67–1.01)
VHAS	5/707	4/707		1.25 (0.34–4.64)
Subtotal NHP	*164/6117*	*200/6178*		*0.83 (0.68–1.02)*
Overall	456/11685	529/11769		0.87 (0.77–0.98)
(*P* homog=0.91)				
Coronary heart disease				
INSIGHT	100/3157	91/3164		1.10 (0.83–1.46)
NICS-EH	2/215	2/214		1.00 (0.14–7.00)
STOP-2	221/2196	199/2213		1.12 (0.93–1.34)
Subtotal DHP	*323/5568*	*292/5591*		*1.11 (0.96–1.30)*
NORDIL	235/5410	208/5471		1.14 (0.95–1.37)
VHAS	9/707	10/707		0.90 (0.37–2.20)
Subtotal NHP	*244/6117*	*218/6178*		*1.13 (0.95–1.35)*
Overall	567/11685	510/11769		1.12 (1.00–1.26)
(*P* homog=0.99)				
Total mortality				
INSIGHT	176/3157	172/3164		1.03 (0.84–1.26)
NICS-EH	2/215	2/214		1.00 (0.14–7.00)
STOP-2	362/2196	369/2213		0.99 (0.87–1.13)
Subtotal DHP	*540/5568*	*543/5591*		*1.00 (0.89–1.12)*
NORDIL	231/5410	228/5471		1.02 (0.86–1.23)
VHAS	5/707	5/707		1.00 (0.29–3.44)
Subtotal NHP	*236/6117*	*233/6178*		*1.02 (0.86–1.22)*
Overall	776/11685	776/11769		1.01 (0.92–1.11)
(*P* homog=0.099)				

0.5   1.0   2.0

Relative risk

Favours   Favours
calcium   diuretics or
antagonists   ß-blockers

Fig. 6.8 Comparisons of calcium-antagonist-based therapy with diuretic-based or beta-blocker-based therapy. Source: Blood Pressure Lowering Treatment Trialists' Collaboration (2001).

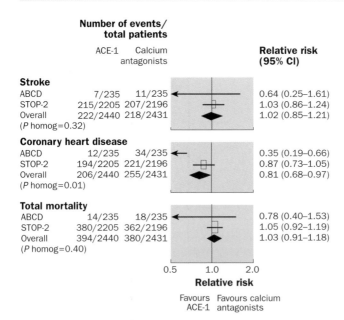

Number of events/
total patients

Fig. 6.9 Comparisons of ACEI-based therapy with calcium-antagonist-based therapy
Source: Blood Pressure Lowering Treatment Trialists' Collaboration (2001).

Cardiovascular protection and blood pressure reduction: a meta-analysis.

Staessen JA, Wang JG, Thijs L. *Lancet* 2001; **358**(9290): 1305–15.

BACKGROUND. Whether antihypertensive drugs offer CV protection beyond BP lowering has not been established. This meta-analysis aimed to investigate whether pharmacological properties of antihypertensive drugs or reduction of systolic pressure accounted for CV outcome in hypertensive or high-risk patients.

INTERPRETATION. The findings emphasise that BP control is important. All antihypertensive drugs have similar long-term efficacy and safety. CCBs might be especially effective in stroke prevention. There was no suggestion that ACEIs or α-blockers affect CV prognosis beyond their antihypertensive effects.

Comment

According to this meta-analysis, new antihypertensives (e.g. ACEIs and CCBs) are as effective in reducing BP as old agents (e.g. diuretics and beta-blockers). The

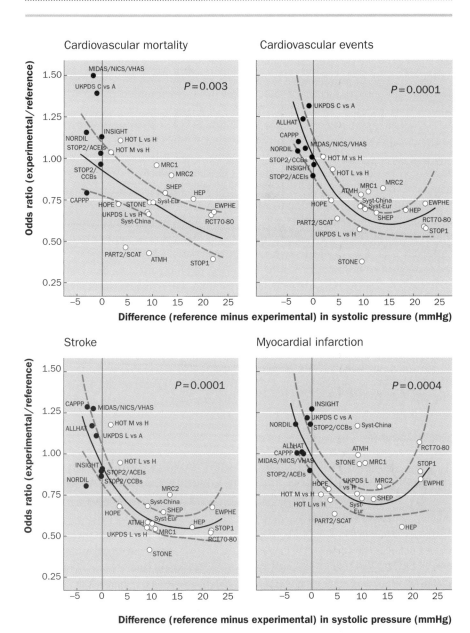

Fig. 6.10 Relation between odds ratios for: (a) and (b) CV mortality and all CV events; (c) and (d) fatal and non-fatal stroke and fatal and non-fatal MI; and corresponding differences in SBP. Source: Staessen *et al.* (2001).

authors extracted summary statistics from published reports, and calculated pooled odds ratios for experimental *versus* reference treatment. Then, correlated across-trials odd ratios for differences in systolic pressure between groups. The first part of the study consisted of a meta-analysis of nine randomized outcome trials, comparing old and new hypertensive therapies in more than 62 605 hypertensive patients. The second part was a meta-regression (a technique used to explore the relationship between study characteristics and study results) across 27 trials (136 124 patients) to assess the influence of differences in BP in treatment and control arms on odds ratios. The results showed no significant difference between old and new antihypertensives in overall CV protection. Although CCBs might give greater protection against stroke, they are however; less effective in reducing the risk for AMI compared to patients receiving other antihypertensives. In addition, neither drug class appears to have any additional cardioprotective effects beyond their BP lowering effect as the meta-regression showed that odds ratios, for the most part, could be explained by differences in SBP between randomized groups. However, as pointed out by the authors, the overview should be interpreted within the context of its limitations as several issues could have affected their results, e.g. wide confidence intervals, patients' characteristics (selective recruitment), or the definition and validation of end-points in individual trials. Indeed, the study population had been criticised as only a relatively small number of patients with proteinuria were evaluated who would perhaps be more beneficial on an ACEI or ARB than CCB. This may have biased the results.

The meta-analysis by Staessen *et al.* does not suggest that calcium antagonists are an inferior class of drugs, having demonstrated that calcium antagonists reduced the risk of stroke by 13.5%, and the risk of MI by 19.2%.

Clinical implications of recent findings from the Antihypertensive and Lipid-lowering Treatment to prevent Heart Attack Trial (ALLHAT) and other studies of hypertension.

Furberg CD, Psaty BM, Pahor M, Alderman MH. *Ann Intern Med* 2001; **135**: 1074–8.

BACKGROUND. Several recent comparative trials in hypertension have reported that similar BP reductions may not necessarily translate into similar reductions in risk for CV complications. Thus, the method used to lower BP may be important. In the ALLHAT, low-dose chlorthalidone as the first-line drug was superior to doxazosin. The 25% higher risk for major CV events associated with doxazosin was attributed primarily to a doubling in the risk for heart failure (HF). A meta-analysis of patients with type 2 DM suggested that despite achieving similar BP reductions, ACEIs are superior to other antihypertensive drugs in reducing the risk for acute myocardial infarction (AMI) and CV events, but not stroke. Although individual comparative trials have failed to show conclusively that CCBs differ from other antihypertensive drugs, a

meta-analysis that included all published trials concluded that CCBs are inferior to other classes of drugs in reducing the risk for AMI and HF.

INTERPRETATION. Recent findings from clinical trials have made clinicians rethink the way they look at the treatment of mild and moderate hypertension. Since BP lowering appears to have a limited predictive value as a surrogate marker, selecting and approving drugs based on their BP–lowering effect may not be optimal. Comparative trials that are of sufficient scope and duration and include relevant health outcomes are needed to guide clinicians in drug selection. ALLHAT and other studies have demonstrated important differences in the abilities of drugs to reduce the risk for CV complications, such as HF and AMI, and major renal disease.

CONCLUSION. These observations suggest not only that antihypertensive drugs may have important mechanisms of action apart from BP lowering but also that effective treatment is not a matter of simply lowering BP. These findings have potential implications for the regulatory approval of antihypertensive agents, revisions of treatment guidelines, the design of future randomized trials comparing different antihypertensive drugs and, most importantly, the selection of drugs for the treatment of hypertensive patients.

Comment

With 42 448 patients and a mean planned follow-up of six years, ALLHAT has adequate statistical power for comparing the risk for major disease outcomes in the diuretic (chlorthalidone) control group with that in groups receiving each of three alternative treatments: a CCB (amlodipine), an ACEI (lisinopril), and an α-adrenergic blocker (doxazosin). The doxazosin arm was stopped early in February 2000 because of a 25% increased risk for combined CVD outcomes, and these patients were twice as likely to be hospitalized for HF when compared with patients receiving standard diuretic treatment with chlorthalidone. However, despite their most recent much disputed meta-analysis on CCBs, Furberg *et al.* (Chair of the ALLHAT) once again stirred up more controversies by voicing the ALLHAT conclusions, months before trial end in March 2002! Three main questions were addressed in this paper: 1) Is BP reduction a reliable marker for health benefits of antihypertensive drugs? 2) Does it matter how elevated BP is lowered? 3) What type of antihypertensive clinical trial is needed in the future? Indeed, the main focus was on the choice of drug classes. The message is: 'effective antihypertensive therapy is not a matter of simply lowering BP'. Indeed, this may vary according to the severity of hypertension, class of drug, type of disease outcome and patient characteristics and comorbidity. With the pooled findings, the authors suggested that ACEIs are more effective than other drugs in reducing the risk for AMI and CV events, but not stroke. Moreover, they also criticised the Blood Pressure Lowering Treatment Trialists' Collaboration, asserting that most of the multiple comparisons used lacked adequate statistical power and that when the database in this meta-analysis was used to compare CCBs with all other antihypertensive agents, the results were very similar to those of the previous meta-analysis and were statistically significant: persons who used CCBs had a 26% higher rate of AMI and a 19% higher rate of HF. The clinical significance of early termination of the amlodipine arm in the AASK (*see page 149*) was also cited in this paper. Their conclusions may be correct but it is highly contentious to speculate conclusions and to publish them before the end of the trial. The value of CCBs as antihypertensive cannot be totally discarded as they have a good record of safety profiles. Indeed, the dihydro-pyridine-CCBs are the drugs of choice of compelling indication in elderly patients with isolated systolic hypertension in the JNC VI, WHO-ISH 1999 as well as the BHS guidelines for management of hypertension. The emergence of recent evidence seems to edge out the role of CCBs in hypertension, but until the publication of the full results of ALLHAT, the findings from the International Verapamil SR/Trandolapril (INVEST) trial and the Anglo-Scandinavian Cardiac Outcomes Trial (ASCOT), which together involve more than 80 000 patients are available, the fate of CCBs is still unclear.

Baseline characteristics of participants in the Antihypertensive and Lipid lowering Treatment to prevent Heart Attack Trial (ALLHAT).

Grimm RH Jr, Margolis KL, Papademetriou V *et al. Hypertension* 2001; **37**: 19–27.

BACKGROUND. Diuretics and ß-blockers have been shown to reduce the risk of CV morbidity and mortality in people with hypertension in long-term clinical trials. No study has compared newer, more costly antihypertensive agents (calcium antagonists, ACEIs and adrenergic blockers) with diuretics for reducing the incidence of CVD in an ethnically diverse group of middle-aged and elderly hypertensive patients.

INTERPRETATION. ALLHAT will add greatly to our understanding of the management of hypertension by providing an answer to the following question: are newer antihypertensive agents similar, superior or inferior to traditional treatment with diuretics?

Comment

The study is a randomized, double-blind, active-controlled clinical trial designed to determine whether the incidence of the primary outcome, fatal coronary heart disease or non-fatal MI, differs between treatment initiation with a diuretic *versus* each of three other antihypertensive drugs. This report describes only the baseline characteristics of the 42 448 ALLHAT participants. We have seen many debates about the trial since it began. Debates seemed to escalate even more when the doxa-zosin arm was stopped early, and when the most controversial meta-analysis by Furberg *et al.* (the Chairman of ALLHAT) was presented and published, the debates became even more vigorous. All researchers in the field of hypertension are eagerly awaiting the main outcomes results of ALLHAT, and although some questions will be answered, it is likely that there will be even more questions raised.

This will be exciting and doubtless many excellent ideas will be generated for further research.

Beta-blockers in hypertension

Introduction

The beta-blockers are now considered to be the first-line choice of treatment in hypertension along with diuretics. CVD and stroke are the major causes of mortality both of insulin-dependent (type 1) and non-insulin-dependent (type 2) diabetic patients. Beta-blockers are effective antihypertensive agents in these patients, which in long-term studies have proven beneficial effect in reducing a variety of important clinical end-points, as seen in the UK Prospective Diabetes Study (UKPDS). It has been well established that treatment of hypertension in patients with type 2 DM significantly reduce the incidence of stroke, heart failure, progression of diabetic complications and mortality both of patients with systolic and/or diastolic hypertension. Co-existant disease may influence the choice of a beta-blocker to treat hypertension. Beta-blockers are valuable agents in ischaemic heart disease in both diabetics and non-diabetics, notably the control of chronic angina pectoris and improved prognosis after MI. Indeed, in the Swedish Trial in Old Patients with Hypertension-2 (STOP-2) diabetic subpopulation, the incidence of end-points on conventional treatment, diuretics and beta-blockade did not differ significantly from ACE inhibition or calcium antagonist treatment. Moreover, in the UKPDS type 2 diabetic hypertensives, tight control of the BP with atenolol and captopril compared with less tight control achieved with other drugs, deaths related to diabetes were reduced, as were strokes, microvascular complications and end-points related to diabetes. The hypoglycaemic problems were not different between those on atenolol and captopril. Furthermore, with careful dose titration, beta-blockers are also strongly indicated for the treatment of heart failure.

However, there is considerable variation in the pharmacological actions of the various beta-blockers. Some evidence shows that the beta-1-selective agents are more efficacious than the non-selective beta-blockers in terms of lowering BP. In addition, non-selective beta-blockers may adversely disturb lipid profiles and contribute to hypoglycaemic unawareness or even worse, glucose imbalance, which may influence clinicians' decision to prescribe to some patients with DM. It had been considered a relative contraindication for beta-blockade. Indeed, this view has been challenged as we will discuss in the papers below.

Furthermore, the arrival of newer and more selective beta-blockers may overcome many of these problems. Some of these newer agents have novel properties, such as the release of nitric oxide, which would theoretically make them more attractive for patients with DM. Overall, the adverse metabolic effects of beta-blockers do not appear to be important in clinical practice and these agents should no longer be contraindicated in patients with type 2 DM.

Hypertension and antihypertensive therapy as risk factors for type 2 diabetes mellitus: Atherosclerosis Risk in Communities Study.

Gress TW, Nieto FJ, Shahar E, Wofford MR, Brancati FL. *N Engl J Med* 2000; **342**(13): 905–12.

BACKGROUND. Previous research has suggested that thiazide diuretics and beta-blockers may promote the development of type 2 DM. However, the results of previous studies have been inconsistent, and many studies have been limited by inadequate data on outcomes and by potential confounding.

INTERPRETATION. Concern about the risk of diabetes should not discourage physicians from prescribing thiazide diuretics to non-diabetic adults who have hypertension. The use of beta-blockers appears to increase the risk of diabetes, but this adverse effect must be weighed against the proven benefits of beta-blockers in reducing the risk of CV events.

Comment

Beta-blockers and diuretics are one of the preferred first-line therapies in the treatment of hypertension consistently recommended by all the international treatment guidelines. However, despite these guidelines, the use of beta-blockers is not widespread. Recent evidence has in fact indicated that the use of thiazide diuretics is on the decline though they are the most cost-effective antihypertensive drugs. There are a variety of factors affecting the prescribing habits of physicians. One of these factors is the adverse metabolic effect that is not uncommonly seen with both beta-blocker and diuretics.

Data from the Atherosclerosis Risk in Communities Study (ARIC), including information on 12 550 non-diabetic adults aged 45–64 years, suggest that the presence of hypertension and its treatment with beta blockers seem to increase the subsequent risk of developing type 2 DM in subjects free of diabetes at baseline. No such association was seen with ACEIs, calcium channel antagonists or with diuretics.

After adjustment for a variety of factors, subjects with hypertension were found to have a significantly increased risk of developing diabetes, with a relative risk of 2.43 (95% CI 2.16–2.73), over subjects without hypertension. Examination of the risks associated with the four classes of antihypertensive medications – thiazide diuretics, ACEIs, beta-blockers and calcium channel antagonists – showed that treatment with all of these were associated with increased risk of diabetes over time. However, once the researchers controlled for the presence of hypertension, only beta-blockers continued to show a significant increase, associated with a 28% higher risk of diabetes (relative hazard 1.28, 95% CI 1.04–1.57).

Despite the potentially adverse metabolic effects of beta-blockers, they have proved to have significant long-term protective effects against CV disease in hypertensive patients, including those with DM.

These observations from ARIC are in contrast to data from the HOPE study which found that the ACEI ramipril reduced the occurrence of new diabetes by about 30% among patients with CV risk factors.

Betablocker treatment in diabetes mellitus.
Sawicki PT, Siebenhofer A. *J Intern Med* 2001; **250**(1): 11–17.

BACKGROUND. **Beta-blockers have been convincingly shown to reduce total and CV morbidity and mortality of hypertensive diabetic patients. In diabetic patients, after MI, these agents confer a twice as high protective effect when compared to non-diabetic patients. However, most paradoxically, beta-blocking agents are used less frequently in diabetes. Control of hypertension is insufficient in most of the diabetic patients, probably because a combination of antihypertensive agents including beta-blockers is frequently needed to sufficiently control BP but is not used in these patients. The fear of beta-blocker-associated side effects in diabetes may be partly responsible for the frequent antihypertensive mono-therapy and the resulting poor quality of BP control among diabetic patients.**

INTERPRETATION. The unnecessary less frequent prescription of beta-1-selective beta-blockers in DM may contribute to the higher CV mortality among these patients.

Comment

This thorough review of the literature does not indicate that beta-1-selective beta-blocking agents have important adverse effects on glucose metabolism, prolong hypoglycaemia or mask hypoglycaemic symptoms. In diabetic nephropathy, beta-blockers are as nephroprotective as ACEIs. Thus, given the proven primary and secondary cardioprotective effect in antihypertensive treatment and after MI, there is no evidence-based reason to withhold prescription of beta-blockers from diabetic patients.

Alpha blockers

Introduction

Alpha blockers as an antihypertensive agent had received little attention from clinicians up until the point when the doxazosin arm was terminated two years early in the ALLHAT trial. The alpha-blocker arm was stopped early; doxazosin was shown to be clearly inferior to low-dose chlorthalidone not only in preventing CHF, but also stroke, in spite of similar BP reduction. Indeed, the data indicate that the risk of CHF with doxazosin was more than 100% (relative risk 2.04; 95% CI 1.79–2.32) higher than the risk in patients who were treated with chlorthalidone. Since then, it is supported by many that until more safety data are available, doxazosin, and probably all alpha blockers, should no longer be used as first-line antihypertensive therapy.

On the other hand, it is of note that several randomized double-blind placebo controlled studies have consistently demonstrated the safety and effectiveness of selective alpha 1 blockers for the treatment of clinically benign prostatic hyperplasia (BPH). Selective alpha 1 blockers relieve the symptoms of prostatism and decrease bladder outlet obstruction. To this end, however, these drugs should be used with caution, if at all, even as add-on therapy in hypertension or for symptomatic relief of prostatic hyperplasia in patients at risk of CHF. In women, alpha blockers may cause urinary incontinence.

ALLHAT – diuretics rule, OK

Major cardiovascular events in hypertensive patients randomized to doxazosin *vs* chlorthalidone: the Antihypertensive and Lipid-lowering Treatment to prevent Heart Attack Trial (ALLHAT).

The ALLHAT Officers and Coordinators for the ALLHAT Collaborative Research Group. *JAMA* 2000; **283**: 1967–75.

BACKGROUND. Hypertension is associated with a significantly increased risk of morbidity and mortality. Only diuretics and beta-blockers have been shown to reduce this risk in long-term clinical trials. Whether newer antihypertensive agents reduce the incidence of CVD is unknown.

INTERPRETATION. The data indicate that compared with doxazosin, chlorthalidone yields essentially equal risk of coronary heart disease (CHD) death/non-fatal MI but significantly reduces the risk of combined CVD events, particularly CHF, in high-risk hypertensive patients.

Comment

The doxazosin arm of the ALLHAT trial was suspended earlier in January 2000 after an interim analysis indicated that patients randomized to receive the alpha blocker doxazosin had a 25% increase in CV events, and were twice as likely to be hospitalized for CHF when compared to patients receiving standard diuretic treatment with chlorthalidone.

The ALLHAT trial also managed to randomize 4873 African-Americans to the chlorthalidone arm and 2984 to the doxazosin arm. (A total of 42 448 patients > age 55 were initially included in the ALLHAT study.) While chlorthalidone outperformed doxazosin in terms of lowering SBP when the whole study cohort was analyzed, the BP-lowering effects were much more pronounced in African-Americans, with differences of 5–6 mmHg in the first year. The difference in BP control between chlorthalidone and doxazosin for the entire study population was 3 mmHg.

While the relative risk of CHF for the entire cohort was 2.04, the relative risk of CHF in African-Americans hovered at 2.17 ($P < 0.0001$ for both). The risk of developing CV disease was also slightly higher for African-Americans on the alpha blocker than it was for the group as a whole, at 37% *versus* 35%. There was also a higher risk of stroke in the African-American patients in the doxazosin arm when compared to Caucasians, at 1.36 *vs* 1.19.

Many commentaries have been written about the doxazosin findings. The more persuasive ones conclude that alpha blockers should no longer be considered first-line agents for hypertension in high-risk, elderly adults. Mechanisms of action are always difficult to prove. We may never know with certainty why doxazosin had unfavourable cardiovascular effects in ALLHAT.

Doxazosin added to single-drug therapy in hypertensive patients with benign prostatic hypertrophy.

Martell N, Luque M, on Behalf of the HT-BPH Group. *J Clin Hyperten*s 2001; **3**(4): 218–23.

BACKGROUND. The purpose of this study was to evaluate the efficacy and safety of the addition of doxazosin in the treatment of hypertensive patients who are being treated on another antihypertensive drug.

INTERPRETATION. The results of this open-label study suggest that the addition of doxazosin to another antihypertensive drug in hypertensive patients with benign prostatic hypertrophy is well tolerated and leads to a reduction in prostatic symptoms. The additional beneficial effects on BP suggest that the use of doxazosin may provide a rational approach to this category of patients.

Comment

See below

Alpha-adrenoceptor blocking drugs and female urinary incontinence: prevalence and reversibility.

Marshall HJ, Beevers DG. *Br J Clin Pharmacol* 1996; **42**(4): 507–9.

BACKGROUND. There have been occasional reports of female stress incontinence related to prazosin therapy for hypertension. This drug is now rarely used but recently longer acting alpha-adrenoceptor blocking drugs have been introduced. The authors have, therefore, investigated the prevalence of urinary incontinence in all their female patients who were receiving alpha-adrenoceptor blockers in comparison with women, matched for age and parity, who were receiving other drugs.

INTERPRETATION. The results suggest that there is a significantly higher prevalence of urinary incontinence in women taking alpha-adrenoceptor antagonists with reversibility on withdrawal of these drugs. As both female urinary incontinence, hypertension and the use of alpha-adrenoceptor blocking drugs are common, this distressing side effect should be borne in mind so that gynaecological or urological treatment may be avoided in some women.

Comment

We occasionally resort to the alpha blockers as additional therapy for hypertensives, but concerns from ALLHAT aside (see above), they are effective and generally well tolerated – or so it would seem in men at least.

As the paper by Martell *et al.* would suggest, the use of alpha blockers may result in improved symptoms of prostatism in men, and occasional amelioration of impotence. The older study by Marshall *et al.* would emphasise that women do not necessarily feel the same, with an excess of incontinence whilst on alpha blockers. This distressing adverse effect is not usually volunteered, and awareness and discreet enquiry may be necessary.

Meta-analysis of studies using selective alpha1-blockers in patients with hypertension and type 2 diabetes.

Glanz M, Garber AJ, Mancia G, Levenstein M. *Int J Clin Pract* 2001; **55**(10): 694–701.

BACKGROUND. This meta-analysis of published studies evaluated the effect of selective alpha 1-blockers on lipid and carbohydrate profiles and BP as well as tolerability in patients with hypertension and type 2 diabetes.

INTERPRETATION. This meta-analysis demonstrates a number of favourable effects of therapy with selective alpha 1-blockers in hypertensive patients with type 2 diabetes. These agents provide an effective modality for reducing BP, with favourable effects on lipid, no deterioration in glycaemic control, and little risk of orthostatic hypotension.

Comment

Glanz *et al.* included 22 clinical trials with a randomized comparative and other controlled studies into their meta-analysis. The mean pooled results showed beneficial effects of selective alpha 1-blockers on total serum cholesterol (TC), high-density lipoprotein (HDL) cholesterol, and systolic and diastolic BP. The results also showed doxazosin had beneficial effects on fasting glucose levels, insulin sensitivity, TC, HDL cholesterol, low-density lipoprotein (LDL) cholesterol, HDL/TC ratio, and systolic and diastolic BP. The risk difference was equivalent between the alpha 1-blocker group and the control group for postural hypotension or syncope.

7

New developments in pharmacological therapy

New drugs

Introduction

Vasopeptidase inhibitors (VPIs) are innovative drugs that inhibit two key enzymes, neutral endopeptidase (NEP) and angiotensin-converting enzyme (ACE). The result is an increase in vasodilatory peptides (atrial natriuretic peptide [ANP], brain natriuretic peptide [BNP], bradykinin, and adrenomedullin) and inhibition of the production of the vasoconstrictor angiotensin II.

The physiological effects of ANP and BNP include vasodilation and inhibition of the renin–angiotensin–aldosterone system (RAS). The metabolism of ANP and BNP involves two main pathways: an enzymatic degradation by NEP 24.11 and a receptor-mediated clearance process via the clearance receptor. Inhibition of NEP produces increases in plasma ANP concentrations and urine sodium and volume excretion and a decrease in blood pressure (BP) in deoxycorticosterone acetate–salt uninephrectomized rats.

NEP inhibitors, when given alone, have not been effective as long-term anti-hypertensive agents in humans, probably because of compensatory reflex activation of the renin–angiotensin–aldosterone system. These limitations may be over-come by VPIs through their additional ability to inhibit ACE and to potentiate the kallikrein–kinin system, resulting in additional vasodilation.

An impairment in nitric oxide (NO) bioactivity or endothelial dysfunction involving resistance arteries may increase the systemic BP in susceptible individuals, thus giving rise to hypertension. Indeed, angiographically normal epicardial coronary arteries in hypertensives have been shown to have endothelial dysfunction, an abnormality that is now known to precede atherosclerosis. Hence, reversing endothelial dysfunction in hypertension is an attractive pharmacological aim if the natural history of the hypertension disease process is to be altered. One candidate drug is nebivolol, a new selective beta-1-receptor blocker that has vasodilating properties.

Omapatrilat *versus* lisinopril: efficacy and neurohormonal profile in salt-sensitive hypertensive patients.

Campese VM, Lasseter KC, Ferrario CM, *et al. Hypertension* 2001; **38**(6): 1342–8.

BACKGROUND. Omapatrilat, a vasopeptidase inhibitor, simultaneously inhibits NP and ACE. The efficacy and hormonal profile of omapatrilat and lisinopril were compared in salt-sensitive hypertensive patients.

INTERPRETATION. In salt-sensitive hypertensive patients, omapatrilat demonstrated the hormonal profile of a vasopeptidase inhibitor and lowered ambulatory diastolic (DBP) and systolic blood pressures (SBP) more than lisinopril.

Comment

See below

Comparison of vasopeptidase inhibitor, omapatrilat and lisinopril on exercise tolerance and morbidity in patients with heart failure: IMPRESS randomized trial.

Rouleau JL, Pfeffer MA, Stewart DJ, *et al. Lancet* 2000; **356**(9230): 615–20.

BACKGROUND. To assess in patients with congestive heart failure (CHF) whether dual inhibition of neutral endopeptidase and ACE with the vasopeptidase inhibitor omapatrilat is better than ACE inhibition alone with lisinopril on functional capacity and clinical outcome.

INTERPRETATION. The findings suggest that omapatrilat could have some advantages over lisinopril in the treatment of patients with CHF. Thus, use of vasopeptidase inhibitors could constitute a potentially important treatment for further improving the prognosis and well being of patients with this disorder.

Comment

Patients with salt-sensitive hypertension (SSH) do not respond as well to an ACE inhibitor (ACEI) monotherapy as hypertensive patients who are not salt sensitive. In response to a high dietary salt intake, SSH patients exhibit salt retention and an increase in renal vascular resistance compared with salt-resistant hypertensive patients. Moreover, black SSH patients manifest a paradoxical decrease in ANP plasma levels after a sodium load.

Campese *et al.* report a study in salt-sensitive hypertensive patients, where omapatrilat lowered ambulatory diastolic and SBPs more than lisinopril. This new class of drugs was also tested in the IMPRESS trial, which was a randomized, double-blind, parallel trial of 573 patients with New York Heart Association (NYHA) class II–IV CHF, left-ventricular ejection fraction of 40% or less, and receiving an ACEI. Patients were randomly assigned omapatrilat at a daily target dose of 40 mg ($n = 289$) or lisinopril at a daily target dose of 20 mg ($n = 284$) for 24 weeks. This study was not powered for clinical end-points, but Week 12 ETT increased similarly in the omapatrilat and lisinopril groups, with fewer cardiovascular (CV)-system serious adverse events in the omapatrilat group than in the lisinopril group (7% vs 12%, $P = 0.04$). There was a trend in favour of omapatrilat on the combined end-point of death or admission for worsening heart failure ($P = 0.052$; hazard ratio 0.53 [95% confidence internal (CI) 0.27–1.02]) and a significant benefit of omapatrilat in the composite of death, admission, or discontinuation of study treatment for worsening heart failure ($P = 0.035$; 0.52 [0.28–0.96]). Omapatrilat improved NYHA class more than lisinopril in patients who had NYHA class III and IV ($P = 0.035$), but not if patients with NYHA class II were included.

Nebivolol reverses endothelial dysfunction in essential hypertension: a randomized, double-blind, crossover study.
Tzemos N, Lim PO, MacDonald TM. *Circulation* 2001; **104**(5): 511–4.

BACKGROUND. Vascular endothelial dysfunction may predict future atherosclerosis. Hence, an antihypertensive agent that reverses endothelial dysfunction and lowers BP might improve the prognosis of patients with hypertension. The authors hypothesized that nebivolol, a vasodilating beta-blocker, could improve endothelial dysfunction. They tested this hypothesis by comparing the effects of nebivolol and atenolol on endothelial function.

INTERPRETATION. Nebivolol/bendrofluazide increased both stimulated and basal endothelial NO release, whereas for the same degree of BP control, atenolol/bendrofluazide had no effect on nitric oxide bioactivity. Thus, nebivolol may offer additional vascular protection in treating hypertension.

Comment

Tzemos *et al.* report a study of 12 hypertensive patients with a mean ambulatory BP of 154/97 mmHg who were randomized after a 2-week placebo run-in period (baseline) in a double-blind, crossover fashion to 8-week treatment periods with either 5 mg of nebivolol with 2.5 mg of bendrofluazide or 50 mg of atenolol with 2.5 mg of bendrofluazide. Forearm venous occlusion plethysmography and intra-arterial infusions of acetylcholine and N(G)-monomethyl-L-arginine (L-NMMA) were used to assess stimulated and basal endothelium-dependent nitric oxide release, respectively. Sodium nitroprusside was used as an endothelium-independent control. Nebivolol/bendrofluazide increased both stimulated and basal endothelial NO release, whereas for the same degree of BP control, atenolol/bendrofluazide had no effect on NO bioactivity. Thus, nebivolol may offer additional vascular protection in treating hypertension.

 Angiotensin II suppression in humans by the orally active renin inhibitor Aliskiren (SPP100): comparison with enalapril.
Nussberger J, Wuerzner G, Jensen C, Brunner HR. *Hypertension* 2002; **39**(1): E1–8.

BACKGROUND. Renin is the main determinant of angiotensin (Ang) II levels. It, therefore, always appeared desirable to reduce Ang II levels by direct inhibition of renin. So far, specific renin inhibitors lacked potency and/or oral availability.

INTERPRETATION. The renin inhibitor Aliskiren dose-dependently decreases Ang II levels in humans following oral administration. The effect is long-lasting and, at a dose of 160 mg, is equivalent to that of 20 mg enalapril. Aliskiren has the potential to become the first orally active renin inhibitor that provides a true alternative to ACE-inhibitors and Ang II receptor antagonists in therapy for hypertension and other CV and renal diseases.

Comment

Over the last three decades, inhibition of RAS was successfully used in the treatment of hypertension and heart failure. Reduced activation of the Ang II receptor appears to be a key event to counteract increased BP and sympathetic tone as well as harmful CV hypertrophy and renal lesions. Pharmacological blockade of the Ang II receptors of the AT1-subtype so far turns out to be clinically equally effective to the less specific ACE-inhibition, but the generation of Ang II remains unopposed during AT-blockade and leaves the potential for stimulation of other Ang II receptor subtypes.

Specific inhibitors of renin reduce Ang II generation, but unlike ACEIs they do not cumulate other peptides like substance P or bradykinin and consequently untoward drug effects like cough and angioedema are not to be expected. Several specific renin inhibitors were synthesized as of the 1970s, but low efficacy or the lack of oral availability or high cost of synthesis always prevented renin inhibitors from becoming successful drugs.

A new orally active non-peptidic renin inhibitor, Aliskiren, is undergoing Phase II clinical trials. The paper by Nussberger *et al.* investigates in healthy volunteers the effect of repeated ingestion of four oral doses of Aliskiren on the renin-angiotensin-aldosterone system and on BP, heart rate, and plasma and urinary drug levels and in comparison to the ACEI enalapril. They conclude that the renin inhibitor Aliskiren dose-dependently decreases Ang II levels in humans following oral administration and, at a dose of 160 mg, is equivalent to that of 20 mg enalapril. Aliskiren has the potential to become the first orally active renin inhibitor

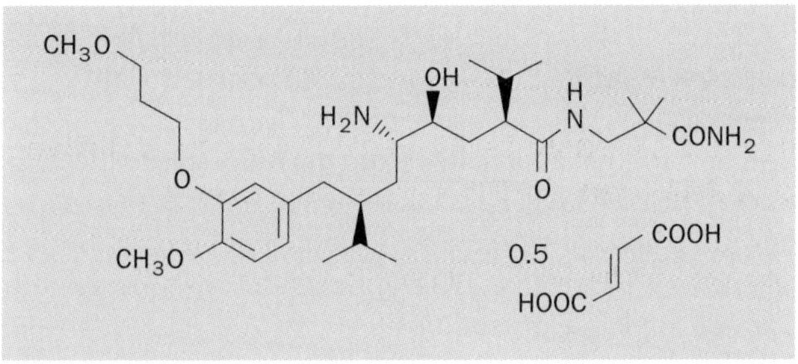

SPP 100 (Aliskiren)

Fig. 7.1 Structural formula of the renin inhibitor SPP100 (Aliskeren) or 2(S),4(S),5(S),7(S)-N-(carbamoyl-2-methylpropyl)-5-amino-4-hydroxy-2,7-diisopropyl-8-[4-methoxy-3-(3-methoxypropoxy-)phenyl]-octanamid hemifumarate. Source: Nussberger *et al.* (2002).

that provides a true alternative to ACEIs and Ang II receptor antagonists in therapy for hypertension and other CV and renal diseases.

HOT HOPE or hype over blood pressure

Introduction

Many commentaries have been published since the main data of the Heart Outcomes Prevention Evaluation Study (HOPE) was first reported. The study was performed on patients with high CV risk, 80% of whom had coronary heart disease (CHD), with an average entry BP of 139/79 mmHg, so that both normotensive and hypertensive subjects were randomized. After 4.5 years of treatment with the ACEI ramipril, there was only an overall 3/2 mmHg greater fall in BP on active treatment than placebo but remarkably highly significant reduction in all the main CV end-points including death. The overall benefits were similar in hypertensive and non-hypertensive subjects (25% and 21% reduction in the composite vascular end-point). The benefits achieved were reported to be far greater than that which can be predicted by the modest BP reduction alone. This strongly suggests a mechanism for the beneficial effects of ramipril unrelated to BP and presumably related to interruption of the renin–angiotensin axis at the tissue level. It was postulated that the non-haemodynamic effects of ACE inhibition such as those actions on reactive oxygen species, lipoprotein oxidation and transport, and bradykinin may be responsible for the extra benefits achieved beyond that of BP lowering. However, whether these observed findings in the HOPE study are a 'class effect' for all ACEIs remains to be determined.

Interestingly, it is of note that ramipril is also reported to be the first ACEI shown to prevent ischaemic events in high-risk patients without left ventricular (LV) dysfunction. This observation highly suggestive of a specific vasculoprotective effect of ramipril above and beyond that anticipated from the modest BP reduction observed in the HOPE study. The mechanism for such vasculoprotection is speculative. Undoubtedly, some contribution to the positive outcome derived from a negation of cellular effects of Ang II, which include intimal and vascular smooth muscle cell proliferation as well as plaque instability.

Overwhelming evidence has been reported that BP lowering is beneficial and mandatory in diabetic subjects regardless of their hypertensive status, as reinforced in the UK Prospective Diabetes Study (UKPDS), the Hypertension Optimal Treatment (HOT) and Systolic Hypertension in Europe (Syst-Eur) studies. However, the evidence is now growing stronger of the benefit of ACEIs treatment in those with normotensive BP range, especially in the diabetic populations. Indeed, it is now clear that BP lowering is beneficial in any patients with CHD, stroke, or diabetes regardless of their hypertensive status. This raises the question of the validity of BP reduction as an effective guide of any antihypertensive therapies. This issue and many others is being addressed in the Antihypertensive and Lipid Lowering Treatment to Prevent Heart Attack Trial (ALLHAT), in which patients with hypertension and at least one additional risk factor are currently randomized to either an ACEI, a calcium channel blocker (CCB), or a thiazide diuretic. To this end, wherever possible the choice of antihypertensive agents, treatment should be evidence-based.

Effects of an angiotensin-converting-enzyme inhibitor, ramipril, on cardiovascular events in high-risk patients: the Heart Outcomes Prevention Evaluation Study Investigators.

Yusuf S, Sleight P, Pogue J, Bosch J, Davies R, Dagenais G. *N Engl J Med* 2000; **342**(3): 145–53.

BACKGROUND. ACEIs improve the outcome among patients with LV dysfunction, whether or not they have heart failure. This study assessed the role of an ACEI, ramipril, in patients who were at high risk for CV events but who did not have LV dysfunction or heart failure.

INTERPRETATION. Ramipril significantly reduces the rates of death, myocardial infarction (MI) and stroke in a broad range of high-risk patients who are not known to have a low ejection fraction or heart failure.

Comment

See below

Major cardiovascular events in hypertensive patients randomized to doxazosin *vs* chlorthalidone: the Antihypertensive and Lipid-Lowering treatment to prevent Heart Attack Trial (ALLHAT).

ALLHAT Collaborative Research Group. *JAMA* 2000; **283**(15): 1967–75.

B A C K G R O U N D . **Hypertension is associated with a significantly increased risk of morbidity and mortality. Only diuretics and beta-blockers have been shown to reduce this risk in long-term clinical trials. Whether newer antihypertensive agents reduce the incidence of cardiovascular disease (CVD) is unknown.**

I N T E R P R E T A T I O N . The data indicate that compared with doxazosin, chlorthalidone yields essentially equal risk of CHD death/nonfatal MI but significantly reduces the risk of combined CVD events, particularly CHF, in high-risk hypertensive patients.

Comment

In the Heart Outcomes Prevention Evaluation (HOPE) which was a large trial of 9541 patients at high risk for CVD, treatment with 10 mg/day of the ACEI, ramipril, was associated with large reductions in CV events. Cardiovascular deaths were reduced by 25%, stroke by 32%, and non-fatal MI by 20%. Patients at baseline had normal BP, since those with uncontrolled hypertension were excluded, and all were receiving the best treatment with a variety of agents. Over the course of the trial, 'office' SBP dropped by only 3.3 mmHg, and DBP by only 2 mmHg, although a subsequent ambulatory BP measurement substudy in a small proportion of patients suggests that night time BPs were significantly reduced to the levels in keeping with the event rate reductions, since ramipril was given at night.

SECURE was a substudy of the HOPE trial, and included 750 patients. The patients were divided evenly into three groups (250 patients per group), each one randomized to either 2.5 mg/day of ramipril, 10 mg/day of ramipril, or placebo. The researchers used carotid ultrasound to measure progression of intima-medial thickening among the three groups over the 4.5 years of follow-up. They found progression of carotid thickening was slowed by both doses of ramipril, but the difference from placebo reached statistical significance only for the 10 mg/day group

Table 7.1 HOPE: expected *vs* actual decreases in outcome

Benefits	Stroke	MI
Expected decreases from epidemiological studies	13%	5%
Actual decreases in HOPE	31%	20%

Source: ALLHAT Collaborative Research Group (2000).

Table 7.2 Increases in intima-medial thickness (mm) over 4.5 years in SECURE

Treatment group	Placebo	Ramipril (2.5 mg/day)	Ramipril (10 mg/day)
Increase in intima-medical thickness (mm)	0.022	0.018	0.014*

*$P = 0.028$ vs placebo
Source: ALLHAT Collaborative Research Group (2000).

even though the BP lowering achieved was not different between the 2.5 and 10 mg groups.

In the HOT study, a hypertension trial of about 19 000 patients comparing outcomes with three different target DBP targets, 1501 patients were diabetic. In those randomized to the most aggressive target, 80 mmHg DBP and below, the risk of events was reduced to 0.2 times the risk of those with hypertension alone.

In the doxazosin arm of the ALLHAT trial, there was also a difference in BP control between the alpha blocker and the diuretic of about 3 mmHg, favouring the diuretic. Nevertheless, this small difference was associated with an increase in CV events in the doxazosin group of about 25%, largely but not exclusively driven by an excess of congestive heart failure.

A clue to HOPE's benefit – might lie under the nocturnal BP drop

Comparative effects of ramipril on ambulatory and office blood pressures: a HOPE substudy.

Svensson P, de Faire U, Sleight P, Yusuf S, Östergren J. *Hypertension* 2001; **38**: E28–32.

BACKGROUND. In the HOPE-trial, the ACEI ramipril significantly reduced CV morbidity and mortality in patients at high risk for CV events. The benefit could only partly be attributed to the modest mean reduction of office BP (OBP) during the study period (3/2 mmHg). However, because according to the HOPE protocol ramipril was given once daily at bedtime and BP was measured during the day, the 24-hour reduction of BP may be underestimated based on OBP.

INTERPRETATION. Although, OBP is the correct comparator when comparing with previous large intervention trials and epidemiological studies, the effects on CV morbidity and mortality seen with ramipril in the HOPE study may, to a larger extent than previously ascribed, relate to effects on BP patterns over the 24-hour period.

Comment

Given the overwhelming claims from the company on the superiority of ramipril in CV events reduction (with only modest BP reduction, based on OBP measurements) seen in the main study, the results of this HOPE substudy are particularly

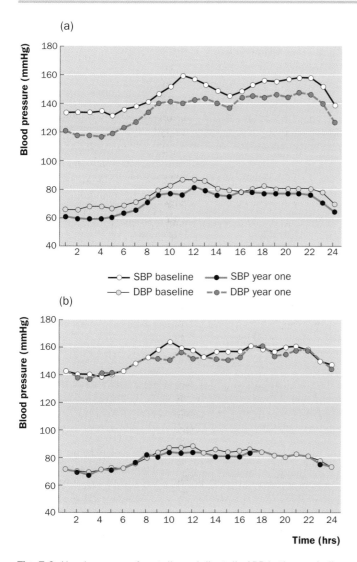

(a)

(b)

Fig. 7.2 Hourly means of systolic and diastolic ABP in the ramipril group ((a) $n = 20$) and placebo group ((b) $n = 18$) at baseline and 1 year. x-axis indicates time in hours starting at 0:00 a.m. Source: Svensson *et al.* (2001).

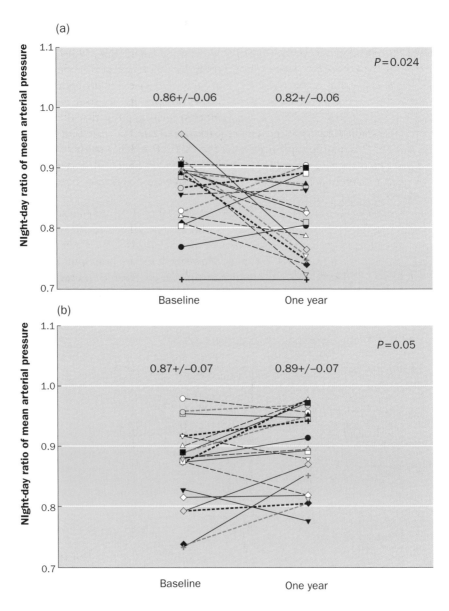

Fig. 7.3 Night/day ratio of ambulatory mean arterial pressure (MAP) in patients randomized to ramipril ((a) $n = 20$) and placebo ((b) $n = 18$) at baseline and 1 year. Reduction of night-day ratio of ambulatory MAP at 1 year in patients randomized to placebo ($n = 18$) and ramipril ($n = 20$). Source: Svensson *et al.* (2001).

interesting. The results showed that, night ambulatory BP (ABP), 1 year after randomization, was significantly lowered during treatment with ramipril 10 mg once daily at bedtime compared with placebo. OBP and mean day ABP showed a modest and insignificant fall, which was of the same order as the significant but modest BP fall observed in the overall HOPE study population. However, the failure to achieve statistical significance during daytime might well be due to the small numbers in this substudy. Because of the marked effect on night BP by ramipril the night/day ratio decreased in the ramipril group compared with placebo ($P < 0.01$). Such observation is rather surprising given that other anti-hypertensive studies usually found a more pronounced effect of treatment on OBP than on ABP. This may be explained by the fact that in the HOPE study and in this substudy, patients were not selected on the basis of having high OBP and may thus be regarded to represent a more 'normal' OBP distribution and thus more closely related to ABP.

More importantly, based on the findings of this substudy, it may be suggested that more of the benefits of ramipril in HOPE may be related to BP reduction (especially during night time) than that which was explained by the effects on OBP seen in both the main study and this study. However, it should be emphasised that the knowledge of BP as a CV risk factor is mainly based on epidemiological and intervention trials in which BP was recorded in the office. On the other hand, in several cohort studies, ABP has been shown to predict CV risk better than OBP. In

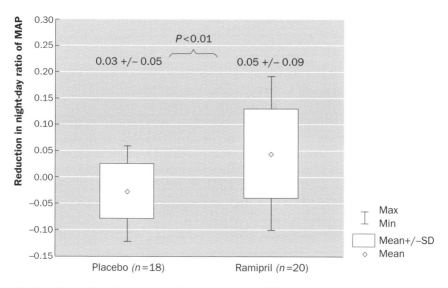

Fig. 7.4 Reduction of night-day ratio of ambulatory MAP at 1 year in patients randomized to placebo ($n = 18$) and ramipril ($n = 20$). Source: Svensson *et al.* (2001).

addition, because previous trials are based on OBP, it is difficult to relate a reduction of ABP to a reduction of CV risk. One novel suggestion from the authors is that the mode of BP measurement and the timing of drug intake in relation to BP measurement are important factors to consider when assessing BP effects and relating these to clinical outcomes.

HOPE – perseverance on modest BP benefit

Blood-pressure reduction and cardiovascular risk in the Heart Outcomes Prevention Evaluation (HOPE) study.
Sleight P, Yusuf S, Pogue J, *et al. Lancet* 2001; **358**: 2130–31.

BACKGROUND. In the HOPE study, use of the ACEI ramipril was associated with a 22% relative risk reduction in CV death, MI, or stroke, despite only a modest reduction in BP (-3·3 mmHg systolic).

INTERPRETATION. These analyses of HOPE, together with data from other HOPE substudies, show that the modest BP decrease from ramipril is unlikely to explain all the benefits seen. Clear benefit was apparent after adjustment for baseline BP and for reduction in BP. Benefit was also seen in those with a normal baseline BP. To confine this preventive therapy only to hypertensive patients in this high-risk group would therefore be a mistake.

Comment

To test the hypothesis that the benefits seen were not due to reduced BP alone, the present paper further presents analyses of the relation between the observed benefit and baseline BP, and degree of BP reduction, together with estimates of what might be expected from previous data on BP and risk, as well as from estimates derived from the placebo group of the HOPE trial. It turned out that the benefits seen in HOPE were around three times greater than predicted from these calculations. It appears that in this well-treated and largely normotensive population with coronary disease, but good left-ventricular function, the benefits from ramipril were additive to other proven therapies in normotensive patients and in those with higher baseline BP. As pointed out by the authors, the choice of any specific combination of drugs for a high-risk patient will be influenced by that patient's concomitant disease.

However, the message is clear from the authors: ramipril achieved CV events reductions beyond its BP lowering benefit in high-risk patients, hence, strongly support the notion that antihypertensive drugs may have important mechanisms of action apart from BP lowering but also that effective treatment is not a matter of simply lowering BP.

Table 7.3 Estimates of risk reduction for stroke and MI for a given difference in SBP

Data source	Difference in systolic blood pressure (mmHg)	Relative risk reduction	
		Myocardial infarction	**Stroke**
WHO/ISH* guidelines HOPE	10–15	15	40
Ramipril group estimated†	3.3	5	13
Observed placebo group	3.3	20	32
Estimated	3.3	5.5	7

* International Society of Hypertension.
† Derived from WHO/ISH.
Estimates of risk reduction for stroke and myocardial infarction for a given difference in systolic blood pressure.

Source: [Sleight] *et al.* (2001).

Table 7.4 Primary outcome (CVD, non-fatal MI, or stroke) by median baseline BP

	Placebo	Ramipril	Difference/relative risk (95% CI)	P
Systolic blood pressure				
Above median (≥138 mmHg)				
Average over trial (mmHg)	146.8	143.3	−3.5 (−4.3 to −2.7)	<0.0001
Events/patients	456/2329 (19.6%)	338/2294 (14.7%)	0.73 (0.64 to 0.84)	<0.0001
Below median (<138 mmHg)				
Average over trial (mmHg)	129.5	126.2	−3.3 (−4.0 to −2.6)	<0.0001
Events/patients	370/2322 (15.9%)	313/1251 (13.3%)	0.83 (0.71 to 0.96)	0.015
Diastolic blood pressure				
Above median (≥80 mmHg)				
Average over trial	83.6	81.4	−2.2 (−2.7 to −1.6)	<0.0001
Events/patients	301/1624 (18.5%)	220/1662 (13.2%)	0.69 (0.58 to 0.83)	<0.0001
Below median (<80 mmHg)				
Average over trial	74.7	73.1	−1.6 (−1.9 to −1.2)	<0.0001
Events/patients	525/3025 (17.4%)	431/2983 (14.4%)	0.82 (0.82 to 0.93)	0.003

Interaction *P* values for above/below median analysis for primary outcome are as follows: systolic interaction *P* = 0.2504, diastolic interaction *P* = 0.1179.

Source: Sleight *et al.* (2001).

The Heart Outcomes Prevention Evaluation (HOPE) Study: limitations and strengths.

Sica DA. *J Clin Hypertens* 2000; **2**(6): 406–9.

BACKGROUND. The HOPE study was a landmark study employing the ACEI, ramipril, in a patient population predestined for vascular events. The improvement in outcomes strongly suggests a mechanism for the beneficial effects of ramipril unrelated to BP and presumably related to interruption of the renin–angiotensin axis at the tissue level.

INTERPRETATION. Whether the observed findings in the HOPE study are a 'class effect' for all ACEIs remains to be determined. Ramipril is the first ACEI shown to prevent ischaemic events in high-risk patients without LV dysfunction. Until results become available from other ACEI trials currently underway, which involve populations similar to those included in the HOPE study, it is premature to assume that the benefits of ramipril in the HOPE trial are a class effect.

Comment

This is excellent overview of the entire HOPE study, a study that prompted the American Heart Association to include this study in its top ten list of research advances for the year 1999. The author critically reviewed the trial's strengths and limitations. The study findings provided the factual underpinnings for conducting additional studies, employing different pharmacological approaches to interruption of the renin–angiotensin system in at-risk patients. It should be noted that, however, HOPE was not designed to determine whether ACEIs are the optimal agents for preventing CV events in high-risk hypertensive patients. This issue is being addressed in the ALLHAT trial in which patients with hypertension and at least one additional risk factor are currently randomized to either an ACEI, a CCB, or a thiazide diuretic.

How long should angiotensin-converting enzyme inhibitors be given to patients following myocardial infarction: implications of the HOPE trial.

Bonarjee VVS, Dickstein K. *Curr Control Trials Cardiovasc Med* 2001; **2**: 151–5.

BACKGROUND. Long-term treatment with ACEIs reduces post-infarction morbidity and mortality in patients with LV systolic dysfunction or symptomatic heart failure. Until recently, the effect of such treatment in patients with preserved LV function has not been known.

INTERPRETATION. The results from the HOPE trial have indicated that long-term treatment with ramipril leads to a significant reduction in CV events in patients with atherosclerotic disease, including those with prior MI and preserved LV function. These results suggest that long-term ACE inhibition should also be considered in post-infarction patients with normal cardiac function.

Comment

Whether the results of the HOPE trial could be generalized to other ACEIs or Ang II receptor blockers is currently being addressed by several on-going major trials.

All antihypertensive drugs can reduce cardiovascular events in diabetics

High blood pressure and diabetes mellitus: are all antihypertensive drugs created equal?

Grossman E, Messerli FH, Goldbourt U. *Arch Intern Med* 2000; **160**(16): 2447–52.

BACKGROUND. The coexistence of diabetes mellitus (DM) and hypertension in the same patient is devastating to the CV system. The risk of stroke or any CV event is almost doubled when the hypertensive patient has DM. Lowering of BP markedly decreases the rate of CV events and renal deterioration in these patients. However, it is unclear whether all antihypertensive agents are equipotent in this regard.

INTERPRETATION. Intensive control of BP reduced CV morbidity and mortality in diabetic patients regardless of whether low-dose diuretics, beta-blockers, ACEIs, or calcium antagonists were used as a first-line treatment. A combination of more than one drug is frequently required to control BP and may be more beneficial than monotherapy.

Comment

Intensive measures to control BP in diabetic patients will pay off in terms of reduced CV mortality and morbidity, regardless of which treatment is used. Most diabetics, however, will require more than one drug to achieve target BP lowering. In all cases, CV benefit appears to be better when BP is reduced to the lowest possible target level. In the four prospective, randomized double-blind studies comparing an ACEI, beta-blocker, diuretic or calcium antagonist to placebo, treatment, in all cases, was associated with reduced CV events and mortality.

To achieve a BP of less than 130/85 mmHg, more than 60% of patients will require combination therapy. In the HOT study and the UKPDS study, the proportion of patients in these studies who required combination therapy to reach lowest target BP levels set in each trial was 76% and 62% respectively.

Blood pressure control and benefits of antihypertensive therapy: does it make a difference which agents we use?
Ruilope LM, Schiffrin EL. *Hypertension* 2001; **38**(3 Pt 2): 537–42.

BACKGROUND. This article debates the important question of whether BP lowering alone is responsible for the benefits accrued from antihypertensive therapy as demonstrated in many multicentre randomized clinical trials with different antihypertensive agents or whether there is evidence that some agents have special properties that result in benefits that go beyond those resulting from lowering BP.

INTERPRETATION. Over the past ≥ 30 years, it has been demonstrated beyond any doubt that lowering BP in severe forms of hypertension, and more recently in systolic and even mild hypertension, will result in reduced incidence of stroke and slower progression of heart and renal failure. These effects have been easier to demonstrate in sicker patients, because enough end-points may be counted in the 3–5 years that these clinical trials last. However, risk attributable to high BP comes, to a greater degree, from the much larger group of hypertensive individuals who have less severe forms of hypertension. BP lowering offers less protection from CHD, which is highly prevalent in hypertensive patients, than from stroke. With the introduction of agents such as the renin–angiotensin system inhibitors or CCBs, it has been demonstrated that hypertensive vascular remodelling and endothelial dysfunction may be corrected. It has therefore been suggested that benefits beyond BP lowering may be achieved with the use of specific drugs to lower BP. Although some evidence suggests that this may be the case, it is difficult to extrapolate from mechanistic studies to prevention of hard end-points in outcome trials and *vice versa*. The question remains for the time being largely unanswered.

Comment
See below

Debate: does it matter how you lower blood pressure?
McInnes GT. *Curr Control Trials Cardiovasc Med* 2001; **2**: 63–6.

BACKGROUND. The evidence base for drug treatment of hypertension is strong. Early trials using thiazide diuretics suggested a shortfall in prevention of CHD. The superiority of newer drugs has been widely advocated but trial evidence does not support an advantage of beta-blockers, ACEIs, CCBs or alpha-blockers for this outcome.

INTERPRETATION. Even meta-analyses have failed to clarify matters. If this issue is to be settled, bigger and better trials of longer duration in high-risk patients are needed. Meanwhile, the importance of rigorous BP control using multiple drugs has been established. This should be the focus of our attention rather than agonising over differences in cause-specific outcomes that may not be generalizable to all patient populations.

Comment

It is generally agreed by many that 'the lower the BP in hypertensive patients, the better the cardiovascular (CV) outcomes'. The usual level of cholesterol, just like BP, is continuously related to the risk of CHD. Hence, it might follow that 'the lower the cholesterol level, the lower the CV events rate in patients with established CHD'.

The role of statins in secondary prevention has been well established. Indeed, most of us now recognize that the beneficial effects of statins on early CV events reduction in major clinical trials may involve mechanisms that may be unrelated, or indirectly related, to their lipid-lowering abilities i.e. the so-called 'pleiotropic effects' of statins. Similarly, few would disagree that ACE inhibitor is the first drug of choice in diabetic hypertensives with or without proteinuria. The benefits gained in these high-risk patients are probably beyond that which can be achieved by its BP lowering property alone i.e. the so-called 'cardiovascular protective effects' of ACE inhibitions.

The Heart Protection Study (HPS), recently presented at the American Association meeting at the end of 2001 has provided compelling evidence that 'statins' when given to high-risk patients, but with a serum cholesterol in the normal range, resulted in an overall reduction of about 24% in total CHD, total stroke and revascularization procedures. Once again, these benefits were equally seen across the whole range of entry cholesterol. Thus the benefits of cholesterol lowering, like those of BP lowering, are present in high-risk patients, whether or not the cholesterol (or the BP) is elevated. In the HOPE study, treatment with ramipril, an ACEI, resulted in a highly significant reduction in all the main CV end-points including death, both in high-risk normotensive and hypertensive subjects, achieved even when there was only modest BP reduction.

Aspirin for hypertension?

Introduction

The Thrombosis Prevention Trial showed a benefit of aspirin in men at particularly high CHD risk, and the HOT study showed benefits of aspirin in treated hypertensive patients whose BP is well controlled.

The Italian Primary Prevention Project (PPP) study included both men and women who were mainly recruited from general practice and who had one or more major CV risk factors. The PPP trial evaluated low-dose aspirin (100 mg/day) and vitamin E (300 mg/day) in a randomized, open 2 × 2 factorial design in 4495 people (2583 female, mean age 64.4 years), mainly recruited in general practice. They all had one or more major CV risk factor (hypertension, hypercholesterolaemia, diabetes, obesity, family history of premature MI, or old age).

The trial was prematurely stopped after a mean follow-up of 3.6 years when evidence from the two other trials became available showing a benefit of aspirin in primary prevention. The PPP results showed that aspirin lowered the frequency of all the end-points, being significant for CV death (from 1.4 to 0.8%; relative risk [RR] 0.56) and total CV events (from 8.2 to 6.3%; RR 0.77).

Severe bleeding was more frequent in the aspirin group than the non-aspirin group (1.1% *vs* 0.3%). Only one of the bleeding complications was fatal, and that among the roughly 8000 person-years of aspirin treatment there was no suggestion of an excess risk for haemorrhagic cerebrovascular events.

Some authorities would thus recommend low doses of aspirin (80–100 mg daily) for primary prevention in individuals who have one or more risk factors, but whose BP is contained within the normal range. All three studies conducted so far highlight the fact that in hypertensive patients, BP must be well controlled, since the higher the BP the greater the risk of haemorrhagic strokes. In addition, aspirin should be prescribed in low doses to avoid bleeding complications.

Low-dose aspirin and vitamin E in people at cardiovascular risk: a randomized trial in general practice.

Collaborative Group of the Primary Prevention Project. *Lancet* 2001; **357**(9250): 89–95.

B A C K G R O U N D. In addition to the treatment of specific CV risk factors, intervention that interferes with the general mechanisms of atherosclerosis could further reduce the incidence of CV events. We aimed to investigate in general practice the efficacy of antiplatelets and antioxidants in primary prevention of CV events in people with one or more major CV risk factors.

I N T E R P R E T A T I O N. In women and men at risk of having a CV event because of the presence of at least one major risk factor, low-dose aspirin given in addition to treatment of specific risk factors contributes an additional preventive effect, with an acceptable safety profile. The results on vitamin E's CV primary preventive efficacy are not conclusive *per se*, although our results are consistent with the negative results of other large published trials on secondary prevention.

Comment

See below

Effects of intensive blood-pressure lowering and low-dose aspirin in patients with hypertension: principal results of the Hypertension Optimal Treatment (HOT) randomized trial. HOT Study Group.

Hansson L, Zanchetti A, Carruthers SG, *et al. Lancet* 1998; **351**(9118): 1755–62.

B A C K G R O U N D. Despite treatment, there is often a higher incidence of CV complications in patients with hypertension than in normotensive individuals. Inadequate reduction of their BP is a likely cause, but the optimum target BP is not known. The impact of acetylsalicylic acid (aspirin) has never been investigated in patients with hypertension. This study aimed to assess the optimum target DBP and the potential benefit of a low dose of acetylsalicylic acid in the treatment of hypertension.

INTERPRETATION. Intensive lowering of BP in patients with hypertension was associated with a low rate of CV events. The HOT Study shows the benefits of lowering the DBP down to 82.6 mmHg. Acetylsalicylic acid significantly reduced major CV events with the greatest benefit seen in all MI. There was no effect on the incidence of stroke or fatal bleeds, but non-fatal major bleeds were twice as common.

Comment

The investigation of the effects of a small dose of acetylsalicylic acid *versus* placebo in treated patients with hypertension, as in this study, provides very clear evidence of a substantial beneficial action of acetylsalicylic acid on fatal and non-fatal acute MIs, the incidence of which was reduced by as much as 36% (with the possibility of a benefit between 15 and 51%), and the prevention of 1·5 MIs per 1000 patients treated for 1 year (and 2·5 MIs per 1000 patient-years in patients with diabetes mellitus) in addition to the benefit achieved by antihypertensive therapy *per se*.

Importantly, this benefit was achieved without any additional risk of strokes, which occurred at the same rates in patients with hypertension receiving acetylsalicylic acid or placebo. The study suggested that acetylsalicylic acid is beneficial in hypertensives, provided that BP is well controlled and the risk of gastrointestinal and nasal bleeding is carefully assessed.

However, there was fear that aspirin may interfere with the BP lowering effect of various antihypertensive agents and attenuate the beneficial effects of angiotensin-converting enzyme inhibitors in patients with congestive heart failure. Data from the reanalysis of the 18 790 intensively treated hypertensive patients in this study will soon be available to clarify the issue.

Aspirin for primary prevention of coronary heart disease: safety and absolute benefit related to coronary risk derived from meta-analysis of randomized trials.
Sanmuganathan PS, Ghahramani P, Jackson PR, Wallis EJ, Ramsay LE.
Heart 2001; **85**(3): 265–71.

BACKGROUND. To determine the CV and coronary risk thresholds at which aspirin for primary prevention of CHD is safe and worthwhile.

INTERPRETATION. Aspirin treatment for primary prevention is safe and worthwhile at coronary event risk ≥ 1.5%/year; safe but of limited value at coronary event risk 1% per year; and unsafe at coronary event risk 0.5% per year. Advice on aspirin for primary prevention requires formal accurate estimation of absolute coronary event risk.

Comment

In this meta-analysis by Sanmuganathan *et al.* of four randomized controlled trials of aspirin for primary prevention to define the threshold of absolute CHD risk at which aspirin treatment is safe, and to quantitate benefit and harm from aspirin treatment at different levels of CHD risk. The four trials included were the US Physicians Health Study, the UK Doctors study, the Thrombosis Prevention Trial and the HOT study. They found that at a CHD event risk of 1.5% per year, aspirin appears to give an acceptable outcome, with one MI prevented without any important bleeding for every 77 patients treated. At this level of risk, benefit exceeds harm even if all non-minor bleeds are included. However, at a lower CHD event risk level of 0.5% per year, aspirin is unattractive, the researchers note. At this level of risk, the chance of having a significant bleed is higher than that of preventing an MI.

Thus, aspirin cannot be prescribed safely for primary prevention without formal estimation of CHD event risk in the individual. They emphasize that aspirin treatment should be guided by formal estimation of CHD risk using epidemiological studies such as the Framingham approach.

The risk levels at which they are recommending treatment (1.5% per year) would apply to 17% of the UK adult population. The UK risk prevalence is higher than most countries and thus a smaller percentage of the US population would probably fit into this category. Women under 50 or men under 40 would not reach this risk unless they had at least one major risk factor such as diabetes, hypertension or smoking. In men in their 50s, quite a high proportion would be candidates for aspirin, even if they have no clear risk factors.

The use of antithrombotic therapy in hypertensive patients should always be in addition to rigorous and aggressive BP control. The importance of the latter is illustrated by the recent Medical Research Council Thrombosis Prevention Trial, which compared low-intensity oral anticoagulation with warfarin and low-dose aspirin in the primary prevention of ischaemic heart disease in men at increased vascular risk, where mean BP was highest in those sustaining cerebral haemorrhage, intermediate in those with non-haemorrhagic strokes, and lowest amongst those who did not have strokes.

In the recently published subgroup analysis of the Thrombosis Prevention Trial, aspirin reduced coronary events by 20%, which was mainly for non-fatal events, and importantly, was significantly greater the lower the SBP at entry ($P = 0.0015$). The relative risk at BPs of 130 mmHg was 0.55 compared with 0.94 at BPs > 145 mmHg. Aspirin also reduced strokes at low but not high BPs, the relative risks being 0.41 and 1.42 ($P = 0.006$) respectively. The relative risk of all major CV events that is, the sum of CHD and stroke was 0.59 at pressures < 130 mmHg, when compared with 1.08 at BPs > 145 mmHg ($P = 0.0001$) (Table 7.5). This analysis therefore suggests that the benefit of low dose aspirin in primary prevention may occur mainly in those with lower SBPs, although it is not clear even in these men that the benefit outweighed the potential hazards. In particular, men with higher BPs may be exposed to excess risks of bleeding whilst deriving little or no benefit through reductions in CHD and stroke.

Aspirin administration to patients with established CVD is common practice. Data from the meta-analysis of the Antiplatelet Trialists Collaboration suggests that this practice is probably correct. The evidence for the benefit of aspirin in primary prevention in hypertensive patients is less clear and the risks of aspirin administra-

Table 7.5 Major CV events (CHD and stroke) by SBP at entry according to treatment with aspirin in the Thrombosis Prevention Trial

Systolic blood pressure mmHg	numbers of events (rates per 1000 person years)		
	Aspirin	No aspirin	Relative risk*
<130	42 (7.7)	64 (12.2)	0.59
130–145	4 8 (9.0)	75 (14.0)	0.68
>145	111 (20.5)	99 (17.9)	1.08

*corrected for other risk factors

Source: Sanmuganathan *et al.* (2001).

Table 7.6 Practical guidelines for antithrombotic therapy use in the hypertensive patient

- **High risk hypertensives requiring secondary prevention:** These are the hypertensive patients with a previous heart attack or stroke, or other vascular disease. These patients should receive antithrombotic therapy with aspirin 75mg daily, in the absence of contraindications.
- **Hypertensives with atrial fibrillation:** Warfarin (INR 2.0–3.0) is recommended in the older patient (age >75 years), especially if structural heart disease or vascular risk factors are present. Aspirin 75–300mg daily can be considered for younger hypertensive patients with AF who have no other risk factors, or if warfarin is contraindicated.
- **Hypertensives with other vascular risk factors:** Hypertensives at moderate risk of thrombotic complications may include those with target organ damage (e.g. LVH, renal impairment, or proteinuria), diabetes, hyperlipidaemia or a strong family history of adverse vascular outcomes or smokers. These patients may benefit more than the low risk group from aspirin therapy but these additional risk factors need to be identified in a multivariate analysis. The risk-benefit ratio in these patients is still uncertain to recommend widespread prescription of aspirin and individual circumstances should thus be considered.
- **"Lone-hypertension":** There is little evidence at present that low risk individuals with "lone-hypertension", especially those aged under 50 years with no hypertensive target organ damage, will significantly benefit from aspirin therapy and any benefit seen may possibly be out-weighed by an increase in bleeding risk. More evidence is needed before aspirin therapy can be recommended for these patients.

NOTE: blood pressure should be reduced to below 150/90mmHg, and kept well-controlled, with regular clinical surveillance if antithrombotic therapy is to be given.

Source: Sanmuganathan *et al.* (2001).

tion, namely increased incidence of major bleeding events, may possibly out-weigh the benefits.

With the available information, we suggest the simple guidelines for antithrombotic therapy use in the hypertensive patient (Table 7.6), which should always be in addition to rigorous and aggressive BP control. Indeed, risk stratification is never static and should always be regularly reviewed, especially in the older patient with associated comorbidity, structural heart disease or other risk factors for stroke.

8

Non-pharmacological therapy

Exercise

Introduction

Although pharmacological treatment for hypertension significantly reduces morbidity and mortality from cardiovascular (CV) diseases, long-term pharmacological therapy can have undesirable side effects and requires the expense of continuing medical supervision. Thus, lifestyle interventions for primary prevention and initial treatment of high blood pressure (BP) remain a vital strategy for controlling hypertension. The positive lifestyle changes may include increased regular exercise or physical activity, increased fish consumption, stopping smoking, reduction of alcohol or fat intake and restriction of sodium intake. All these could have additive effects on lowering BP achieved with weight loss. Aerobic exercise training is often recommended as an effective non-pharmacological approach to modulation of CV risk factors.

Evidence from various well control randomized trials, reviews and meta-analyses support regular aerobic exercise as an effective mean to lower BP. This effect has been demonstrated in almost all subjects, in normotensives as well as hypertensives, in women and men, in the obese and also the elderly. Although what level of exercise intensity is optimal for lowering BP is debatable, there is growing evidence that lower intensity exercise (40–50% maximum oxygen consumption, VO_{2max}) may be as effective as higher intensity exercise (60–70% VO_{2max}). Current evidence has also suggested that a daily regular lifestyle physical activity such as walking is at least as effective as structured aerobic exercise sessions in lowering BP. However, the evidence for resistance training programmes in lowering BP is inconsistent. A meta-analysis has suggested no statistically significant BP-lowering effects with resistance training, but there have been too few studies to firmly conclude this. Furthermore, sudden severe strenuous exercise may be harmful, particularly in hypertensive patients who have marked coronary artery disease.

What is the magnitude of blood pressure response to a programme of moderate intensity exercise? Randomized controlled trial among sedentary adults with unmedicated hypertension.

Cooper AR, Moore LA, McKenna J, Riddoch CJ. *Br J Gen Pract* 2000; **50**(461): 958–62.

BACKGROUND. Current guidelines for the management of hypertension recommend regular, moderate intensity aerobic exercise such as brisk walking as a means of BP reduction. However, there is a lack of consistent evidence regarding the magnitude of BP response to such a prescription. In particular, no well-designed studies have investigated the efficacy of a programme of exercise meeting current guidelines.

INTERPRETATION. Despite high compliance with the exercise programme, the magnitude of the hypotensive effect of moderate intensity exercise was not as great as that found in studies of higher intensity exercise among hypertensives. Expectations of general practitioners and patients that a programme of moderate intensity exercise will lead to a clinically important reduction in the individual's BP are unlikely to be realised.

Comment

Current guidelines for the management of hypertension recommend regular, moderate intensity exercise. Nevertheless, it has never been really clear how much BP reduction is achieved due to a paucity of well-designed studies.

This paper by Cooper *et al.* investigates the effect of a six-week programme of moderate intensity exercise on daytime ambulatory BP among untreated, sedentary hypertensives aged 25 years to 63 years. However, the net hypotensive effect of exercise was not statistically significant (systolic BP [SBP] −3.4 mmHg, 95% confidence interval [CI] −7.4 to 0.6; diastolic BP [DBP] −2.8 mmHg, 95% CI −5.8 to 0.2).

Despite high compliance with the exercise programme, the BP lowering effect of moderate intensity exercise among hypertensives was modest.

Long-term effects of exercise on blood pressure and lipids in healthy women aged 40–65 years: the Sedentary Women Exercise Adherence Trial (SWEAT)

Cox K, Burkea V, Morton AR, *et al. J Hypertens* 2001; **19**: 1733–43.

BACKGROUND. To evaluate the long-term effects of regular moderate or vigorous intensity exercise on BP and blood lipids in previously sedentary older women.

INTERPRETATION. In this largely normotensive population of older women, a moderate, but not vigorous exercise programme, achieved sustained falls in resting SBP and DBP over 18 months. The study demonstrates that, in older women, moderate intensity exercise is well accepted, sustainable long-term and has the health benefit of reduced BP.

Comment

In most studies on the effects of regular exercise on BP, women have been under-evaluated and under-represented. Indeed, in a review of 25 exercise and BP studies in hypertensives, only three were identified that reported on women alone. In women, exercise has been shown to improve lipid profiles in some studies but not all. The mode of exercise, its intensity and the amount of exercise needed to improve lipid profiles in women also remains poorly defined.

In this study by Cox *et al.*, 126 sedentary women aged 40–65 years were randomized to either a supervised centre-based (CB) or a minimally supervised home-based (HB) exercise programme, initially for 6 months. Subjects exercised three times per week for 30 min. They were evaluated at baseline, 6, 12 and 18 months. Within each programme, subjects were further randomized to exercise either at moderate (40–55% heart rate reserve, HRres) or vigorous intensity (65–80% HRres). After 6 months, all groups continued a HB moderate or vigorous exercise programme for another 12 months.

The results demonstrated that a moderate rather than vigorous-intensity exercise programme, not only optimized the initiation and maintenance of physical activity in previously sedentary women, but also resulted in modest but significant long-term falls of approximately 3 mmHg in both SBP and DBP. This effect is independent of both improvements in fitness, as measured by maximal oxygen uptake, and changes in body composition, diet or other lifestyle factors, each of which were carefully monitored throughout. Small relative reduction in total cholesterol and low density lipoprotein with vigorous-intensity exercise were seen only in the short term but not maintained.

From a public health perspective these results have important implications for physical activity promotion in older women, with clear evidence that a minimally supervised home-based regular moderate exercise programme is not only well accepted and sustainable, but also results in improved CV risk through a reduction in BP.

Walking and resting blood pressure in adults: a meta-analysis.
Kelley GA, Kelley KS, Tran ZV. *Prev Med* 2001; **33**(2 Pt 1): 120–7.

BACKGROUND. The purpose of this study was to examine the effects of walking on resting SBP and DBP in adults.

INTERPRETATION. Walking exercise programmes reduce resting BP in adults.

Comment

The above meta-analyses were carried out based on a total of 24 primary outcomes from 16 studies and 650 subjects (410 exercise, 240 control) who met the criteria for inclusion: 1) randomized and non-randomized controlled trials, 2) walking as the only intervention, 3) subjects apparently sedentary, 4) adult humans ≥ 18 years of age, 5) English-language studies published between January 1966 and December 1998, 6) resting BP assessed, 7) training studies ≥ 4 weeks. Using a random effects model, the results demonstrated a statistically significant decreases of approximately 2% for both resting SBP and DBP (systolic, mean $\pm$ SEM = –3 $\pm$ 1 mmHg, 95% CI –5 to –2 mmHg; diastolic, mean $\pm$ SEM = –2 $\pm$ 1 mmHg, 95% CI –3 to –1 mmHg).

Aerobic exercise and resting blood pressure among women: a meta-analysis.
Kelley GA. *Prev Med* 1999; **28**(3): 264–75.

BACKGROUND. The aim of this study was to use the meta-analytic approach to examine the effects of aerobic exercise on resting SBP and DBP among adult women.

INTERPRETATION. Aerobic exercise results in small reductions in resting SBP and DBP among adult women. However, a need exists for additional, well-designed studies on this topic, especially among hypertensive adult women.

Comment

Again, the same author included ten studies representing 732 subjects and 36 primary outcomes (19 systolic, 17 diastolic) which met the criteria for inclusion: 1) randomized trials, 2) aerobic activity as the primary exercise intervention, 3) comparative non-exercise control group included, 4) changes in resting SBP and/or DBP assessed for women ages 18 and older, and 5) studies published in English-language journals between January 1966 and January 1998. Overall, the result showed an approximate 2% decrease in resting systolic and 1% decrease in resting DBP were (systolic, x $\pm$ SD = –2 $\pm$ 2.6 mmHg, 95% bootstrap CI –3 to –1 mmHg; diastolic, x $\pm$ SD = –1 $\pm$ 1.9 mmHg, 95% bootstrap CI –2 to –1 mmHg).

Exercise and weight loss reduce blood pressure in men and women with mild hypertension: effects on cardiovascular, metabolic, and haemodynamic functioning.
Blumenthal JA, Sherwood A, Gullette EC, *et al. Arch Intern Med* 2000; **160**(13): 1947–58.

BACKGROUND. Lifestyle modifications have been recommended as the initial treatment strategy for lowering high BP. However, evidence for the efficacy of exercise and weight loss in the management of high BP remains controversial.

INTERPRETATION. Although exercise alone was effective in reducing BP, the addition of a behavioral weight loss programme enhanced this effect. Aerobic exercise combined with weight loss is recommended for the management of elevated BP in sedentary, overweight individuals.

Comment

In this study, Blumenthal *et al.* recruited 133 sedentary, overweight men and women with unmedicated high-normal BP or stage 1 to 2 hypertension and randomized them into 3 groups: aerobic exercise only; a behavioural weight management programme, including exercise; or a waiting list control group. They showed that although participants in both active treatment groups exhibited significant reductions in BP relative to controls, those in the weight management group generally had larger reductions. Weight management was associated with a 7 mmHg systolic and a 5 mmHg diastolic clinic BP reduction, compared with a 4 mmHg SBP and DBP reduction associated with aerobic exercise; the BP for controls did not change. Participants in both treatment groups also displayed reduced peripheral resistance and increased cardiac output compared with controls, with the greatest reductions in peripheral resistance in those in the weight management group. Weight management participants also exhibited significantly lower fasting and postprandial glucose and insulin levels than participants in the other groups.

Psychological factors in hypertensive patients

Introduction

Hypertension has long been considered a psychosomatic disorder in that psychosocial variables may influence the onset or course of the disease process. Lifestyle factors known to influence BP and linked with stress, such as smoking, alcohol intake, exercise patterns and obesity, may mediate associations between BP and stress. While there are some apparent inconsistencies in the evidence linking life stress and hypertension, these inconsistencies can be reasonably explained by different psychological state and trait effects. It is generally agreed that BP is acutely elevated in response to mental stress. Longer-term effects of stress on BP, however, are less clear. But the evidence is now accumulating and overall these support some causal relationship between life event stress, especially occupational stress and later hypertension. Job strain, defined as a combination of high psychological demand and low decision attitude, is related to higher levels of BP both at work and at home, and marital stress is associated with higher BP, particularly in women. These findings in many studies remain significant after controlling possible confounders.

High CV responses to active coping mental stressors have been shown to predict greater BP increases at follow-up. Similarly, hyperreactivity of SBP to the cold pressor test was also related to increased development of hypertension after an average of 24 and 28 years of follow-up. It is also known that acute vascular reactivity to stress can predict left ventricular mass. Animal models suggest that genetic susceptibility to hypertension and frequent stress exposure are important modulating factors in stress-related hypertension. Indeed, one human study has suggested that stress responsivity as a long-term predictor is modulated by both genetic and environmental factors.

Relaxation strategies e.g. biofeedback, transcendental meditation, yoga, sleep therapy, Tai Chi and psychotherapy, have been recommended by some to lower stress thus lowering BP. However, these therapies are not evidence-based as few trials have been controlled adequately and only few have shown positive results. Only one well-conducted randomized study showed a fall in BP in both normotensive and hypertensive patients after relaxation therapy.

Depression and risk of heart failure among older persons with isolated systolic hypertension.
Abramson J, Berger A, Krumholz HM, Vaccarino V. *Arch Intern Med* 2001; **161**(14): 1725–30.

BACKGROUND. Investigators have shown that depression is associated with an increased risk of coronary heart disease (CHD) in general and myocardial infarction (MI) in particular. However, it is unknown whether depression, independent of its association with myocardial infarction, is a risk factor for heart failure (HF).

INTERPRETATION. Depression is independently associated with a substantial increase in the risk of heart failure among older persons with isolated systolic hypertension (ISH). This association does not appear to be mediated by myocardial infarction.

Comment

Previous research has found depression associated with risk of CHD, and has shown that depression is a negative prognostic factor in patients with existing CHD or HF. What are the likely mechanism(s) linking depression to HF in hypertensives? First, depression increases the risk of MI. Secondly, depression is believed to induce excessive activation of the sympathetic nervous system.

Of the 4538 participants of the Systolic Hypertension in the Elderly Program (SHEP), 221 were clinically depressed at baseline according to a CES-D self-report scale. These depressed patients were twice as likely as their non-depressed counterparts to develop HF over follow-up (average 4.5 years): 18 of 221 depressed patients (8.1%) experienced HF, as compared to 138 of 4317 non-depressed patients (3.2%). After adjusting for demographic factors, baseline health status, and other potential confounders, the association between depression and risk of HF remained significant, with a hazard ratio of 2.59 (95% CI 1.57–4.27, $P < 0.001$).

Individualized stress management for primary hypertension: a randomized trial.

Linden W, Lenz JW, Con AH. *Arch Intern Med* 2001; **161**(8): 1071–80.

BACKGROUND. **To test the efficacy of individualized stress management for primary hypertension in a randomized clinical trial with the use of ambulatory BP measures.**

INTERPRETATION. Individualized stress management is associated with ambulatory BP reduction. The effects were replicated and further improved by follow-up. Reductions

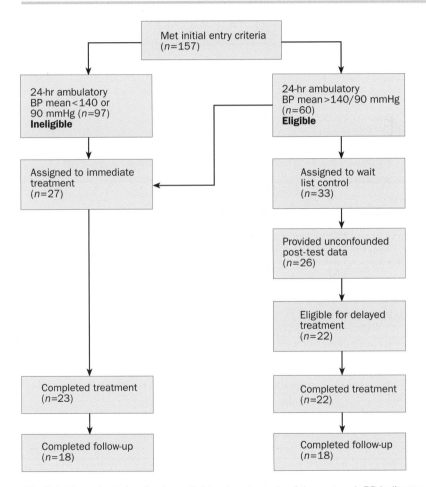

Fig. 8.1 Flow chart of patients available at each stage of the protocol. BP indicates blood pressure. Source: Linden *et al.* (2001).

in psychological stress and improved anger coping appear to mediate the reductions in BP change.

Comment

Psychological intervention in the management of hypertension has received little recognition. This study is the first of its kind to show that psychological intervention without drugs can in fact produce 'meaningful' BP reductions in people with hypertension. Using 24-hour ambulatory BP monitoring, 45 men and women with BP > 140/90 were randomized to wait list controls or to receive 10 hours of individualized stress management over a 30-day period, then followed for 60 days. BP was significantly reduced in the immediate treatment group, but not in the wait-listed controls during the same period. The interesting feature of this study is that when the control group underwent stress-management subsequently, they, too, experienced significant reductions in BP. However, it would be even more interesting to see if certain group of patients may benefit more from such intervention, and to compare stress management approaches to drug therapy in hypertensive patients.

Psychosocial predictors of hypertension in men and women.

Levenstein S, Smith MW, Kaplan GA. *Arch Intern Med* 2001; **161**(10): 1341–6.

BACKGROUND. Psychosocial stressors have been shown to predict hypertension in several cohort studies; patterns of importance, sex differences, and interactions with standard risk factors have not been fully characterized.

INTERPRETATION. In the general population, low occupational status and performance and the threat or reality of unemployment increases the likelihood of developing hypertension, especially among men, independent of demographic and behavioral risk factors. Psychological distress and social alienation may also increase hypertension incidence, especially in women, chiefly through an association with health risk behaviours.

Comment

Increasing evidence points towards a role for psychological factors in the pathogenesis of CV disease. For example, abnormal psychological morbidity leads to an increase in mortality amongst patients with myocardial infarction and heart failure. In light of the relationship between the sympathetic system and high BP, it is plausible that psychological factors have a role in the pathogenesis of hypertension. Indeed, laboratory stressors and real-life difficulties such as job strain and job dissatisfaction can lead to elevations in BP, and stress or distress have been reported in some cohorts to predict the subsequent incidence of sustained hypertension.

The paper by Linden *et al.* reports that individualized stress management is associated with reductions in ambulatory BP. They suggest that reductions in psychological stress and improved anger coping appear to mediate the reductions in BP change.

In the general population, data from the Alameda County Study as described in this paper, a longitudinal investigation of behavioural, social, psychological and economic influences on health, found that low occupational status and performance and the threat or reality of unemployment increased the likelihood of developing hypertension, especially among men, independent of demographic and behavioural risk factors. Thus, psychological distress and social alienation may increase the incidence of hypertension, especially in women, chiefly through an association with health risk behaviours.

Salt and hypertension: recent insights

Introduction

Numerous epidemiological and clinical studies have demonstrated a clear relationship between high salt intake and BP. Meta-analyses from controlled trials have shown consistently that BP decreases with sodium restriction, although estimates of the magnitude of fall vary.

The publication of the Dietary Approaches to Stop Hypertension (DASH)-Sodium Study in January 2001 may well have marked the end of the controversy surrounding the role of salt in hypertension. The study has showed convincingly that the DASH diet (which focuses on fruits, vegetables, low fat dairy products, whole grain, poultry, fish and nuts) lowers BP and that on top of the dietary sodium restriction lowers the BP further. The result was impressive and has great implications from the public health perspective. We will discuss this in more detail below.

Effects on blood pressure of reduced dietary sodium and the Dietary Approaches to Stop Hypertension (DASH) diet. DASH-Sodium Collaborative Research Group.
Sacks FM, Svetkey LP, Vollmer WM, *et al. N Engl J Med* 2001; **344**(1): 3–10.

BACKGROUND. The effect of dietary composition on BP is a subject of public health importance. This study was designed to test the effect of different levels of dietary sodium, in conjunction with the DASH diet, which is rich in vegetables, fruits, and low-fat dairy products, in persons with and in those without hypertension.

INTERPRETATION. The reduction of sodium intake to levels below the current recommendation of 100 mmol per day and the DASH diet both lower BP substantially, with greater effects in combination than singly. Long-term health benefits will depend on

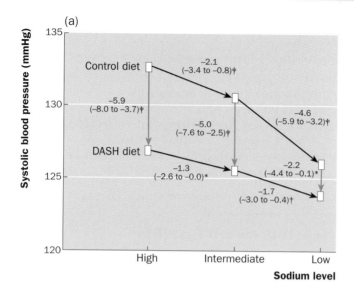

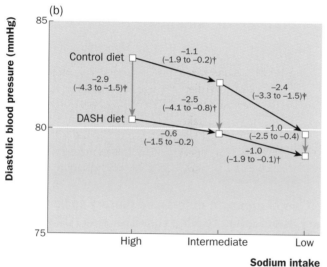

Fig. 8.2 Effects of differing levels of dietary sodium on BP against a background of a usual North American diet or a DASH combination diet, rich in fruit and vegetables and low fat dairy foods. BP fell with lower levels of sodium with both diets.
Source Sacks *et al.* (2001).

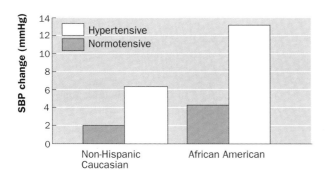

Fig. 8.3 Net reduction in systolic BP from DASH combination diet. Source: Sacks *et al.* (2001).

the ability of people to make long-lasting dietary changes and the increased availability of lower-sodium foods.

Comment

The DASH study was a multicentre randomized trial involving 412 hypertensive participants who consumed either a control diet (average American) or the DASH diet. In both diet groups, subjects received three different mixtures of foodstuffs, resulting in three predetermined total salt intakes: high sodium (about 150 mmol per day; 8.7 g NaCl), intermediate (100 mmol per day; 5.8 g NaCl) or low (50 mmol per day; 2.9 g NaCl). Each of the three dietary periods was 30 days in length; all food and drink was provided to the subjects; and caloric intake was adjusted to maintain body weight.

Major results

The DASH diet lowered BP relative to the control diet as had previously been demonstrated. Independent of diet group, reducing the sodium content of the diet resulted in a progressive stepwise reduction in BP. The benefit of decreasing sodium intake was greater in the control than in the DASH diet. The combined effects of the DASH diet and sodium restriction were smaller than they would have been if the effects of each intervention were strictly additive. However, the combined effects were greater than either intervention alone. SBP and DBP differences between the DASH and control groups were greatest at the higher sodium levels. The sodium effect was observed in: both normotensive and hypertensive subjects; both female and male subjects; both blacks and subjects of other races.

Effects of diet and sodium intake on blood pressure: subgroup analysis of the DASH-Sodium Trial.

Vollmer WM, Sacks FM, Ard J, *et al. Ann Intern Med* 2001; **135**(12): 1019–28.

BACKGROUND. Initial findings from the DASH-Sodium Trial demonstrated that reduction of sodium intake in two different diets decreased BP in participants with and without hypertension.

INTERPRETATION. The DASH diet plus reduced sodium intake is recommended to control BP in diverse subgroups.

Comment

This DASH paper has demonstrated that the DASH diet plus reduced sodium intake is equally effective in reducing BP in diverse groups of patients with high systolic BP. The greatest effect was achieved by this combination than either alone. Among non-hypertensive participants who received the control diet, lower (*vs* higher) sodium intake decreased BP by 7.0/3.8 mmHg in those older than 45 years of age ($P < 0.001$) and by 3.7/1.5 mmHg in those 45 years of age or younger ($P < 0.05$).

Effects on blood lipids of a blood pressure-lowering diet: the Dietary Approaches to Stop Hypertension (DASH) Trial.

Obarzanek E, Sacks FM, Vollmer WM, *et al. Am J Clin Nutr* 2001; **74**(1): 80–9.

BACKGROUND. Effects of diet on blood lipids are best known in white men, and effects of type of carbohydrate on triacylglycerol concentrations are not well defined.

INTERPRETATION. The DASH diet is likely to reduce coronary heart disease risk. The possible opposing effect on coronary heart disease risk of high-density lipoprotein (HDL) reduction needs further study.

Comment

The results further support the multifaceted beneficial effects of the DASH diet in subgroups by sex, race, and baseline lipid concentrations. The results showed that relative to the control diet, the DASH diet resulted in lower total cholesterol, low-density lipoprotein (LDL)-C and HDL-C concentrations (all $P < 0.0001$), without significant effects on triacylglycerol. The net reductions in total and LDL cholesterol in men were greater than those in women. Furthermore, changes in lipids did not differ significantly by race or baseline lipid concentrations, except for HDL, which decreased more in participants with higher baseline HDL-cholesterol concentrations than in those with lower baseline HDL-cholesterol concentrations. The fruit and vegetable diet produced few significant lipid changes.

DASH (Dietary Approaches to Stop Hypertension) diet is effective treatment for stage 1 isolated systolic hypertension.

Moore TJ, Conlin PR, Ard J, Svetkey LP, for the DASH Collaborative Research Group. *Hypertension* 2001; **38**: 155–8.

BACKGROUND. Use of the DASH diet, which is rich in fruits, vegetables, and low-fat dairy foods, significantly lowers BP. Among the 459 participants in the DASH Trial, 72 had stage 1 ISH (SBP, 140 to 159 mmHg; DBP, 90 mmHg).

INTERPRETATION. The results indicate that the DASH diet, which is rich in fruits, vegetables and low-fat dairy foods, is effective as first-line therapy in stage 1 ISH.

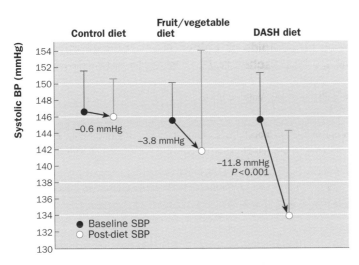

Fig. 8.4 SDP before and after 8 weeks on each of the 3 experimental diets (mean, SD). Only the DASH diet group had a significant BP decrement; the response in the DASH diet group was significantly greater than that in the control and fruits/vegetable diet groups ($P < 0.001$ and $P < 0.01$, respectively). Source: Moore *et al.* 2001.

Comment

The results demonstrated that, compared with the control diet, use of the DASH diet lowered SBP by 11.2 mmHg in participants with stage 1 ISH. This was sufficient to control SBP to < 140 mmHg in 18 of 23 participants in the DASH diet group. Although there were only 72 individuals in this ISH analysis, the results are quite robust. This treatment effect size is comparable to the BP reduction seen with a typical antihypertensive drug.

Additional comment

The relationship between salt and hypertension has been subject to accusations of conspiracy and disinformation. Some have even suggested that a low-salt diet might be harmful. Aside from these, most clinicians accept some causal relationship between salt and hypertension. Recent papers from the DASH-Sodium study group have defined this relationship further. The DASH diet emphasizes fruits, vegetables and low-fat dairy foods, and includes whole grains, poultry, fish and nuts. It is reduced in, but does not exclude, red meat, sweets and sugary beverages. The result is a diet high in potassium, calcium and magnesium, protein, and fibre. Sodium in the first DASH study was constant at a level slightly below American average consumption.

In the DASH-Sodium subgroup analysis, decreases in BP associated with reduced sodium intake were present in all hypertensive or non-hypertensive; African-

Table 8.1 Blood reduction with low sodium intake and the DASH diet: hypertensives *vs* non-hypertensives

Blood pressure	Hypertensive subjects	Non-hypertensive subjects
Systolic (mmHg)	−11.5 ± 1.3	−7.1 ± 1.1
Diastolic (mmHg)	−5.7 ± 0.9	−3.7 ± 0.8

*P values < 10(−6)

Source: Moore *et al.* (2001).

Table 8.2 Blood reduction among control subjects in DASH: hypertensives *vs* non-hypertensives

Blood pressure	Hypertensive subjects	Non-hypertensive subjects
Systolic (mmHg)	−8.3 ± 0.9	−5.6 ± 0.7
Diastolic (mmHg)	−4.4 ± 0.6	−2.8 ± 0.5

*P values < 10(−8)

Source: Moore *et al.* (2001).

American or non-African-American; female or male; and aged under 45 or over 45; subgroups and were clinically relevant. It is accepted that antihypertensive drug therapy typically lowers BP more than simple salt restriction, and low-salt diets have adjunctive BP-lowering effects of about 2 to 4 mmHg when combined with beta-blockers, diuretics, or angiotensin-converting enzyme inhibitors (ACEIs). However, salt restriction probably does not enhance the blood-pressure lowering effects of calcium channel blockers (CCBs).

Nevertheless, there is the difficulty of achieving and maintaining very low-salt diets, the uncertain clinical benefits of either low-salt or very low-salt diets, and the fact that other therapies have clearer proven benefits.

In another analysis, reductions in BP were seen with reduced sodium between both those following a diet similar to that consumed by many Americans, considered the control diet, and among those consuming the DASH diet, which has been previously shown to reduce BP itself. In this study, a total of 412 participants were enrolled; about 57% were women, and 57% were African Americans. (Breakdowns by race and gender have been analysed separately.) Subjects had systolic pressures ranging from 120 to 159 mmHg, and diastolic pressures between 80 and 95 mmHg. About 41% were hypertensive. The combination of the DASH diet and low sodium, about 1.5 g per day – well below the current recommended intake of 2.4 g – produced the best results, where lower sodium resulted in reduced systolic and diastolic pressures in both diet groups, but best results were seen with the combination of low sodium intake and the DASH diet. Overall, this combination reduced systolic BP by 8.9 mmHg and diastolic BP by an average of 4.5 mmHg. The reduction was even greater among those who were hypertensive.

It is important for the generalization of this finding, however, that reduced sodium also resulted in substantial BP reductions among those consuming the control diet.

Toning down the sodium in the older individuals

Effects of reduced sodium intake on hypertension control in older individuals. Results from the trial of non-pharmacologic interventions in the elderly (TONE).
Appel LJ, Espeland MA, Easter L, *et al. Arch Intern Med* 2001; **161**: 685–93.

BACKGROUND. Few trials have evaluated the effects of reduced sodium intake in older individuals, and no trial has examined the effects in relevant subgroups such as African Americans.

INTERPRETATION. A reduced sodium intake is a broadly effective, non-pharmacologic therapy that can lower BP and control hypertension in older individuals.

Comment

Sodium reduction has been widely advocated as a means to reduce BP and control hypertension especially in older persons. This large randomized controlled trial demonstrated that older people with hypertension can reduce their sodium intake and that a reduced sodium intake can lower BP and the need for antihypertensive drug therapy. The effects were consistent in subgroups defined by sex, ethnicity, and weight status. Specifically, from a mean baseline BP of 128/71 mmHg, a reduced sodium intake lowered SBP and DBPs by 4.3 and 2.0 mmHg, respectively. However, the effects of the intervention on BP and end-points in the age group 70–80 years did not achieve statistical significance, perhaps as a result of small sample size. In dose-response analyses, progressively greater reductions in sodium intake were associated with a reduced risk of a trial end-point. However, TONE did not assess the impact of sodium reduction in persons with high BP. Nevertheless, it is plausible that the extent of BP reduction would be greater if not similar to that observed in this trial.

There are two main reasons why sodium reduction should be particularly effective in older persons. First, because arterial compliance decreases with age, any change in intravascular volume related to sodium intake should result in a greater BP change in older persons than in younger individuals. Secondly, because of the decline in kidney function associated with aging, older individuals may retain sodium to a greater extent than younger persons.

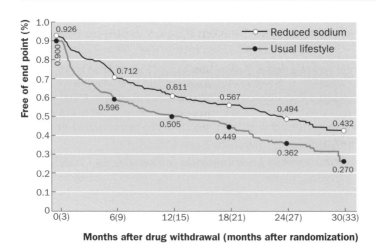

Fig. 8.5 Proportion of participants who remained free of elevated BP during follow-up. Cardiovascular events were censored. Source: Appel *et al.* (2001).

Smoking

Introduction

Overwhelming evidence supports the causal relationship between cigarette smoking and various adverse CV events and acts synergistically with hypertension and hyperlipidaemia to increase the risk of coronary heart disease. Smoking causes an acute increase in BP and heart rate and has been found to be associated with malignant hypertension. Indeed, several studies have reported that smokers have a greater prevalence of severe uncontrolled hypertension in otherwise medication-compliant patients.

Nicotine acts as an adrenergic agonist, mediating local and systemic catecholamine release and possibly the release of vasopressin. Paradoxically, several epidemiological studies have found that BP levels among cigarette smokers were the same as or lower than those of non-smokers. But such 'paradox' observations may be attributable to several confounders such as weight differences: smokers are generally lighter than non-smokers, probably as a consequence of the anorectic effects of regular inhalation of cigarette smoke.

The earliest prospective population studies suggested effects of smoking cessation to increase the level of BP independently of the increases in body weight characteristically observed after quitting smoking.

Effects of smoking cessation on changes in blood pressure and incidence of hypertension: a 4-year follow-up study.
Lee DH, Ha MH, Kim JR, Jacobs DR Jr. *Hypertension* 2001; **37**(2): 194–8.

BACKGROUND. Some epidemiological studies have reported lower BP in smokers than in non-smokers. This finding is regarded as a paradox, because nicotine has potent sympathomimetic effects, which affects BP levels and heart rate. Furthermore, ex-smokers tend to have BPs similar to those of people who never smoked. The results of follow-up studies on the effects of smoking or the cessation of smoking on the changes of BP are equivocal.

INTERPRETATION. This study implies that the cessation of smoking may result in increases in BP, hypertension, or both.

Comment

The aim of the present study was to investigate the effect of smoking cessation on the changes of BP and incidence of hypertension in male workers at a steel manufacturing company.

Smoking is an important CV risk factor, and much of the efforts at CV risk factor modification have been directed at smoking cessation. However, many patients paradoxically report an increase in weight with smoking cessation, which may itself bring adverse effects.

Lee *et al.* report on a cohort of 8170 healthy male employees at a steel manufacturing company who had received occupational health examinations at the company's health care centre in 1994 and were reexamined in 1998. This 4-year prospective study suggests that the increases in BP among the quitters and current non-smokers, especially the quitters, were generally larger than those of the current smokers. More interestingly, the increments of BP in the quitters for < 1 year were very similar to those of the current smokers. Quitters for ≥ 1 year, however, showed larger increases in BP than did the current smokers.

This was observed consistently in all groups classified by weight changes. Furthermore, the incidence of hypertension was also higher in the group of subjects who had stopped smoking for ≥ 1 year, whereas the incidence was lower in the quitters for < 1 year. Relative risks increased in direct relationship with the increasing periods of smoking cessation.

Association between smoking and blood pressure: evidence from the health survey for England.

Primatesta P, Falaschetti E, Gupta S, Marmot MG, Poulter NR. *Hypertension* 2001; **37**(2): 187–93.

BACKGROUND. Cigarette smoking causes acute BP elevation, although some studies have found similar or lower BPs in smokers compared with non-smokers.

INTERPRETATION. The data show that any independent chronic effect of smoking on BP is small. Differences between men and women in this association are likely to be due to complex interrelations among smoking, alcohol intake and body mass index (BMI).

Comment

In this study from the Health Survey for England, older male smokers had higher SBP adjusted for age, BMI, social class and alcohol intake than did non-smoking men. Among women, light smokers (1 to 9 cigarettes/d) tended to have lower BPs than heavier smokers and never smokers. Thus, any independent chronic effect of smoking on BP is small, especially in view of complex interrelations among smoking, alcohol intake and BMI. These results were consistent with the previous German reports of an interaction between alcohol and smoking to increase BP in regular drinker.

Weight loss

Introduction

Being overweight or weight gain is associated with hypertension in many populations. Indeed, being overweight increases the prevalence of hypertension three-fold

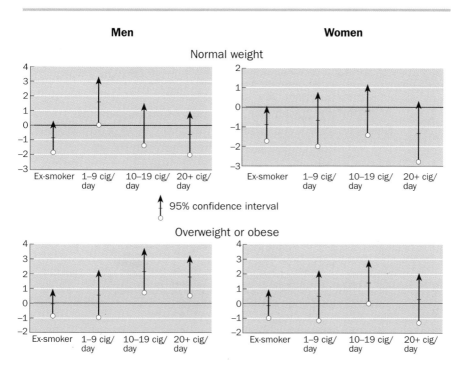

Fig. 8.6 Differences (and 95% CI) in mean SBP between the smoking groups (reference, non-smoking) in persons with normal weight and overweight or obese. Source: Primatesa *et al.* (2001).

and the incidence of weight related hypertension is growing in parallel with the epidemic of obesity especially in developed countries. Indeed, excess body fat remains the biggest single contributor to BP elevation. It can be estimated from the Nurses' Health Study that for every 1 kg gain in weight, there is a 5% increase in the risk of hypertension. It is of note that the relationship between CV risk and weight is a continuous one and weight gain increases risk even when BMI is in the 'normal range'. There is growing body of evidence that weight loss is effective in reducing BP in obese humans. All hypertension treatment guidelines support that weight reduction is a worthwhile objective for people who are overweight, or who are at risk for hypertension and certainly those whose BP is already high. One meta-analysis of controlled clinical trials estimated that loss of 4–8% body weight is associated with a reduction of 3/3 mmHg systolic/diastolic BP and a decreased requirement for antihypertensive drugs. Thus, weight control is a key strategy in preventing and managing hypertension and has additional CV benefits. However, the practical problem is that of individual's motivation and the need for intensive weight counselling sessions over a long period of time in order to maintain substantial weight loss and to achieve prognostically relevant BP reduction, as shown in the Phase II of the Trials of Hypertension Prevention (TOHP II) below. The main question which follows is: is it cost-effective?

AHA dietary guidelines, AHA Scientific Statement Revision 2000; a statement for healthcare professionals: the Nutrition Committee of the American Heart Association.
Krauss RM, Eckel RH, Howard B, *et al. Circulation* 2000; **102**: 2284–99.

INTERPRETATION. This document presents guidelines for reducing the risk of cardiovascular disease by dietary and other lifestyle practices. Since the previous publication of these guidelines by the American Heart Association (AHA), the overall approach has been modified to emphasize their relation to specific goals that the AHA considers of greatest importance for lowering the risk of heart disease and stroke. The revised guidelines place increased emphasis on foods and an overall eating pattern and the need for all Americans to achieve and maintain a healthy body weight

Long-term weight loss and changes in BP: results of the Trials of Hypertension Prevention, phase II (TOHP II). Trials for the Hypertension Prevention Research Group.
Stevens VJ, Obarzanek E, Cook NR, *et al. Ann Intern Med* 2001; **134**(1): 1–11.

BACKGROUND. **Weight loss appears to be an effective method for primary prevention of hypertension. However, the long-term effects of weight loss on BP have not been extensively studied.**

INTERPRETATION. Clinically significant long-term reductions in BP and reduced risk for hypertension can be achieved with even modest weight loss.

Comment
Weight loss has been shown to reduce BP in overweight hypertensive patients and in overweight persons with high-normal BP. Most of these trials were small, with only one having more than 500 participants, and most had short-term follow-up (1 year or less). In almost all trials, SBP and DBP were reduced with weight reduction.

Stevens *et al.* reports data from the participants assigned to the weight loss ($n = 595$) and usual care control ($n = 596$) groups in TOHP II. Mean weight change from baseline in the intervention group was –4.4 kg at 6 months, –2.0 kg at 18 months, and –0.2 kg at 36 months (*vs* control group 0.1, 0.7, and 1.8 kg, respectively). The risk ratio for hypertension in the intervention group was 0.58

(95% CI, 0.36 to 0.94) at 6 months, 0.78 (CI, 0.62 to 1.00) at 18 months, and 0.81 (CI, 0.70 to 0.95) at 36 months. In subgroup analyses, intervention participants who lost at least 4.5 kg at 6 months and maintained this weight reduction for the next 30 months had the greatest reduction in BP and a relative risk for hypertension of 0.35 (CI, 0.20 to 0.59).

In TOHP II, Stevens *et al.* focused on the changes seen in the most adherent participants. The target weight reduction was 4.5 kg (10 lb), and the quintile of participants who lost the most weight (> 4.4 kg) had a reduction of 5 mmHg in SBP and 7 mmHg in DBP. A linear relationship was observed between reduction in weight and reduction in BP: for every 2 pounds of body weight lost, SBP and DBP were reduced by 1 mmHg and 1.4 mmHg, respectively. Thus, this trial suggests that clinically significant long-term reductions in BP and reduced risk for hypertension can be achieved with even modest weight loss.

However, one problem with lifestyle interventions on BP reduction is that patients' adherence to weight loss is often poor. Despite more than 20 hours of group counselling sessions with experienced dieticians or health educators, only 13% of participants in the weight loss group in TOHP II were able to maintain substantial weight loss over 3 years. Nevertheless, as in the DASH trial, it is no doubt that lifestyle intervention is a worthwhile objective for those who are at risk for hypertension.

Weight reduction and pharmacologic treatment in obese hypertensives.
Masuo K, Mikami H, Ogihara T, Tuck M. *Am J Hypertens* 2001; **14**(6 Pt 1): 530–38.

BACKGROUND. This study was conducted to evaluate the mechanisms of weight loss-induced BP reduction focusing, in particular, on the contributions of sympathetic nervous system activity, fasting plasma insulin, and leptin to BP levels, and to delineate the additional influence of antihypertensive drug therapy.

INTERPRETATION. The study showed that weight loss is associated with favourable metabolic improvements and these improvements are amplified when combined with pharmacological treatment. Therefore, weight loss should be regarded as an essential component of any treatment programme for obesity-related hypertension. A novel finding from this study is that ACE inhibition had a striking effect to lower plasma leptin. Suppression of sympathetic activity, insulinaemia and leptinaemia appeared to play a role in the BP reduction accompanying weight loss.

Comment

In this study, each of five groups of obese hypertensives was treated with the long-acting CCB amlodipine, the ACEI enalapril with or without a weight reduction programme, or a weight reduction programme alone. The goal BP was less than

140/90 mmHg for the pharmacological treatment groups. The weight reduction programme groups with or without pharmacological treatment were divided into two groups; weight loss groups who succeeded in weight reduction ($\geq$ 10%) and non-weight loss groups who failed in weight reduction ($<$ 10%) in the first 6 months. The final dose of CCB and ACEI were less in the combined pharmacological and weight loss groups than in the pharmacological treatment alone groups or in the pharmacological and non-weight loss groups. In the weight reduction groups regardless of pharmacological treatment, the per cent reductions from baseline in plasma insulin, leptin and norepinephrine (NE) were greater in the weight loss groups ($\geq$ 10%) than in the non-weight loss groups ($<$ 10%). The reductions in plasma NE, insulin and leptin were significantly greater and earlier in combined pharmacological and weight loss groups than in the pharmacological treatment alone groups. In ACEI groups, the reductions in plasma NE, in insulin, and especially in leptin were greater than the other groups. In the CCB alone group, reductions in insulin and leptin occurred, but there was no change in plasma NE. Reductions in insulin and leptin in CCB groups were less and occurred later than in the ACEI groups or the weight reduction alone group.

Alcohol reduction

Introduction

Light-to-moderate alcohol consumption ($<$ 30g/day i.e. one to two drinks/day) is associated with 10–40% lower risks of MI and CV death than those who abstain; however, heavy alcohol consumption or binge drinking increases such risk, especially of haemorrhagic stroke. The latter may well be related to an acute rise in BP in binge or sustained heavy drinkers. On the other hand, the reduction in CV risks with light to moderate alcohol intake may be attributable to an increase of high density lipoprotein cholesterol or a decrease in fibrinogen levels.

Over the last 30 years a large number of cross-sectional studies and a smaller number of prospective cohort studies have demonstrated a dose relationship between increase alcohol intake and BP. However, the threshold dose for hypertension, and plausible pathophysiological mechanisms at which such effects are clearly manifest still remain unclear. Nevertheless, it is clear that a causal association exists between chronic intake of $\geq$ 30–60 g alcohol per day and BP elevation in men and women as well as in hypertensive and non-hypertensives. Such causal relationship have been consistently shown in several well conducted intervention studies which not only support the data from observational studies but also has shown a remarkable consistency in demonstrating a potentially valuable decrease in BP when heavy drinkers abstain or restrict their alcohol intake. From the different studies a rule of thumb can be derived: above 30 g of alcohol intake per day an increment/decrement of 10 g of alcohol per day increases/decreases on average systolic BP (SBP) by 1–2 mmHg and DBP by 1 mmHg.

With respect to pattern of drinking, similar BP raising effects have been reported with binge drinking or drinking on a regular basis. The risk of haemorrhagic stroke is equally high in both, with estimates from a meta-analysis of nine studies; the relative risk for haemorrhagic stroke increases by 50% in those who drink 25 g alcohol per day and there is a 4.5-fold increase in risk in those drinking 100 g alcohol per day.

Effects of alcohol reduction on blood pressure: a meta-analysis of randomized controlled trials.

Xin X, He J, Frontini MG, Ogden LG, Motsamai OI, Whelton PK. *Hypertension* 2001; **38**(5): 1112–7.

B a c k g r o u n d . **Alcohol drinking has been associated with increased BP in epidemiological studies.**

I n t e r p r e t a t i o n . The study suggests that alcohol reduction should be recommended as an important component of lifestyle modification for the prevention and treatment of hypertension among heavy drinkers.

Summary of results

This is a meta-analysis of 15 randomized controlled trials (total of 2234 participants) to assess the effects of alcohol reduction on BP. The study included randomized control trials published before June 1999 in which alcohol reduction was the only intervention difference between active and control treatment groups. By means of a fixed-effects model, findings from individual trials were pooled after results for each trial were weighted by the inverse of its variance. Overall, alcohol reduction was associated with a significant reduction in mean (95% confidence interval) SBP and DBP of −3.31 mmHg (−2.52 to −4.10 mmHg) and −2.04 mmHg (−1.49 to −2.58 mmHg), respectively. A dose-response relationship was observed between mean percentage of alcohol reduction and mean BP reduction. Effects of intervention were enhanced in those with higher baseline BP.

Different alcohol drinking and blood pressure relationships in France and Northern Ireland: the PRIME Study.

Marques-Vidal P, Arveiler D, Evans A, Amouyel P, Ferrieres J, Ducimetiere P. *Hypertension* 2001; **38**(6): 1361–6.

B a c k g r o u n d . **Alcohol consumption is positively associated with BP. In France, alcohol consumption is regular throughout the week, whereas in Northern Ireland, most of the alcoholic consumption occurs on Fridays and Saturdays, with little consumption during the other days. Furthermore, it has been shown that the effects of an acute intake of alcohol are somewhat different than that of regular intake.**

INTERPRETATION. The binge-drinking pattern observed among Northern Irish drinkers leads to physiologically disadvantageous consequences regarding BP levels, whereas no such fluctuations in BP levels are found for regular consumption.

Summary of results

The PRIME study included 6523 male subjects who drank at least once a week (5156 in France and 1367 in Northern Ireland). In France, alcohol consumption was rather homogeneous throughout the week, with a slight increase during weekends, whereas in Northern Ireland, Fridays and Saturdays accounted for 66% of total alcohol consumption. After adjustment for age, BMI, heart rate, tobacco smoking, educational level, marital status and professional activity, BP levels were higher in Northern Irish drinkers on Monday and decreased until Thursday, whereas BP levels were constant throughout the week for French drinkers (day x country interactions, $P < 0.05$). Conversely, no between-day differences were found regarding teetotalers in both countries. In drinkers, between-day differences and day x country interactions were suppressed after adjustment for the average alcohol consumption of the third day before measurement.

Comment

The association between alcohol and hypertension has been recognized for several years. A large number of cross-sectional and prospective epidemiological studies have repeatedly demonstrated that alcohol consumption is one of the most important modifiable risk factors for hypertension among populations from a variety of geographic regions. The positive association between alcohol intake and BP generally persists after adjustment for important confounders such as age, body mass, smoking, exercise, and sodium and potassium intake.

However, it remains a paradox that if alcohol does cause hypertension there is little convincing evidence that alcohol is related to the CV complications of hypertension such as stroke and heart attack. The relationship between alcohol and strokes also remains inconclusive and there is evidence that moderate alcohol consumption may be protective against heart attack. It is possible, therefore, that alcohol does not so much cause hypertension, but rather a rapidly reversible rise in BP that does not cause CV damage.

When managing hypertensive patients, however, relevant counselling can bring about a useful fall in BP. A number of clinical trials have been conducted to examine the effects of a reduction in alcohol consumption on BP. In general, these studies have had a small sample size and have reported inconsistent findings.

Xin *et al.* report a meta-analysis of randomized controlled trials to assess the effects of alcohol reduction on BP. They included 15 randomized control trials (total of 2234 participants) published before June 1999 in which alcohol reduction was the only intervention difference between active and control treatment groups. Overall, alcohol reduction was associated with a significant reduction in mean SBP

Table 8.3 Randomized, controlled trials of the effect of alcohol reduction on BP

Study, year	n	Age in years (mean ± SD OR range)	Duration (weeks)	Baseline BP (mmHg)	Alcohol intake difference (drinks/day)*	BP difference (mmHg)	P value
Puddey, 1985	46	35 ± 8	6	133/76	3.7	3.8/1.4	<0.001/<0.05
Howes, 1985	10	25–41	0.6	120/66	5.7	8/6	<0.025/<0.001
Puddey, 1987	44	53 ±16	6	142/84	4.0	5/3	<0.001/<0.001
Ueshima, 1987	50	46 ± 7	2	148/93	2.6	5.2/2.2	<0.005/ns
Wallace, 1988	641	42 ± 20	52	136/82	1.0	2.1/?	<0.05/ns
Parker, 1990	59	52 ± 11	4	138/85	3.8	5.4/3.2	<0.01/<0.01
Cox, 1990	72	20–45	4	132/73	3.4	4.1/1.6	<0.05/<0.05
Maheswaran, 1992	41	40s	8	144/90	3.1	Not reported	ns
Puddey, 1992	86	44	18	137/85	3.0	4.8/3.3	<0.01/<0.01
Ueshima, 1993	54	44 ± 8	3	144/96	1.7	3.6/1.9	<0.05/ns
Rakic, 1998							
• Weekend (pattern)	14	41	4	122/72	3.1	1/0	ns/ns†
• Daily	41	48	4	124/77	2.6	2/2	<0.05/<0.01**
Cushman, 1998	641	57 ± 11	104	140/86	1.3	0.9/0.6	0.16/0.10

BP = blood pressure

*A standard drink is defined as 14 g of ethanol and is contained in a 12-oz glass of beer, a 5-oz glass of table wine, or 1.5 oz of distilled spirits.

**Supine office BP; 24-hour ambulatory SBP (but not DBP) was lowered by 3.1 mmHg ($P < 0.001$) and 2.2 mmHg ($P < 0.001$) in weekend and daily drinkers, respectively.

Source: Marques-Vidal et al. (2001).

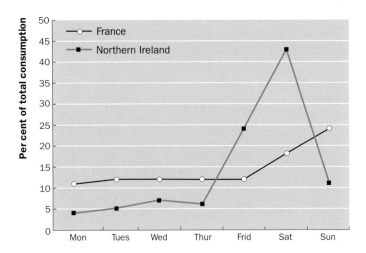

Fig. 8.7 Distribution of alcohol consumption (expressed as percentage of total alcohol consumption) throughout the week in France and Northern Ireland.
Source: Marques-Vidal *et al.* (2001).

and DBP of –3.31 mmHg (95% CI –2.52 to –4.10 mmHg) and –2.04 mmHg (–1.49 to –2.58 mmHg), respectively. A dose-response relationship was observed between mean percentage of alcohol reduction and mean BP reduction. Effects of intervention were enhanced in those with higher baseline BP. This emphasizes that alcohol reduction should be recommended as an important component of lifestyle modification for the prevention and treatment of hypertension among heavy drinkers.

The effects of an acute intake of alcohol are somewhat different than that of regular intake. For instance, consistent regular drinking is a more important determinant of the alcohol/BP relationship than intake in the previous 24 hours; additionally, a single intake of alcohol has a depressor effect on BP that lasts for several hours after drinking, whereas repeated intakes for 7 days have both depressor and pressor effects according to the differences in time intervals after the last drink. The study by Marques-Vidal *et al.* investigates 6523 male subjects who drank at least once a week (5156 in France and 1367 in Northern Ireland). In France, alcohol consumption was rather homogeneous throughout the week, with a slight increase during weekends, whereas in Northern Ireland, Fridays and Saturdays accounted for 66% of total alcohol consumption. After adjustment for age, body mass index, heart rate, tobacco smoking, educational level, marital status, and professional activity, BP levels were higher in Northern Irish drinkers on Monday and decreased until Thursday, whereas BP levels were constant throughout the week for French drinkers (day x country interactions, $P < 0.05$). Thus, the binge-drinking pattern observed among Northern Irish drinkers leads to physiologically disadvantageous consequences regarding BP levels, whereas no such fluctuations in BP levels are found for regular consumption.

Hypertension and sexual dysfunction

Introduction

With more effective pharmacological therapy recently available for the treatment of sexual dysfunction, there has been renewed interest in the effect of hypertension itself, as well as its treatment, on sexual function. Recent survey data suggest that the prevalence of sexual dysfunction among women in the United States is approximately 40%. With almost one half of all treated hypertensives being women, the effect of antihypertensive treatment, as well as the condition of hypertension itself, is of extreme importance to the practitioner. Although considerable research has been done on sexual function in the male hypertensive, there has been a lack of research on sexual function in women with hypertension.

Hypertension *per se*, regardless of drugs, has been suggested to affect sexual function. Several factors may be involved. These may include hormonal and psychogenic influences, and neurovascular disturbance in men, where defective nitric oxide may lead to erectile dysfunction (ED). Such defect may be a manifestation of hypertensive vascular or target organ damage. Indeed, hypertension is a predictor of ED. There is further evidence supporting a link between the pathogenesis of atherosclerotic disease and ED. In the Treatment of Mild Hypertension Study (TOMHS) involving hypertensive patients, the incidence of ED was 14.4%.

Moreover, sexual dysfunction secondary to antihypertensive drugs in particular beta-blockers and diuretics have been well documented. Since sexual function is an important aspect of quality of life for the individual, it is important in treating hypertension to ensure that the drugs used have the lowest possible potential for causing sexual problems. This ensures the best balance between therapeutic efficacy and quality of life, which is essential for compliance.

Does hypertension and its pharmacotherapy affect the quality of sexual function in women?
Duncan LE, Lewis C, Jenkins P, Pearson TA. *Am J Hypertens* 2000; **13**(6 Pt 1): 640–7.

B A C K G R O U N D . Considerable research has been conducted into the effects of antihypertensive drugs on male sexual functioning. This remains underexplored in women, even though almost half of treated hypertensives are women. An ambulatory medical record-based, case-control study was designed to study sexual function in treated and untreated hypertensive women and healthy controls.

INTERPRETATION. The quality of female sexual functioning was quantified in an ambulatory outpatient setting. Hypertensive women, regardless of type of treatment, reported age-adjusted decrease in vaginal lubrication, less frequent orgasm, and more frequent pain when compared to non-hypertensive women. Emotional aspects of sexual functioning in hypertensive women do not appear to be impaired. These areas require further investigation. An incidental finding indicated diminished orgasm reported in current smokers, compared to non-smokers, which was not associated with age or hypertension.

Comment

Although a number of studies have documented a link between hypertension and sexual dysfunction in men, little research has been conducted about this association in women. Hypertensive women appear to suffer from sexual dysfunction caused by high BP, just like hypertensive men.

Duncan *et al.* report a study of 67 hypertensive women who received various types of drug therapy, 37 women with unmedicated hypertension, and 107 normotensive controls, where those women with mildly elevated BP (> 140/90 mmHg and < 160/110 mmHg) reported an age-adjusted decrease in vaginal lubrication and orgasm frequency, and an increase in pain, compared to women with normal BP.

Women who were taking angiotensin-converting enzyme inhibitors, beta-blockers, calcium channel blockers, diuretics, or a combination of drugs against their high BP did not have significantly different sexuality scores from those with unmedicated hypertension. All hypertensives, however, had significantly decreased lubrication and orgasm and increased pain compared to non-hypertensive women.

In these premenopausal women, whose oestrogen status would appear to be ideal, we should ask about vaginal dryness and achievement of orgasm and offer lubricating agents for use prior to intercourse. It appears that it is the hypertensive state itself and not the medications we use that are responsible for these effects. In addition, emotional aspects of sexual functioning do not appear to be impaired. Furthermore, all women who smoke should be counselled about its effect on sexual performance. While we await further research to explain these findings, all hypertensive women should be routinely assessed with a careful sexual history and problems should be managed appropriately.

Sexual dysfunction is common and overlooked in female patients with hypertension.
Burchardt M, Burchardt T, Anastasiadis AG, *et al. J Sex Marital Ther* 2002; **28**(1): 17–26.

BACKGROUND. The objective was to investigate sexual activity, behaviour, dysfunction, and satisfaction in hypertensive women.

INTERPRETATION. The study revealed highly prevalent untreated sexual dysfunction of long duration. It also showed low frequency of sexual activity in spite of the high availability of partners. There was low frequency of initiation of sexual activity. In spite of the high prevalence of sexual dysfunction, more than a third of patients reported sexual activity to be less than desired, and more than half of patients reported sexual activity as important.

Comment

This survey has again highlighted the high prevalence of sexual dysfunction among the hypertensive female. The study included 67 patients with a mean age of 60.4 years and completed a detailed questionnaire. Of these women, 81.3% had a sex partner; 42.6% had untreated sexual dysfunction, with a duration of more than 5 years in 70.9% and a duration of more than 10 years in 41.7%; 5.3% initiated sexual activity; 36.6% reported less sexual activity than desired; and 54.8% reported sexual activity as important.

Use of Angiotensin II blockers in hypertensives may improve sexual function

Sexual activity in hypertensive men treated with valsartan or carvedilol: a crossover study.
Fogari R, Zoppi A, Poletti L, *et al. Am J Hypertens* 2001; **14**(1): 27–31.

BACKGROUND. The aim of this study was to compare the effect of antihypertensive treatment with valsartan or cavedilol on sexual activity in hypertensive men who were never treated for hypertension.

INTERPRETATION. The findings suggest that carvedilol induces a chronic worsening of sexual activity, whereas valsartan not only does not significantly worsen sexual activity but may even improve it.

Comment

Fogari *et al.* report that the angiotensin blocker valsartan was associated with an increase in sexual intercourse rate whereas patients on the alpha/beta blocker carvedilol showed a dramatic decline in intercourse rate. There is a myth that impotence is caused by hypertension drugs, although certain drugs such as beta-blockers and diuretics can aggravate it. In contrast, it is possible that sexual dysfunction is part of the hypertension disease process. Angiotensin blockers may improve sexual function in two ways: by acting on blood vessels in the penis that have been damaged by high BP, and by acting in the brain to improve well-being.

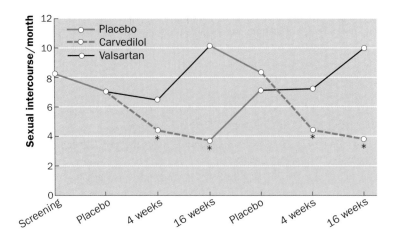

Fig. 8.8 Mean number of sexual intercourse episodes per month during treatment with valsartan and carvedilol (*P < 0.01 *versus* screening). Source: Fogari *et al.* (2001).

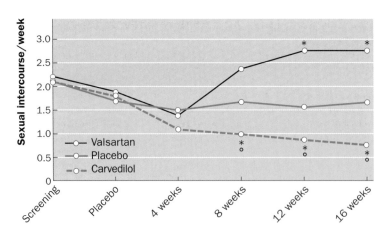

Fig. 8.9 Mean number of sexual intercourse episodes per week in the two treatment groups and in the placebo group (*P < 0.05 *versus* placebo, °P < 0.01 *versus* valsartan). Source: Fogari *et al.* (2001).

Erectile dysfunction is a marker for cardiovascular complications and psychological functioning in men with hypertension.

Burchardt M, Burchardt T, Anastasiadis AG, *et al. Int J Impot Res* 2001; **13**(5): 276–81.

BACKGROUND. The aim of this study was to investigate the incidence of CV complications in hypertensive patients with erectile dysfunction.

INTERPRETATION. Erectile dysfunction in hypertensive patients can be considered as a marker for CV complications in this patient group.

Comment

From the mailed anonymous questionnaires completed by 104 hypertensive male patients, Burchardt *et al.* reported the following findings: 70.6% of the patients who responded suffered from erectile dysfunction. The hypertensive patients with erectile dysfunction had significantly higher prevalence of CV complications ($P < 0.05$). The correlation between depression and low quality of life as well as between erectile dysfunction and low sexual satisfaction was also statistically significant ($P = 0.05$). Such observations are interesting but the response rate from the mailed anonymous questionnaires was only 22%, and thus the data analysed may not be from a representative population.

Sexual dysfunction in hypertensive patients treated with losartan.

Llisterri JL, Lozano Vidal JV, Aznar Vicente J. *Am J Med Sci* 2001; **321**(5): 336–41.

BACKGROUND. Impaired erectile function in men is a component of the dysmetabolic syndrome of high BP as well as a sequela of antihypertensive therapy. This prospective interventional study in men with uncontrolled hypertension (BP $\geq$ 140/90 mmHg) used a survey instrument to assay sexual dysfunction before and after therapy with losartan.

INTERPRETATION. The data suggest that losartan improved erectile function and both satisfaction and frequency of sexual activity. Because side effects are one of the most influential factors in the management of hypertension, an added benefit of losartan therapy may be its positive impact on quality of life.

Comment

This case controlled study evaluated the influence of a 12-week therapy with losartan (50–100 mg/day) in 164 hypertensive subjects (aged 30 to 65 years) with

(n = 82) and without (n = 82) a diagnosis of erectile dysfunction using a self-administered questionnaire validated in another 60 subjects with hypertension. The results demonstrated that losartan treatment improved sexual satisfaction from an initial 7.3 to 58.5% (χ^2; P = 0.001). Subjects reporting a high frequency of sexual activity also improved from 40.5% initially to 62.3% after drug treatment, whereas the number of patients with low or very low frequency of sexual activity decreased significantly (χ^2; P = 0.001). At the completion of the 12-week losartan regimen, only 11.8% of the treated subjects reported an improvement in sexual function. However, improvement on quality of life was demonstrated in 73.7% of subjects medicated with losartan, 25.5% reported no change, and only 0.8% felt worse. In the group without sexual dysfunction, losartan had a non-significant effect on sexual function.

Part IV

Current practical issues

9

Clinical features

'White-coat' hypertensives are not 'normal'

Introduction

White-coat hypertension, or more appropriately termed as isolated office hypertension (IOH), is somewhat generic to the medical professions. The exact underlying mechanism is not known though it has been traditionally attributed to a 'pressor effect' induced by attending the 'doctor's office'. Its detection is most reliably assessed by ambulatory blood pressure (BP) monitoring (ABPM) as indicated in consensus documents. Depending on the definitions (of normal daytime ambulatory BP levels) used and on patient selection, the prevalence of this condition may be as high as 10–20%.

The clinical significance of white-coat hypertension continues to be debated, with cross-sectional studies providing conflicting results. However, it seems that more evidence is suggesting that it is not an innocent entity. Careful follow-up of these patients has shown development into sustained hypertension at an equal rate to an age-matched group. However, cross-sectional studies examining the effect of white-coat hypertension on hypertensive organ damage show conflicting results. The reasons for this are likely to be due to the fact that various definitions are used and different patient populations have been studied. Various cut-off values are used to define the upper normal limits of both ambulatory and clinic/office BPs. One possible classification is as follows:

- White-Coat Hypertension (WCH): daytime average systolic BP (SBP) of < 140 mmHg by ABPM, no antihypertensive drugs, and an abnormal office SBP of > 150 mmHg
- White-Coat Syndrome Normotensive (WCSN): daytime average SBP of < 140 mmHg by ABPM, taking antihypertensive drugs; and an abnormal office SBP of > 150 mmHg
- White-Coat Syndrome Hypertensive (WCSH): daytime average SBP of > 140 mmHg by ABPM with or without antihypertensive drugs, and an office SBP of > 150 mmHg and > 15 mmHg higher than the average daytime SBP

Whether white-coat hypertension simply represents a physical manifestation of mental anxiety, or actual pathology has not been firmly established. On current weight of evidence, white-coat hypertension probably carries an overall cardiovascular (CV) risk that is intermediate between that of sustained hypertension and normotension. Thus, those with white-coat hypertension, detected by ABPM, should have other CV risk factors assessed and treated since transition to the persistent-hypertensive state may be overlooked.

White-coat hypertension as a cause of cardiovascular dysfunction.

Glen SK, Elliott HL, Curzio JL, Lees KR, Reid JL. *Lancet* 1996; **348** (9028): 65–7.

BACKGROUND. The increasing use of 24-h ambulatory BP monitoring has allowed diagnosis of white-coat hypertension, in which BPs are higher on clinic measurements than on ambulatory monitoring. Treatment is not generally thought to be necessary for this disorder. However, there is evidence that patients with white-coat hypertension develop renal impairment and left ventricular(LV) hypertrophy (LVH). We undertook this study to assess whether white-coat hypertension, in the absence of CV structural abnormalities, is associated with CV functional abnormalities.

INTERPRETATION. Functional CV abnormalities were identified in white-coat hypertensive patients who had no identifiable structural abnormalities. Such functional abnormalities can be reversed by antihypertensive treatment. We propose that patients with white-coat hypertension might benefit from antihypertensive treatment as well as those with persistent hypertension. This hypothesis should be addressed in prospective clinical trials.

Comment

In this study, the indices of cardiac structure and function and carotid arterial compliance were compared among groups of normotensive, white-coat hypertensive, and persistent-hypertensive (on the basis of ABPM) patients of similar age, weight and sex distribution. Both white-coat and persistent-hypertensive groups showed similar reduction of mean indices for arterial elasticity, compliance and stiffness. These two groups also had similar reductions in E:A ratios on echocardiogram, indicative of diastolic dysfunction. However, only the persistent-hypertensive group showed an increase in left ventricular mass (LVM). Thus it seems that white-coat hypertension may represent an early stage in the evolution of structural CV abnormalities.

Left ventricular changes in isolated office hypertension: a blood pressure-matched comparison with normotension and sustained hypertension.

Grandi AM, Broggi R, Colombo S, *et al. Arch Intern Med* 2001; **161**(22): 267–81.

BACKGROUND. Isolated office (IO) hypertension is a benign condition according to some researchers, whereas others believe it is associated with CV abnormalities and

increased CV risk. The aim of this study is to compare morphofunctional characteristics of the LV in IO hypertensive subjects, normotensive subjects, and never-treated sustained hypertensives.

INTERPRETATION. Comparing matched BP groups, IO hypertensives have LV morphofunctional characteristics considerably different from normotensives and qualitatively similar to sustained hypertensives. Therefore, IOH should not be considered as simply a benign condition.

Comment

Elevations of casual BPs seem to correlate with changes in vascular resistance and the presence of LV diastolic dysfunction, and frequently have been associated with obesity and insulin resistance syndrome. However, opinion is still sharply divided on whether to initiate therapy to these patients based primarily on office BP readings. In this study LV morphologic features and function were assessed using digitized M-mode echocardiography in 42 IO hypertensives (clinic BP > 140 and/or 90 mmHg and daytime BP 130/80 mmHg), 42 sustained hypertensives (clinic BP > 140 and/or 90 mmHg and daytime BP 140 and/or 90 mmHg) and 42 normotensives (clinic BP < 135 and/or 85 mmHg and daytime BP 130/80 mmHg). Not surprisingly, sustained hypertensives had the highest LV walls and mass, but similar prevalence of LVH and pre-clinical diastolic dysfunction to IO hypertensives. Conversely, normotensives had the lowest of these parameters. This study by Grandi *et al.* does not settle the argument but such observations, plus long-term epidemiologic data and prospective treatment data, support the concept that white-coat hypertensives should be treated. We await a long-term, carefully conducted prospective trial to obtain a definitive answer.

Alterations of cardiac structure in patients with isolated office, ambulatory, or home hypertension: data from the general population (Pressione Arteriose Monitorate E Loro Associazioni [PAMELA] Study).
Sega R, Trocino G, Lanzarotti A, *et al. Circulation.* 2001; **104**: 1385–92.

BACKGROUND. The prevalence and clinical significance of isolated office (or white coat) hypertension is controversial, and population data are limited.

INTERPRETATION. Isolated office hypertension (IOH) has a noticeable prevalence in the population and is accompanied by structural cardiac alterations, suggesting that it is not an entirely harmless phenomenon. This is the case also for the opposite condition, that is, normal office but elevated home or ambulatory BP, which implies that limiting BP measurements to office values may not suffice in identification of subjects at risk.

Comment

The study population in PAMELA consisted of a large, 3200 randomized subjects (25–74 years of age) with the aim to determine the normality values of ambulatory and home BP in the Milan population. IOH was defined as systolic or diastolic values 140 mmHg or 90 mmHg, respectively. Home and ambulatory normotension were defined according to the PAMELA criteria: < 132/83 mmHg (systolic/diastolic) for home and 125/79 mmHg for 24-hour average BP. The prevalence of IOH ranged from 9–12%. In these subjects, LV mass index (LVMI) and LVH was greater than in subjects with normotension both in and outside the office, independent of age and sex. Unlike other studies, two interesting features noteworthy in the resent study: 1) treated hypertensive subjects were excluded from analysis, thus eliminating possible drugs effects on the ventricles; 2) LVMI and LVH were similarly greater in subjects found to have normal office but elevated home or ambulatory BP (10% of the population, only discovered by home and ambulatory BP measurements). However, it is unclear whether the increased LV mass is prognostically significant and if so, should early treatment be effective. Furthermore, the dissociation between ambulatory and home BP measurements may be clinically important, and its effect on structural LV changes needs further investigation.

White-coat hypertensive patients do not exhibit the same target organ damage over time as those whose hypertension is more sustained, but still show metabolic derangement, including insulin resistance, a known risk factor for CV disease (CVD). These patients, whose BP only appears elevated when they present to the doctor's office, should still be actively assessed for other markers of CV risk.

 ## Is 'isolated home' hypertension as opposed to 'isolated office' hypertension a sign of greater cardiovascular risk?
Bobrie G, Genès N, Vaur L, *et al. Arch Intern Med.* 2001; **161**: 2205–211.

BACKGROUND. Controversy remains on whether isolated office hypertension is a benign clinical condition or is linked with an increased risk of target organ damage and a worse prognosis. Few data are available on the converse phenomenon 'reverse white coat effect' or 'white coat normotension', they support the hypothesis that subjects with these conditions may represent a high-risk group.

INTERPRETATION. This retrospective analysis suggests that patients with 'isolated home' hypertension (IHH) belong to a high-risk subgroup. The 3-year follow-up of these patients will provide prospective data about the CV prognosis of these subgroups.

Comment

The SHEAF (Self-Measurement of Blood Pressure at Home in the Elderly: Assessment and Follow-up) study is a prospective observational study (from February

1998 to early 2002) designed to determine whether home BP measurement (by semiautomatic digitalized device) has a greater CV prognostic value than office BP measurement among 5211 elderly (60 years) French patients with hypertension. The objective of this present work is to describe the baseline characteristics of the treated patients in the SHEAF study from February 1998 to March 1999, placing special emphasis on IOH and IHH. A 140/90 mmHg threshold was chosen to define IOH, and a 135/85 mmHg threshold to define HIGH. Recognising the importance or the impact of BP thresholds on their data, the authors have carefully described two different approaches (clinical and statistical) to evaluate the differences in BP measurements. The results showed that patients with IOH represented 12.5% of this population, while patients with IHH represented 10.8%. The important finding was that the rates of CV risk factors and history of CVD in patients with IHH are similar to those in patients with uncontrolled hypertension. We eagerly await the 3-year follow-up outcome data between the two groups.

Pulse pressure and prognosis in cardiovascular disease

Introduction

There has been an obvious growing interest in 'pulse pressure' (PP) in the year 2001. Clearly, the trend is expanding into the year 2002. While more is being discovered, we shall look back at what actually sparked our interest for PP. Hence, what can the 'gap' between the systolic blood pressure (SBP) and diastolic blood pressure (DBP) tell us? What does the 'gap' mean? Can we narrow the 'gap'? and so on.

Traditionally, we have based our antihypertensive treatment on DBP as previous epidemiological studies had used DBP as a measure of CV risk. This was reinforced by a number of therapeutic trials, showing the benefits of treating hypertension defined on the basis of elevated DBP. At the same time, SBP was considered to be a natural and innocuous effect of increased stiffness of the aorta caused by aging. However, more evidence is now emerging showing that DBP has the least predictive value, and only recently, we turn our emphasis back on SBP, and lately PP is becoming fashionable. This is in part due to a reappraisal of the early studies and the emergence of new insights into the pathophysiological significance of increased arterial stiffness and its influence on BP components, particularly SBP and PP.

Simply, PP is the difference between the SBP and DBP, hence the 'gap'. Numerically, the 'gap' increases when SBP increases and/or DBP decreases. Mechanistically, PP arises from the interaction of cardiac ejection (stroke volume) and the properties of the arterial circulation. Reduction of the compliance (or increased stiffness in qualitative terms) of the great vessels leads to an increase in SBP and a decrease in DBP, hence an increased PP. A number of factors are known to influence arterial wall behaviour and, therefore, PP.

Progressive stiffening of central elastic arteries is a reflection of biological aging of the arterial system. SBP rises continuously throughout life, while DBP levels off or even declines after about the age of 50. Thus, arterial stiffness could be indicative of increased PP and this explained the increased risk and prevalence of isolated systolic hypertension (ISH) in older subjects. This may be due to an accumulative insult to the vascular tree with age, but increased arterial stiffness could also be indicative of on-going vascular disease beside the age-effects. Indeed, the evidence of PP as an independent predictor of CV risk has grown stronger in the past year. In hypertensive patients, higher PP is associated with hypertension-induced target organ damage including LVH, microalbuminuria and arterial remodelling. Data from the articles below are clear and self-explanatory. Thus, the bigger the 'gap', the higher the CV risks. As a readily available index, the predictive value of PP seems to be the strongest, particularly in older populations, follow by systolic, mean arterial BP and DBP. However, the underlying mechanisms that govern its risk are not well understood. Elevated PP, which is often a manifestation of increased arterial stiffness, can lead to adverse CV effects such as increased myocardial work, impaired ventricular relaxation, and ischaemia. There may be two different independent mechanisms involved; increase SBP, increase cardiac afterload and pressure load/burden in the vascular tree; increased DBP may enhance the pressure load of SBP while a decrease of DBP may cause decreased coronary or cerebral blood flow, thus lower myocardial or cerebral perfusion, respectively.

Treatment trials in older patients with essential hypertension have suggested that PP change during antihypertensive treatment may influence prognosis. However, a variety of issues still remain about the use of PP as a target in the clinic. Currently, there are little data on how the clinician might use PP measurements to select candidates for treatment, or how exactly the antihypertensive drugs available compare in reducing PP and arterial stiffness. Preliminary data suggest, for example, that angiotensin-converting enzyme inhibitors (ACEIs) and calcium channel blockers improve arterial stiffness, but diuretics may lead to greater reductions in PP. In addition, a wide PP has also been shown to be closely associated with carotid intima-media (IM) thickness, carotid atherosclerosis, and LVM. Accordingly, direct measurements of the structure and function of key arteries could be an attractive way of evaluating the relationship of arterial compliance with PP and CVD. The age-induced increase in arterial stiffness is classically measured by pulse wave velocity (PWV). In adults aged more than 50 years the increase in PP has been attributed to early wave reflection. However, the concept of using arterial compliance as a marker for CV changes is still evolving; we will see different methods being tested in various settings over the next few years. In the meantime, the articles below will give us some insight for the future.

Pulse pressure – a review of mechanisms and clinical relevance.

Dart AM, Kingwell BA. *J Am Coll Cardiol* 2001; **37**(4): 975–84.

BACKGROUND. **The goal of this study was to review the origin, clinical relevance and treatment of PP. Elevated PP is increasingly being recognized as a risk factor for CV, particularly coronary, disease. Pulse pressure is discussed in terms of both Windkessel and distributive models of the arterial circulation.**

INTERPRETATION. Pulse pressure arises from the interaction of cardiac ejection (stroke volume) and the properties of the arterial circulation. An increased stiffness of the aorta and large arteries leads to an increase in PP through a reduction in arterial compliance and effects on wave reflection. A number of factors are known to influence arterial wall behaviour and, therefore, PP. In addition to the effects of aging and blood pressure on arterial wall elasticity, there is some evidence that atherosclerosis, *per se*, amplifies these effects. Thus, the relationship between PP and coronary disease may be bidirectional. A number of dietary and lifestyle interventions have been shown to modify large artery behaviour. These include aerobic exercise training and consumption of n-3 fatty acids. Conversely, strength training is associated with an increase in arterial

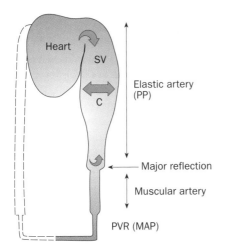

Fig. 9.1 PP arises from the interaction between stroke volume (SV) and the characteristics of the arterial circulation that determine compliance (C) and wave reflection. As discussed in the text, wave reflection occurs at multiple sites but is shown in the diagram as a single site for the sake of simplicity. Cardiac output and peripheral vascular resistance (PVR) determine mean arterial pressure (MAP). Source: Dart *et al.* (2001).

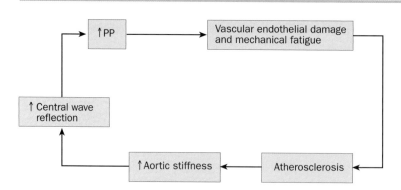

Fig. 9.2 Schematic diagram illustrating the concept of bidirectionality in the relationship between PP and atherosclerosis. Elevated PP promotes vascular damage, an antecedent to atherosclerosis, which results in large-vessel stiffening and increased wave reflection, thus, further amplifying PP. While it is not clear which is the incipient event in this cycle, it is clear that, once initiated, a vicious cycle promoting disease progression ensues. Source: Dart *et al.* (2001).

stiffness and a higher PP. The effects of antihypertensive medication have been extensively studied, but many studies are difficult to interpret because of concomitant change in BP, and to a lesser degree, heart rate. However a number of studies do suggest direct arterial wall effects, particularly for ACEIs. A distributed compliance model of the arterial circulation provides a framework for understanding the causes, effects and potential treatment of elevations in PP.

Comment

This paper provides an excellent review on pulse pressure; its complexity and implications are certainly much bigger than just the 'gap' difference between the SBP and DBP!

Cardiovascular risk assessment using pulse pressure in the First National Health and Nutrition Examination Survey (NHANES I).

Domanski M, Norman J, Wolz M, Mitchell G, Pfeffer M. *Hypertension* 2001; **38**: 793–7.

BACKGROUND. Increased stiffness of the conduit arteries has been associated with increased risk of death and CV death in a number of populations. None of these populations, however, are fully representative of the US population.

INTERPRETATION. In a cohort designed to be representative of the US population, elevated PP has been shown to provide independent prognostic information. This variable may be a marker for the extent of vascular disease and may contribute to the occurrence of clinical events.

Comment

A cohort of 5771 subjects from the First National Health and Nutrition Examination Survey (NHANES I) that was free of overt CVD was used to determine the value of adding PP to standard CVD risk factors for assessment of the risk of death during a mean follow-up period of 16.5 years. Pulse pressure was found to be increased with increasing age, body mass index (BMI), cholesterol level and MAP. Despite these associations with known risk factors, PP was independently predictive of an increased risk of death from CVD, coronary heart disease (CHD), and all-cause mortality. It provides independent prognostic information beyond that provided by known risk factors that were evaluated in this study, including the Sixth Joint National Committee on Prevention, Detection, Evaluation and Treatment of High Blood Pressure (JNC VI) hypertension classification. A 10 mmHg increase in PP in persons 25–45 of age was associated with a 26% increase in risk of CV death and with a 10% increase in persons 46–77 years of age. However, whether this implies a causal or reversible relationship, needs to be evaluated in prospective, randomized clinical trials.

Pulse pressure and risk of cardiovascular events in the systolic hypertension in the elderly program (SHEP).
Vaccarino V, Berger AK, Abramson J, *et al. Am J Cardiol* 2001; **88**(9): 980–6.

BACKGROUND. Pulse pressure has been related to higher risk of CV events in older persons. Isolated systolic hypertension is common among the elderly and is accompanied by elevated PP. Treatment of ISH may further increase PP if DBP is lowered to a greater extent than SBP. Little is known regarding PP as a predictor of CV outcomes in elderly persons with ISH, and the influence of treatment on the PP effect.

INTERPRETATION. These results suggest that PP is a useful marker of risk for heart failure (HF) and stroke among older adults being treated for ISH.

Comment

The present study is unique in the sense that it examined the changing values of PP over time, as well as the baseline values, in the treatment and placebo groups separately. Previous published reports on the relationship of PP with CV events examined the placebo and treatment groups combined, which might not be entirely justified in the SHEP trial given the remarkable differences in outcome in these two groups.

The results showed that in the treatment arm but not in the placebo arm, a higher PP was an independent predictor (after accounted for SBP and DBP) of HF and stroke, and was actually more strongly related to CV outcomes than SBP and DBP. However, the association between PP and CHD risk was not significant in both groups. Although the results may not be generalizable to other population, these results do suggest that PP could provide useful prognostic information among older adults during treatment for ISH and may help optimise treatment regimes. Decreasing PP in addition to SBP may offer additional benefits to these patients.

Association of increased pulse pressure with the development of heart failure in SHEP: Systolic Hypertension in the Elderly (SHEP) Cooperative Research Group.

Kostis JB, Lawrence-Nelson J, Ranjan R, Wilson AC, Kostis WJ, Lacy CR.
Am J Hyperten 2001; **14**(8 Pt 1): 798–803.

BACKGROUND. Patients with isolated systolic hypertension have increased PP and greater risk for CV events including stroke, myocardial infarction (MI), and HF. Although the decreased DBP linked to high PP may trigger thrombotic events such as stroke and MI, it cannot fully explain the relationship between PP and HF without an intervening MI.

INTERPRETATION. In older persons with ISH, high PP is associated with increased risk of heart failure independently of MAP and of the occurrence of acute MI during follow-up.

Comment

This report presents observations on the relationship of PP to the development of HF among 4736 men and women aged $\geq$ 60 years with ISH (mean BP [MBP] 170/77 mmHg and mean PP 93 mmHg) who participated in the SHEP. The main outcome measures were fatal and non-fatal HF. During 4.5 years average follow-up, fatal or non-fatal HF occurred in 160 of 4736 patients. The SBP, PP and MAP were strong predictors of the development of HF. HF was found to be inversely related to DBP but was directly related to PP. Results remained unchanged even when patients who developed MI during follow-up were excluded. The mechanism underlying the increased risk of HF in patients with high PP remains unclear. It may be explained by the association of decreased arterial compliance with both PP and increased afterload. High PP has also been associated with LVH and impaired diastolic LV relaxation, especially in the elderly patients. Furthermore, whether different classes of pharmacotherapy will have different effects on event reduction according to different effect on lowering PP remains speculative. A causal or reversible relationship also remains to be established.

Pulse pressure in normotensives: a marker of cardiovascular disease.
Zakopoulos NA, Lekakis JP, Papamichael CM, *et al. Am J Hypertens* 2001; **14**(3): 195–9.

BACKGROUND. **Pulse pressure is an important predictor of cardiovascular events, including total CVD, CHD, HF and stroke. However, the relation of the systemic arterial PP and other parameters derived from the 24-h arterial BP monitoring to the severity of coronary artery disease (CAD), carotid lesions, and LVMI in patients without arterial hypertension is less well described.**

INTERPRETATION. Systemic arterial PP derived from 24-h arterial BP monitoring is related to CAD, carotid intima-media thickness (IMT) and LVMI independently of age or any other derivative of 24-h arterial BP monitoring, indicating that this parameter could be a marker of global CV risk.

Comment

This study was intended to evaluate PP in normotensive individuals and thus the effect of hypertension, as a known risk factor, is excluded. The data of the present study clearly indicate that in normotensive patients with CAD, PP is more strongly related to severity of CAD, carotid IMT and LV mass than any other derivative of 24-h ABPM. The results also show that the relationship of PP to Gensini score (an index of severity of the CAD), carotid IMT and LVMI is independent of age, BP level (mean BP, BP load) or BP variability. The significant relation between PP and outcome measures without a significant relation between diastolic BP and outcome measures points to the importance of PP in itself and not of diastolic BP. Therefore, PP derived from the 24-h ABPM could be considered as a non-invasive marker of the global CV risk.

Correlates of pulse pressure reduction during antihypertensive treatment (losartan or atenolol) in hypertensive patients with electrocardiographic left ventricular hypertrophy (the LIFE study).
Gerdts E, Papademetriou V, Palmieri V, *et al. Am J Cardiol* 2002; **89**(4): 399–402.

BACKGROUND. **In hypertensive patients, PP has been related to hypertension-induced target organ damage and risk of CV events. However, correlates of PP reduction during antihypertensive treatment have been less extensively investigated.**

INTERPRETATION. In hypertensive patients with electrocardiographic (ECG) LVH, older age, less reduction in MBP, concomitant diabetes mellitus (DM), and shorter stature are associated with attenuated PP reduction during antihypertensive treatment.

Comment

The reduction in PP during antihypertensive treatment does not necessarily parallel that of SBP and DBP. The present study was undertaken to further describe factors (both clinic and echocardiographic variables) associated with PP reduction over two years of antihypertensive treatment in hypertensive patients.

The study identified four clinical variables, besides initial PP, as independent correlates of an attenuated PP reduction in a large series of middle-aged and older hypertensive patients with electrocardiographic LVH: older age, shorter stature, concomitant DM, and less reduction in MBP. This study also demonstrated several ways that PP in hypertensive patients is closely associated with target organ involvement and identified patients at especially high risk for CV events: first, by the relationship between higher PP and older age, concomitant DM, and LVH at baseline – all factors known to influence CV risk adversely in hypertensive patients; secondly, by the relationship between PP and microalbuminuria, another known predictor of renal dysfunction and CV complications in essential hypertension.

Similarly, the negative relation between age and PP reduction in this study is not unexpected given the fact that aging is associated with structural and geometric changes of the aorta, resulting in increased arterial stiffness, earlier wave reflections leading to progressive widening of PP and increased prevalences of isolated or disproportionate systolic hypertension. It should be noted, however, that this study included a highly selected group of patients with ECG LVH, hence higher baseline CV risk.

Reference values for clinic pulse pressure in a non-selected population.

Asmar R, Vol S, Brisac AM, Tichet J, Topouchian J. *Am J Hypertens* 2001; **14**(5 Pt 1): 415–8.

BACKGROUND. A wide PP may constitute an independent predictor of CV morbidity and mortality. To date, normal reference values of PP have not been determined. Therefore, the goal of the present large-scale study was to assess reference values of brachial clinic PP in a general population, according to gender and age.

INTERPRETATION. According to mean values, 50 mmHg is the likely reference value for clinic PP in both men and women. Diagnostic thresholds for clinic PP ($\geq$ 65 mmHg), determined either by adding 2 SD to the means or from the 95th percentiles, are in close agreement with clinic PP values previously reported to be associated with increased CV morbidity and mortality.

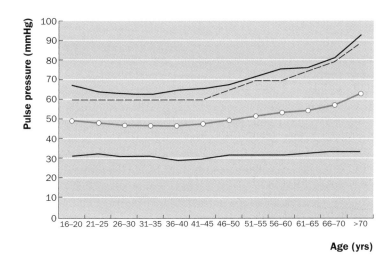

Fig. 9.3 Means, means ± 2 SD limits, and 95th percentiles (dotted line) of the clinic PP in women. Source: Asmar *et al.* (2001).

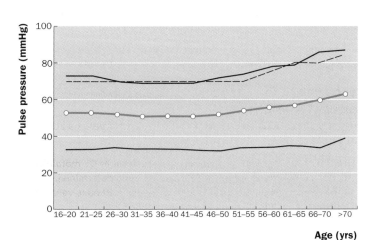

Fig. 9.4 Means, means ± 2 SD limits, and 95th percentiles (dotted line) of the clinic PP in men. Source: Asmar *et al.* (2001).

Comment

This study assessed the reference values of brachial clinic PP, according to age and gender in a non-selected population (61 724 subjects, 51% men, age 16–90) who were undergoing a routine systematic health examination. PP was calculated for each subject as the arithmetic difference between SBP and DBP. The results of this epidemiologic study showed that clinic PP in a non-selected population averaged 49 and 52 mmHg, in women and men, respectively. Because the difference between men and women are within ± 3 mmHg, these data suggest that 50 mmHg may be considered as the normal value of clinic PP. It should be noted that these values are applicable only to brachial clinic BP measurements. Ambulatory PP values would probably be lower than clinic PP. The white coat effect may play an important role. Furthermore, in this study BP measurements were recorded on one visit only. Until all the prospective evidence becomes available, these preliminary results suggest that 50 mmHg could be considered as the normal value of clinic PP in both men and women.

Association between pulse pressure and C-reactive protein among apparently healthy US adults.

Abramson JL, Weintraub WS, Vaccarino V. *Hypertension* 2002; **39**(2): 197–202.

BACKGROUND. Elevated PP has been associated with an increased risk of CVD, which is increasingly being seen as an inflammatory disease. Thus, the mechanism underlying the link between elevated PP and CVD risk may be inflammation. However, investigators have not examined the relationship between PP and C-reactive protein (CRP), an inflammation marker that has been closely linked to CV risk.

INTERPRETATION. The study suggests that increases in PP are associated with elevated CRP levels among apparently healthy US adults, independent of SBP and DBP.

Comment

This study examined the cross-sectional relationship between PP and CRP among 9867 healthy persons 17 years of age or older who participated in the Third National Health and Nutrition Examination Survey (NHANES III). The hypothesis that PP may be related to inflammation, hence elevated CRP, is an interesting one. It has been shown previously that higher levels of PP are associated with greater flow reversals during diastole, and flow reversals can increase the expression of adhesion molecules, which would tend to promote the inflammatory process involved in atherosclerosis.

The primary finding of this study was that an increasing PP was associated with increased odds of having an elevated CRP level (0.66 mg/dl) among apparently healthy adults who were representative of the general US population. Importantly, this association was independent of SBP, DBP, and a number of other factors including demographic factors, cholesterol levels, obesity, smoking status, alcohol consumption and physical activity. The result persisted even when an alternative definition of 'elevated' CRP (0.22 mg/dl) was employed. Of note is that SBP and DBP did not show significant associations with CRP once PP was taken into account.

However, it is also important to be aware that the present study was based on cross-sectional observational data, thus making it impossible to determine the temporal ordering of the association between PP and CRP. The possibility that increases in inflammation lead to higher PP levels cannot be ruled out. Thus, the results should not be taken as evidence of a causal relationship leading from PP to CRP and should therefore be interpreted with caution.

Effect of aging on the prognostic significance of ambulatory systolic, diastolic, and pulse pressure in essential hypertension.

Khattar RS, Swales JD, Dore C, Senior R, Lahiri A. *Circulation* 2001; **104**: 783–9.

BACKGROUND. This study compared the relative prognostic significance of 24-hour intra-arterial ambulatory SBP, DBP, MAP and PP parameters in middle-aged *versus* elderly hypertensives.

INTERPRETATION. The relative prognostic significance of ambulatory BP components depends on age; DBP parameters provided the best prognostic value in middle-aged individuals, whereas PP parameters were the most predictive in the elderly. This may reflect differing underlying haemodynamic mechanisms of hypertension in these age groups.

Comment

There is a growing awareness of the importance of PP, and some of the evidence and potential pathological mechanisms that may underlie this. The present study included 546 middle-aged (< 60 years) and 142 subjects (elderly ≥ 60 years) who had undergone baseline pre-treatment 24-hour intra-arterial ambulatory BP monitoring and were followed for 9.2 ± 4.1 years.

Using multivariate analysis, the predictive values of several AMBP parameters for the occurrence of either death or CV events were identified for the two groups. In the middle-aged subjects, 24-hour, daytime, and night-time DBP, MAP, and SBP, when considered individually, were positively related to morbid events; DBP parameters provided the best predictive values. In the elderly group, 24-hour, day-time, and night-time PP and SBP were the most predictive parameters, whereas ambulatory DBP and MAP measurements failed to provide any prognostic value. When 24-hour values of SBP and DBP were jointly included in the baseline model, DBP but not SBP was related to outcome in younger subjects, whereas in the elderly group, SBP was positively and DBP was negatively related to outcome. Importantly, clinic BP measurements failed to provide any independent prognostic value in either age group.

From a clinical standpoint, Khattar *et al.* pointed out a variety of issues that still remain about the use of PP as a target in the clinic. Even though new guidelines stress the importance of controlling SBP, it is often not as well controlled as DBP,

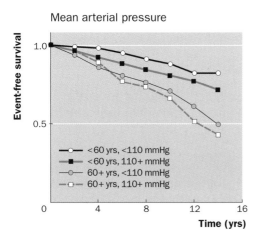

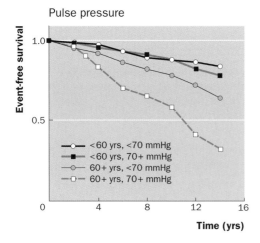

Fig. 9.5 Kaplan–Meier survival curves for each of 4 groups of patients using an age threshold of 60 years and 24-hour MAP and PP cut-off points of 110 mmHg and 70 mmHg, respectively. Source: Khattar *et al.* (2001).

which could actually result in wider PP. It seems likely that lower diastolic pressures may still lull clinicians into a false sense of security when dealing with the elderly patient, whereas in fact CV risk may be increased in this situation.

Currently, there is little data on how the clinician might use PP measures to select candidates for treatment, or how exactly the antihypertensive drugs available compare in reducing PP and arterial stiffness. Preliminary data suggest, for example, that angiotensin converting enzyme inhibitors and calcium channel blockers improve arterial stiffness, but diuretics may lead to greater reductions in PP. Nevertheless, despite caveats in current knowledge, the overwhelming message from the accumulating data is the need for greater attention to SBP and PP control, particularly in the elderly.

Antihypertensive drug therapy in older patients.
Wang JG, Staessen JA. *Curr Opin Nephrol Hypertens* 2001; **10**(2): 263–9.

BACKGROUND. Elevated PP is an important CV risk factor in the elderly, and it remains to be determined whether this can be reversed.

INTERPRETATION. Absolute treatment benefit is greater in men, in patients aged 70 years or more, and in those with previous CV complications or greater PP.

Comment

In the recently published comparative trials, BP gradients largely accounted for most, if not all, of the differences in outcome. In hypertensive patients, calcium-channel blockers (CCB) may offer greater protection against stroke than against MI, resulting in an overall CV benefit similar to that provided by older drug classes. The hypothesis that ACEIs or alpha blockers might influence outcome over and beyond that expected on the basis of their BP lowering effects still remains to be proven.

Elevated pulse pressure is an important cardiovascular risk factor in the elderly, and it remains to be determined whether this can be reversed. Drug treatment is justified in older patients with isolated systolic hypertension whose systolic blood pressure is 160 mmHg or higher on repeated measurement. Absolute benefit is greater in men, in patients aged 70 years or more, and in those with previous cardiovascular complications or greater pulse pressure. In the recently published comparative trials blood pressure gradients largely accounted for most, if not all, of the differences in outcome. In hypertensive patients, calcium-channel blockers may offer greater protection against stroke than against myocardial infarction, resulting in an overall cardiovascular benefit similar to that provided by older drug classes. The hypothesis that angiotensin-converting enzyme inhibitors or alpha-blockers might influence outcome over and beyond that expected on the basis of their blood pressure lowering effects still remains to be proved.

Pulse pressure and human longevity.

Aviv A. *Hypertension.* 2001; **37**: 1060–6.

BACKGROUND. PP is largely determined by progressive stiffening of central elastic arteries, a reflection of biologic aging of the arterial system. Although the age-dependent rise in PP may be the 'price of human longevity', in certain segments of the population, the biological age of the artery actually surpasses the chronological age. The author elucidated three theories that may explain this process.

INTERPRETATION. The implications of these hypotheses serve to draw a critical distinction between biological age (aging) and chronological age and, thereby, offer an answer to the genetic components of essential hypertension and to identify the variant genes responsible for elevated BP in a large segment of the human population.

Comment

Although the rise in PP can be related to chronological age, the situation is different in women, where pre-menopausal PP is lower than for men of the same age – but after menopause, it matches that of men. The review by Aviv examines the association between PP and longevity in humans, suggesting that still little is known about the variant genes that cause hypertension. One hypothesis is that in certain segments of the population, the biologic age of the artery surpasses the chronological age. Indeed, intrauterine growth retardation may drive premature aging in later life. Secondly, telomeres, the TTAGGG repeats at the end of mammalian chromosomes that ultimately limit the number of times that a cell may replicate, potentially serve as a molecular record of biological aging. Although this remains to be proven, two studies have linked PP with telomere length, suggesting that the biological age of people with relatively wide PP is actually more advanced than their chronological age would suggest.

Telomere length as an indicator of biological aging: the gender effect and relation with pulse pressure and pulse wave velocity.

Benetos A, Okuda K, Lajemi M, *et al. Hypertension* 2001; **37**: 381–5.

BACKGROUND. Chronological age is the primary determinant of stiffness of central arteries. Increased stiffness is an independent indicator of cardiovascular risk.

INTERPRETATION. Telomere length provides an additional account to chronological age of variations in both PP and pulse wave velocity among men, such that men with shorter telomere length are more likely to exhibit high PP and PWV, which are indices of large artery stiffness. The longer telomere length in women suggests that for a given chronological age, biological aging of men is more advanced than that of women.

Comment

The hypotheses in this study are interesting and novel. By analysing the length of telomere (the TTAGGG tandem repeats at the ends of mammalian chromosomes is a possible index of biological aging) in both men and women, Benetos *et al.* investigated the biological *versus* chronological aging effects on the variation of arterial stiffness as measured by PP and aortic PVW. Large artery stiffness and its clinical manifestations (PP, PWV) are phenotypes of biologic aging of the arterial system. The study population included 193 French untreated hypertensive subjects (120 men, 73 women), with a mean age of 56 ± 11. Telomere length was evaluated in white blood cells by measuring the mean length of the terminal restriction fragments (TRF). The findings were that age-adjusted telomere length was longer in women than in men and the telomere length was inversely correlated with age in both genders. Multivariate analysis showed that in men, but not in women, telomere length significantly contributed to pulse pressure and pulse wave velocity variations. Given that PP reflects arterial aging, whereas telomere length is an index of biological aging, the authors suggested that the biology of arterial aging is modified by gender. This finding is interesting as it has long been known that premenopausal women are less prone than men to CVD and women tend to catch up with men in the expression of these diseases during the postmenopausal period. It should be noted, however, that their findings do not provide mechanistic links between telomere length and arterial aging. Nevertheless, given that aging is a multifactorial and highly variable entity, the use of telomere length provides a new dimension to the study of cardiovascular disease, as pointed out by the authors.

Pulse pressure and aortic pulse wave are markers of CV risk in hypertensive populations.
Asmar R, Rudnichi A, Blacher J, London GM, Safar ME. *Am J Hypertens* 2001; **14**(2): 91–7.

BACKGROUND. PP and aortic PWV are significant markers of CV risk, but a similar role for central wave reflections has never been investigated.

INTERPRETATION. In cross-sectional hypertensive populations, PP and PWV, but not carotid amplification index (CAI), are significantly and independently associated with CV amplifications.

Comment

This cross-sectional study included a cohort of 1087 patients with essential hypertension (either treated or untreated) to determine the factors influencing PP, PWV, and carotid wave reflections. Atherosclerotic alterations were defined on the basis of clinical events and PWV evaluated from an automatic device. The CAI, a quantitative estimation of the magnitude of central wave reflections, was measured non-invasively from pulse wave analysis using radial and carotid aplanation tonometry. As concluded by the authors, increased PP and PWV, but not altered CAI, are significant and independent identifiers of CV risks. The findings were not influenced by the presence of antihypertensive drug treatment or other confounding variables. Another interesting finding was the influence of plasma glucose on the level of PWV and PP, whereas dyslipidaemia, particularly low high-density lipoprotein cholesterol (HDL-C), had no specific contribution.

Aortic stiffness is an independent predictor of all-cause and cardiovascular mortality in hypertensive patients.

Laurent S, Boutouyrie P, Asmar R, *et al. Hypertension* 2001; **37**(5): 1236–41.

BACKGROUND. Although various studies reported that PP, an indirect index of arterial stiffening, was an independent risk factor for mortality, a direct relationship between arterial stiffness and all-cause and CV mortality remained to be established in patients with essential hypertension.

INTERPRETATION. In multivariate models of logistic regression analysis, PWV was significantly associated with all-cause and CV mortality, independent of previous CVDs, age and diabetes. By contrast, PP was not significantly and independently associated to mortality. This study provides the first direct evidence that aortic stiffness is an independent predictor of all-cause and CV mortality in patients with essential hypertension.

Comment

The study is the first to establish a direct link between aortic stiffness (measured non-invasively by carotid-femoral PWV) and CHD events in people with hypertension. Data were collected from 1980 hypertensive patients whose PWV was measured between 1980 and 1996. The predictive power of PWV was retrospectively compared to that of the Framingham CVD prediction algorithm. While the Framingham Algorithm (FA) appeared to predict CVD in the population as a whole, it did not necessarily predict disease in patients who were CVD-free at baseline. Conversely, the PWV appeared to predict subsequent CHD events, not only in patients with pre-existing CVD, but also in patients who were initially disease-free. Aortic stiffness is associated with hypertension, high cholesterol and diabetes. The predictive power of PWV remained the same after adjustment for FA and PP. The study suggests that consideration of classic CV risk factors may be insufficient to accurately predict the risk of cardiac events in hypertensives, and that the measurement of aortic stiffness may improve the predictive power. Furthermore, it may indicate that classic CVD risk factors increase the risk of CHD events through an increase in aortic stiffness.

Aortic stiffness is an independent predictor of primary coronary events in hypertensive patients: a longitudinal study.

Boutouyrie P, Tropeano AI, Asmar R, *et al. Hypertension* 2002; **39**(1): 10–15.

BACKGROUND. Arterial stiffness may predict CHD beyond classic risk factors. In a longitudinal study, we assessed the predictive value of arterial stiffness on CHD in patients with essential hypertension and without known clinical CVD.

INTERPRETATION. This study provides the first direct evidence in a longitudinal study that aortic stiffness is an independent predictor of primary coronary events in patients with essential hypertension.

Comment

The group further provided data in support of their previous conclusion of the independent predictive value of aortic stiffness for CV events, and in this paper, more specifically predicting for primary coronary events (fatal and non-fatal MI, coronary revascularization and angina pectoris). The risk assessment of CHD was made by calculating the Framingham risk score (FRS) according to the categories

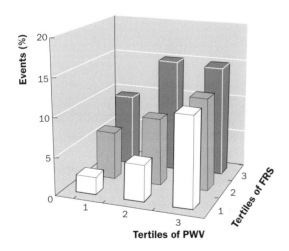

Fig. 9.6 Observed incidence of fatal or non-fatal CHD in patients free of overt CHD at entry *vs* the predicted incidence of CHD calculated with the Framingham equation. Source: Boutouyrie *et al.* (2002).

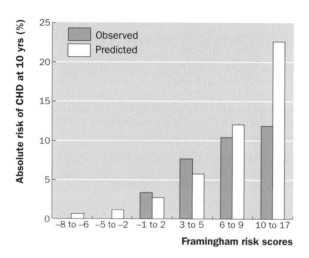

Fig 9.7 Rate of all CV events according to increasing tertiles of PWV and FRS.
Source: Boutouyrie *et al.* (2002).

of gender, age, BP, cholesterol, diabetes and smoking. The Framingham score significantly predicted the occurrence of coronary and all CV events in this population ($P < 0.01$ and $P < 0.0001$, respectively). In multivariate analysis, PWV remained significantly associated with the occurrence of coronary event after adjustment either of Framingham score (for 3.5 m/s: relative risk, 1.345% confidence interval [CI], 1.01 to 1.79; $P = 0.039$) or classic risk factors (for 3.5 m/s: relative risk, 1.395% CI, 1.08–1.79; $P = 0.01$).

Aortic pulse wave velocity predicts cardiovascular mortality in subjects > 70 years of age.

Meaume S, Benetos A, Henry OF, Rudnichi A, Safar ME. *Arterioscler Thromb Vasc Biol* 2001; **21**(12): 2046–50.

BACKGROUND. **Aortic PWV is a significant and independent predictor of CV mortality in subjects with essential hypertension and in patients with end-stage renal disease. Its contribution to CV risk in subjects 70 –100 years old has never been tested.**

INTERPRETATION. Antihypertensive drug treatment and BP, including SBP and PP, had no additive role. In subjects 70 –100 years old, aortic PWV was a strong, independent predictor of CV death, whereas SBP or PP was not. This prospective result will need to be confirmed in an intervention trial.

Comment

A cohort of 141 subjects (mean ± SD age, 87.1 ± 6.6 years) was studied in three geriatrics departments in a Paris suburb. Together with sphygmomanometric BP measurements, aortic PWV was measured with a validated automatic device. During the 30-month follow-up, 56 patients died (27 from CV events). Logistic regressions indicated that age ($P = 0.005$) and a loss of autonomy ($P = 0.01$) were the best predictors of overall mortality. For CV mortality, aortic PWV was the major risk predictor ($P = 0.016$). The odds ratio was 1.19 (95% CI, 1.03–1.37).

Association between arterial stiffness and atherosclerosis: the Rotterdam Study.
van Popele NM, Grobbee DE, Bots ML. *Stroke* 2001; **32**(2): 454–60.

BACKGROUND. Studies of the association between arterial stiffness and atherosclerosis are contradictory. The authors studied stiffness of the aorta and the common carotid artery in relation to several indicators of atherosclerosis.

INTERPRETATION. This population-based study shows that arterial stiffness is strongly associated with atherosclerosis at various sites in the vascular tree.

Comment

This is an interesting study with the aim to examine the association between arterial stiffness and atherosclerosis at different sites in the arterial tree in a large group of elderly subjects (> 3000 elderly subjects aged 60–101 years). Several non-invasive techniques were employed: Arterial stiffness was assessed in the aorta by measuring carotid-femoral PWV and was assessed in the common carotid artery by measuring the distensibility coefficient (DC). Indicators of atherosclerosis were assessed by common carotid IMT, presence of plaques in the carotid artery and in the abdominal aorta, and presence of peripheral arterial disease (PAD). The results showed that aortic stiffness was strongly associated with common carotid IMT, plaques in the carotid artery and in the aorta, and presence of PAD. Common carotid artery stiffness was strongly associated with all indicators of atherosclerosis except for a borderline significant association with peripheral arterial disease. Results were unchanged after additional adjustment for CV risk factors and after exclusion of subjects with prevalent CVD. The strong association of aortic stiffness with atherosclerosis at various sites of the arterial tree suggests that aortic stiffness can be used as an indicator of generalized atherosclerosis. However, whether this also holds for common carotid artery stiffness is less clear. Future longitudinal studies focus on the association between arterial stiffness and CVD must determine whether arterial stiffness is a risk factor for CVD, independent of its association with atherosclerosis.

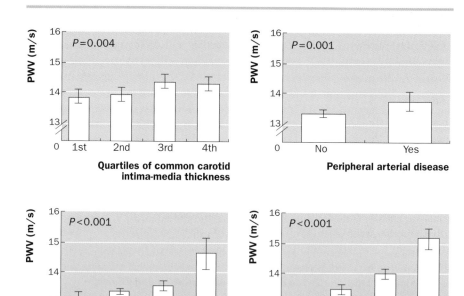

Fig. 9.8 Mean PWV per quartile of common carotid IMT and per category of presence of peripheral arterial disease, plaques in the carotid artery, and plaques in the aorta, adjusted for age, sex, MAP, and heart rate in elderly subjects of the Rotterdam Study. Bars indicate 95% CI; probability value indicates *P* for trend, except for peripheral arterial disease, in which the *P*-value indicates *P* for difference between the groups. Source: van Popele *et al.* (2001).

Office blood pressures, arterial compliance characteristics, and estimated cardiac load.
Izzo JL Jr, Manning TS, Shykoff BE. *Hypertension*. 2001; **38**: 1467–70.

BACKGROUND. Because of rising interest in new methods to detect arterial diseases, this study compared data from three different compliance-related techniques to measure arterial stiffness: systolic pulse contour analysis, diastolic pulse contour analysis (modified Windkessel model), and muscular (brachial) artery compliance by cuff plethysmography.

INTERPRETATION. The weak relationships between BP and compliance-related variables could be due to intrinsic differences in the properties of large and small arteries, theoretical methodological weaknesses, measurement artifacts, or intrinsic haemodynamic differences of the sitting position. At present, compliance-related variables provide little additional advantage over cuff BP in the office estimation of cardiac work.

Comment

This study is timely because of rising interest in new methods to detect arterial disease (or 'stiffness'). The study compared office BPs with data from three different compliance-related techniques to measure arterial stiffness: systolic pulse contour analysis, diastolic pulse contour analysis (modified Windkessel model), and muscular (brachial) artery compliance by cuff plethysmography.

The subjects studied included 63 established hypertensives with 28 age-matched normotensive controls. Variables measured in the sitting position were compared with each other, with clinic BPs, and with the cardiac time-tension integral (an the integral of the central pulse waveform beginning at the pulse upstroke and ending at the dicrotic notch) in subjects. The results, however, demonstrated only low-grade relationships among compliance-related parameters derived from systolic and diastolic pulse contour analysis or cuff plethysmography. Though this was disappointing, it was not too surprising given the fact that the arterial system is not uniform but with clear differences in structure and function between large conduit arteries, mid-sized arteries, and the small pre-capillary vessels.

As pointed out by the authors, other factors such as measurement artefacts may also account for the poor intermethod correlations. Taken together, present results indicate that it is premature to employ the existing compliance methodologies in everyday clinical medicine. However, as quoted in the accompanying editorial: 'we should not be discouraged by the diversity of methods currently being offered for measuring arterial compliance, nor should we be discouraged by apparent inconsistencies among these approaches. As we become more sophisticated in our understanding and use of these methods we will learn how each of them can teach us something different and potentially valuable about the CV system'. We totally concur.

Pulse pressure, arterial stiffness, and drug treatment of hypertension.

Van Bortel LM, Struijker-Boudier HA, Safar ME. *Hypertension.* 2001; **38**: 914–21.

BACKGROUND. Epidemiological studies in the past decade have stressed the importance of PP as an independent risk factor for CV morbidity and mortality.

INTERPRETATION. Increasing evidence from epidemiological and pathophysiological research on the significance of arterial stiffening and raised PP as independent risk factors for CVD creates new challenges for CV therapy. Thus far, pharmacotherapy has focused on BP–lowering properties of antihypertensive drugs. The decrease in arterial stiffness is an attractive additional target.

Comment

The epidemiological evidence, basis pathophysiology of PP and the potential therapeutic consequences were reviewed in detail. As described, both longitudinal and cross-sectional components of the vascular system contribute to the shape of the arterial pressure wave and, thereby, to PP. The primary longitudinal component is the architecture of the arterial tree, which determines the major reflection sites for the pressure wave. The cross-sectional architecture of the vascular system consists of a geometric (diameter) and a structural (composition vessel wall) component. Both diameter and composition of the vessel wall vary greatly when going from central to more peripheral arteries. The implications for the functional properties of various arterial segments were also discussed. Finally, the therapeutic consequences of targeting PP rather than mean BP with various drug classes were also outlined. As pointed out, among the antihypertensive agents, nitrates, nitric oxide donors, and drugs that interfere with the renin–angiotensin–aldosterone system may offer useful tools to lower PP, in addition to mean BP. Future developments may include non-antihypertensive agents that target collagen or other components of the arterial wall matrix. However, large-scale clinical trials will have to confirm the therapeutic value of these agents in the treatment of increased PP and arterial stiffness.

Improvement in blood pressure, arterial stiffness and wave reflections with a very-low-dose Perindopril/Indapamide combination in hypertensive patients: a comparison with atenolol.

Asmar RG, London GM, O'Rourke ME, Safar ME; REASON Project Coordinators and Investigators. *Hypertension* 2001; **38**(4): 922–6.

BACKGROUND. International guidelines recommend that antihypertensive drug therapy should normalize not only DBP but also SBP. Therapeutic trials based on CV mortality have recently shown that SBP reduction requires normalization of both large artery stiffness and wave reflections which are important determinants of SBP and PP and are strong independent CV risk predictors in hypertensive populations. Consequently, the role of drugs or regimens that may selectively reduce SBP and PP assumes importance.

INTERPRETATION. The very-low-dose combination Perindopril/Indapamide (Per/Ind) normalizes SBP, PP and arterial function to a significantly larger extent than does atenolol, a haemodynamic profile that is known to improve survival in hypertensive populations with high CV risk.

Comment

The aim of the present study was to establish whether Per/Ind decreased SBP and PP more than the ß-blocking agent atenolol for the same DBP reduction, and whether any such effect was mediated by a Per/Ind-induced decrease in large artery stiffness (by automatic PWV) and attenuation of wave reflections (pulse wave analysis, applanation tonometry).

In the present study, Per/Ind reduced selectively SBP and PP in association with significant changes in large artery function, involving a decrease in aortic stiffness and mostly an attenuation of wave reflections. Because the results were observed in subjects with relatively mild forms of hypertension, it remains to be seen whether, in the most common forms of human hypertension, Per/Ind is able to reduce CV risk significantly through its action on large artery stiffness and wave reflections.

Pulse pressure changes with six classes of antihypertensive agents in a randomized, controlled trial.

Cushman WC, Materson BJ, Williams DW, Reda DJ. *Hypertension* 2001, **38**: 953–7.

BACKGROUND. Pulse pressure has been more strongly associated with CV outcomes, especially MI and heart failure, than has systolic, diastolic or MAP in a variety of populations, particularly in older individuals. Little is known, however, of the comparative effects of various classes of antihypertensive agents on PP.

INTERPRETATION. These data show that classes of antihypertensive agents differ in their ability to reduce PP. Whether these differences affect rates of CV events remains to be determined.

Comment

This is the first study published on the comparative effects of different classes of antihypertensive agents on PP. In these analyses of the Veterans Affairs Single-Drug Therapy for Hypertension Study, there are significant differences in the effects of six classes of antihypertensive agents (hydrochlorothiazide, atenolol, captopril, clonidine, diltiazem, prazosin, or placebo) on PP. Clonidine was most effective in reducing all BP parameters including PP but was associated with more adverse effects and drug withdrawals. Hydrochlorothiazide, which was well tolerated, came second best but was statistically superior to any other drug after 1 year of maintenance monotherapy. In addition, combinations that included a thiazide diuretic were superior to combinations without a diuretic in reducing PP, giving strength to recommendations to include a diuretic in most multidrug antihypertensive regimens. The mechanisms by which these classes of drugs differ in their effect on

PP were not addressed in this study. It is also not clear whether the differences in PP found in this study are related to differences in vascular compliance. Whether differences in changes in PP by antihypertensive agents affect rates of CV events remains to be demonstrated. However, until we perform trials that evaluate the effects of different antihypertensive agents on the PP, we will continue to target SBP reduction as the primary therapeutic goal.

Conventional antihypertensive drug therapy does not prevent the increase of pulse pressure with age.

Mourad JJ, Blacher J, Blin P, Warzocha U, on behalf of the investigators of the PHASTE study. *Hypertension* 2001; **38**: 958–61.

BACKGROUND. In older subjects with ISH, drug treatment for hypertension markedly reduced CV morbidity and mortality, even to a larger extent than in populations of subjects with systolic-diastolic hypertension. Increased PP (main characteristic feature of ISH patients) is a significant predictor of CV risk, independent of (and in addition to) SBP, DBP, and MBP. In subjects treated for hypertension, particularly those with systolic-diastolic hypertension, DBP is frequently controlled, whereas SBP remains elevated, resulting in an increased prevalence of ISH. Increased PP may be quantified on the basis of the prevalence of ISH in the population at large.

INTERPRETATION. In the studied populations, the increase of PP with age is independent of gender and of the presence of antihypertensive drug treatment, leading to an increased prevalence of ISH and a subsequent increase of CV risk with age.

Comment

The purpose of this study was to estimate the prevalence of ISH and its relationship to age and drug therapy in a large group of outpatient hypertensive subjects in France. About 17 716 consecutive patients with uncontrolled hypertension (SBP > 140 mmHg and/or DBP > 90 mmHg), either treated or not treated were included in the study. Subjects were classified according to five age ranges. In each age range, SBP, DBP, MBP and PP were significantly lower in treated subjects than in untreated subjects, with the exception of PP in subjects >75 years. The latter finding resulted from a significant increase of SBP and PP with age, together with a significant lowering of DBP with age, irrespective of drug treatment. Subsequently, the prevalence of ISH increased with age from 20.4% to 35.2% in men and women. In any given age range, drug therapy for hypertension is associated with marginally lower values of PP.

Thus, the present study has shown that in a French population of hypertensive subjects, an elevated prevalence of patients with ISH is now developing independently of the presence or absence of drug treatment. This population probably results from the increase of longevity in populations at large and from the interactions between the presence of hypertension and of the coexisting age-induced increase in arterial stiffness. The latter is the main haemodynamic mechanism for increased SBP and PP in the aging population. Whether a specific treatment for this alteration should be important to consider at the present time was not determined in the present study and requires further investigation.

Improved arterial compliance by a novel advanced glycation end-product crosslink breaker.

Kass DA, Shapiro EP, Kawaguchi M, *et al. Circulation*. 2001; **104**: 1464–70.

BACKGROUND. Arterial stiffening with increased PP is a leading risk factor for CVD in the elderly. This study tested whether ALT-711, a novel non-enzymatic breaker of advanced glycation end-product crosslinks, selectively improves arterial compliance and lowers PP in older individuals with vascular stiffening.

INTERPRETATION. ALT-711 improves total arterial compliance in aged humans with vascular stiffening, and it may provide a novel therapeutic approach for this abnormality, which occurs with aging, diabetes and ISH.

Comment

As parts of the aging process, collagen and elastin (which maintain CV elasticity) are prone to the formation of advanced glycosylation end-product (AGE) cross-links, leading to stiffening of the blood vessels including the large arteries. This loss of flexibility in the vasculature leads to an increase in the arterial PP and the development of ISH, which substantially increases the risk of CVD and death. As well as being a part of the aging process, the formation of these crosslinks can also be excessive in diabetic patients.

Could this be a new agent for ISH with novel mechanism of action? Indeed, ALT-711 is a novel thiazolium derivative designed to break these AGE crosslinks thus increasing large artery compliance. This Phase IIa pharmacology study of ALT-711 looked promising and safe. In the study, 93 patients aged > 50 years with resting SBP > 140 mmHg and arterial PP > 60 mmHg were randomized on a 2:1 basis to receive oral doses of 210 mg of ALT-711 daily or placebo for 8 weeks. The participants included diabetics and non-diabetics who all had resting large artery compliances of < 1.2 mL/mmHg and who were all maintained on existing anti-hypertensive drugs. BP measurements were taken at frequent intervals and an echodoppler was performed. Patients taking the active drug showed a consistent and significant decline in PP without a concurrent greater decline in MBP, which makes ALT-711 different from current therapies for ISH.

Hence, the drug improves total artery compliance and vascular distensability but does not alter cardiac output or systolic vascular resistance. The drug may also have a role in diastolic dysfunction as it has been shown to increase diastolic dis-tensability of the heart in animals.

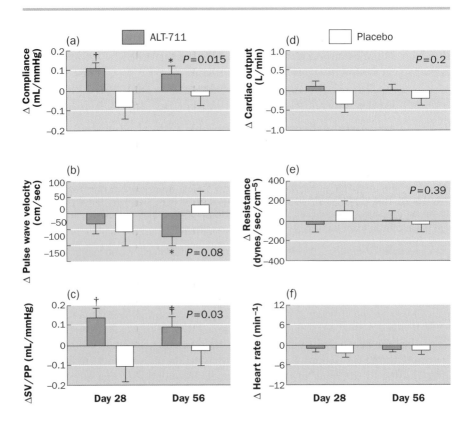

Fig. 9.9 Compliance/stiffness and arterial haemodynamics in ALT-711 and placebo groups. Data are shown as absolute change relative to baseline (± SEM) at both day 28 and day 56, the two post-treatment days when these parameters were assessed. Probability values reflect 2-way RMANOVA for a drug effect. Parameters reflecting total artery compliance or large-vessel stiffness (left panels: (a) through (c) improved with ALT-711 treatment. In contrast, cardiac output, mean arterial resistance, and heart rate did not significantly change in either group (right panels; (d) through (f).
* $P < 0.05$ vs baseline, †$P < 0.01$ vs baseline, ‡$P = 0.09$ vs baseline.
Source: Kass *et al.* (2001).

Systolic and pulse blood pressures (but not diastolic blood pressure and serum cholesterol) are associated with alterations in carotid intima–media thickness in the moderately hypercholesterolaemic hypertensive patients of the Plaque Hypertension Lipid Lowering Italian Study.

Zanchetti A, Crepaldi G, Bond MG, *et al. J Hypertens* 2001; **19**(1): 7–8.

BACKGROUND. There has recently been increasing interest in investigating alterations in the carotid artery wall, mostly for two reasons. 1. Quantitative B-mode ultrasound imaging has been shown to be a valid, sensitive and well-reproducible non-invasive method for measurement of carotid IMT; 2. there is both cross-sectional and prospective evidence that carotid IMT and plaques correlate with coronary events and strokes. Although there is experimental evidence favouring a definite effect of ACEIs on atherosclerosis development and progression, the potential benefit of ACEIs on plaque regression has never been tested in a controlled trial on patients with essential hypertension.

INTERPRETATION. Baseline data from the Plaque Hypertension Lipid Lowering Italian Study (PHYLLIS) indicate that in this population of hypertensive patients with moderate hypercholesterolaemia, SBP and PP are with age among the most significant factors associated with carotid artery alterations. However, the narrow range of inclusion low density lipoprotein (LDL)-cholesterol and DBP values may have obscured an additional role of these variables.

Comment

PHYLLIS is still in progress. This paper described the baseline data of the study to clarify the association of various risk factors with carotid IMT in these medium–high risk hypertensive patients. PHYLLIS is the first and unique study in patients with hypertension, moderate hypercholesterolaemia and initial carotid artery alterations. It is a multicentre, prospective, randomly allocated, double-blind, double-dummy study, with a factorial design (2 × 2) with four treatment groups, comparing two different antihypertensive treatments (hydrochlorothiazide 25 mg once a day *versus* fosinopril, 20 mg once a day) and two different lipid-lowering strategies (American Heart Association step I diet plus placebo *versus* the same diet plus pravastatin 40 mg once a day). Screening was followed by washout of all previous antihypertensive and lipid-lowering medication, and a run-in period of 6 weeks under placebo and diet (American Heart Association step I) preceded randomization. Inclusion criteria were age 45–70 years, men and postmenopausal or surgically sterile women, sitting DBP 95–115 mmHg, sitting SBP 150–210 mmHg, serum LDL cholesterol 4.14–5.17 mmol/l (160–200 mg/dl), serum triglyceride concentration 3.39 mmol/l (300 mg/dl), and asymptomatic early carotid wall alterations (maximum IMT 1.3–4.0 mm at the screening B-mode ultrasound examination). The primary objective of PHYLLIS is investigating whether in these patients administration of an ACEI, fosinopril, and a statin, pravastatin, is more effective than administration of a diuretic and a lipid-lowering diet in retarding or regressing alterations in carotid IMT.

Salt sensitivity, pulse pressure, and death in normal and hypertensive humans.

Weinberger MH, Fineberg NS, Fineberg SE, Weinberger M. *Hypertension* 2001; **37**(2(suppl)): 429–32.

BACKGROUND. **Although factors such as age, BP, and its responsiveness to changes in sodium balance and extracellular fluid volume status (salt sensitivity) are associated with an increased risk of end-organ disease and CV events in hypertensive subjects, no such relationship with mortality has been demonstrated for salt sensitivity in normotensive subjects.**

INTERPRETATION. These observations provide unique evidence of a relationship between salt sensitivity and mortality that is independent of elevated BP.

Comment

This study adds to a growing body of evidence that suggests salt, and an individual's susceptibility to it, plays an important role in the development of hypertension and subsequent adverse health effects.

In this study, the salt sensitivity or resistance status of BP was ascertained in 596 subjects (normo- or hypertensive) about 27 years ago. Of the overall cohort, 338 were found to be salt sensitive and 123 had died. As expected, age, gender, BMI, and all measures of BP, including SBP, DBP, MAP and PP, were associated with significantly increased mortality. However, when survival curves were examined, normotensive salt-sensitive subjects aged > 25 years when initially studied were found to have a cumulative mortality similar to that of hypertensive subjects, whereas salt-resistant normotensive subjects had increased survival.

From their earlier studies, Weinberger *et al.* noted that salt sensitivity is more common in certain groups. These include the elderly, African Americans, first-

Table 9.1 Risk factors and associated odds ratios for CV death

Risk factor	Odds ratio	*P* value
Age	1.06	<0.001
Female gender	0.34	<0.005
Pulse pressure	1.06	<0.001
Salt sensitivity	2.17	<0.003

Source: Weinberger *et al.* (2001).

degree relatives of hypertensives, and those with a family member who is salt-sensitive. The condition is also linked to different end-organ effects than is hypertension. These include an increased risk of LVH, proteinuria, and a blunted decline in nocturnal BP. Among the individuals who were deemed salt-sensitive in their initial study, there was a significantly greater rise in BP with age and time, compared to salt-resistant subjects. The observation suggests that salt-sensitivity in normotensives may presage an increased risk for age-related hypertension. If this turns out to be the case, it is possible that intervention in susceptible individuals, by reducing salt intake, could prevent or delay the subsequent age-related increase in BP, the development of hypertension, and the increased risk of CV events and death.

However, testing for salt-sensitivity remains cumbersome and mass screening is not practicable. Nevertheless, such findings from this study remind the public of a simple message: people with normal BP should stick to the daily-recommended sodium of < 2400 mg! The benefit will be even greater if they reduce their salt intake to 1500 mg a day, as was shown in the Dietary Approaches to Stop Hypertension-Sodium study. In that study, the lower the sodium intake, the lower the BP level.

Pulse wave velocity as end-point in large-scale intervention trial: the Complior Study. Scientific, quality control, coordination and investigation committees of the Complior Study.

Asmar R, Topouchian J, Pannier B, Benetos A, Safar M. *J Hypertens* 2001; **19**(4): 813–8.

BACKGROUND. To evaluate the ability of an antihypertensive therapy to improve arterial stiffness as assessed by aortic PWV in a large population of hypertensive patients.

INTERPRETATION. The Complior Study is the first study to show the feasibility of a large-scale intervention trial using PWV as the end-point in hypertensive patients. Adequate results may be obtained using an automatic device and rigorous criteria for assessment. A long-term controlled intervention study is needed to confirm the results of the present uncontrolled trial.

Comment

In arterial hypertension, aortic wave reflections contribute to determining central systolic and pulse pressures. It is known that ACEIs are able to increase arterial compliance in patients with hypertension as well as in normotensive subjects. The Complior Study group recruited a total of 2187 patients (mean age 50 years) with mild to moderate essential hypertension from 69 healthcare centres in 19 countries.

All patients were treated for 6 months, starting with perindopril 4 mg once daily, increased to 8 mg, and combined to diuretic (indapamide 2.5 mg once daily) if BP was uncontrolled ($> 140/90$ mmHg). Only 703 (52% male) completed the study: mean age $= 50 \pm 12$ years; mean baseline SBP/DBP $= 158 \pm 15/98 \pm 7$ mmHg; mean baseline carotid-femoral PWV $= 11.6 \pm 2.4$ metre/second. The group have shown that measurements of carotid-femoral PWV using the automatic device Complior was feasible at inclusion, 2 and 6 months, along with conventional BP assessments in a population of 1703 patients. The results showed significant decreases ($P < 0.001$) in BP (systolic: $-23.7 +/- 16.8$, diastolic: -14.6 ± 10 mmHg), and carotid-femoral PWV (-1.1 ± 1.4 m/s) at 2 and 6 months on trial medications. The finding of a pressure independent effect of ACEI on arterial wall is interesting as less than 10% of the total reduction in PWV could be explained by the reduction in BP in this study. Whether other agents that block the renin-angiotensin system such as the angiotensin receptor blockers could produce a similar effect is unclear.

Arterial stiffness and cardiovascular risk factors in a population-based study.

Amar J, Ruidavets JB, Chamontin B, Drouet L, Ferrieres J. *J Hypertens* 2001; **19**(3): 381–7.

BACKGROUND. To determine the relationships between PWV, an estimate of arterial distensibility and cardiovascular risk factors.

INTERPRETATION. This study shows that, in a sample of subjects at high risk, the cumulative influence of risk factors, even treated, is an independent determinant of arterial stiffness. These results suggest that PWV may be used as a relevant tool to assess the influence of cardiovascular risk factors on aortic stiffness in high-risk patients.

Comment

This is another cross-sectional population-based study which again supports the fact that PWV could be an indirect measure of arterial stiffness and thus be used in the estimation of CV risk in high-risk patients. The study was carried out from 1995 to 1997 and included a total of 993 subjects, aged 35-64 years (52.7% men), living in the south-west of France. Carotid-femoral PWV was measured using a semi-automatic device (Complior). The relationships between PWV and risk factors were assessed, first in subjects not treated with hypolipidaemic, antidiabetic and antihypertensive drugs and then in treated subjects. The results showed that in subjects not treated for cardiovascular risk factors, age, gender, systolic blood pressure and heart rate ($P < 0.001$) were the variables significantly associated with PWV. In treated patients, age ($P < 0.01$), SBP ($P < 0.001$), heart rate ($P < 0.001$), apolipoprotein B ($P < 0.05$) and the number of treated cardiovascular risk factors ($P < 0.05$) were positively correlated with PWV.

Pulsatile BP component as predictor of mortality in hypertension: a meta-analysis of clinical trial control groups.

Gasowski J, Fagard RH, Staessen JA, *et al. J Hypertens* 2002;
20(1): 145–51.

B A C K G R O U N D . Although current guidelines rest exclusively on the measurement of SBP and DBPs, the arterial pressure wave is more precisely described as consisting of a pulsatile pressure and a steady (mean pressure) component. This study explored the independent roles of pulsatile pressure and mean pressure as predictors of mortality in a wide range of patients with hypertension.

I N T E R P R E T A T I O N . In hypertensive patients PP, not MBP, is associated with an increased risk of fatal events. This appears to be true in a broad range of patients with hypertension.

Comment

Several observational studies have shown that PP may be an independent predictor of CV risk in a wide range of individuals: in general population, in hypertensive subjects, in survivors of myocardial, and patients with left ventricular dysfunction. The collaboration of the INDANA (Individual Data Analysis of Antihypertensive Intervention Trials) project has combined results from the control groups of seven randomized clinical trials conducted in patients with systolo-diastolic or ISH and thus allowed meta-analysis in a much wider age and BP range than previous studies that included mainly older hypertensives with isolated systolic hypertension.

In this study the relative hazard rates associated with PP and mean pressure were calculated using Cox's proportional hazard regression models with stratification for the seven trials and with adjustment for sex, age, smoking and the other pressure. The data revealed that in patients with hypertension a 10 mmHg wider PP is independently associated with an increase in risk by 6% for total mortality ($P = 0.001$), 7% for CV mortality ($P = 0.01$), and 7% for fatal coronary accidents ($P = 0.03$). The corresponding increase in risk of fatal stroke was similar ($+6\%$, $P = 0.27$) but there were too few strokes to reach statistical significance. These risks were consistent throughout a large pool of patients enrolled as controls and assigned to placebo or no medication in seven randomized clinical trials. In similar analyses, mean pressure was not identified as an independent predictor of these outcomes. Furthermore, significant interactions of PP or mean pressure with age suggested that the prognostic power of PP for fatal stroke was more important at higher age ($P = 0.04$), whereas the prognostic power of mean pressure for coronary mortality was greatest in the young ($P = 0.01$).

Thus, the study's results confirm and expand the previously reported findings that PP, rather than mean BP, Is the major risk factor of adverse CV complications. It is of note that early reports from the Framingham Heart Study emphasized that

SBP was a better independent predictor of CV risk than DBP, especially in subjects over the age of 50. Increasing evidence now suggests that PP is a better predictor of CV risk than SBP or DBP. However, the present study does not imply a causal relationship. A well-designed clinical study is needed to clarify the issue of whether or not the lowering of PP would decrease CV morbidity and mortality.

10

Clinical evaluation

Clinical evaluations in hypertension: myocardial ischaemia

Introduction

As in any disease management, objective and accurate clinical assessment is of prime importance for establishing diagnosis, stratifying risk, evaluating therapy, etc.

The diagnosis and management of myocardial ischaemia in hypertensive patients remain a problem in clinical cardiology. Not only are coronary artery disease (CAD) complications the most important causes of morbidity and mortality in hypertensive subjects, such patients can also present with significant myocardial ischaemia without obvious epicardial coronary stenosis. Furthermore, silent myocardial ischaemia has also been reported to be more common in a certain subset of hypertensive patients. Several mechanisms may operate at the same time leading to significant reduction in coronary flow reserve in the absence of significant stenosis of the epicardial coronary arteries. There are several non-invasive techniques available for the assessment of the degree of myocardial ischaemia in these patients, namely, electrocardiographic (ECG) exercise stress test with a treadmill or bicycle ergometer, exercise myocardial perfusion radionuclear imaging looking for perfusion defect, and stress echocardiography (echo) looking for regional wall motion abnormalities or more recently regional perfusion defects using contrast-enhanced tissue Doppler imaging. Certainly, with time, magnetic resonance imaging would also be available. However, all these tests are not meant to be mutually exclusive but be complementary to one another. Exercise ECG may be difficult to interpret if repolarization abnormalities or left bundle branch block (LBBB) are present, but the exercise time, symptoms, and blood pressure (BP) response can still provide useful information.

Diagnosis of myocardial ischaemia in hypertensive patients.
Picano E, Palinkas A, Amyot R. *J Hypertens* 2001; **19**(7): 1177–83.

B a c k g r o u n d . Arterial hypertension can provoke a reduction in coronary flow reserve through several mechanisms that are not mutually exclusive (i.e. epicardial CAD, left ventricular hypertrophy [LVH]) and structural and/or functional microvascular disease). **These different targets of arterial hypertension should be explored with different diagnostic markers.**

INTERPRETATION. The exercise-ECG stress test can be used to screen patients with negative maximal test due to its excellent negative predictive value, which is high and comparable in normotensives and hypertensives. When an exercise-ECG stress test is positive (or uninterpretable or ambiguous), an imaging stress-echo test is warranted for a reliable identification of significant, prognostically malignant epicardial CAD in view of an ischaemia-guided revascularization.

Comment

The diagnosis of CAD in hypertensive subjects is frequently difficult because of the various processes that contribute to myocardial ischaemia like coronary microangiography and LVH especially in the presence of 'strain-pattern' ECG. This paper provides an excellent review on this topic and includes several practical diagnostic flow charts and graphical representations of the basic pathophysiology underlying such clinical problems. As pointed out by the author, stress-induced wall motion abnormalities are highly specific for angiographically assessed epicardial CAD, whereas S-T segment depression and/or myocardial perfusion abnormalities are frequently found with angiographically normal coronary arteries associated with LVH and/or microvascular disease. The following studies illustrate some of the clinical diagnostic modalities used.

Advantages of exercise echocardiography in comparison to dobutamine echocardiography in the diagnosis of coronary artery disease in hypertensive subjects.

Pasierski T, Szwed H, Malczewska B, *et al. J Hum Hypertens* 2001; **15**(11): 805–9.

BACKGROUND. **The diagnosis of CAD in hypertensive subjects is frequently difficult. The positive predictive value of the ECG exercise stress test is low.**

INTERPRETATION. In hypertensive patients with the symptoms of angina, both stress echo methods are significantly more specific than the exercise ECG test. Maximal exercise is associated with less frequent side effects than infusion of dobutamine, so exercise echo may be preferred in the diagnosis of angina in hypertensive patients.

Comment

Efficacy of stress echo has been proved only in small groups of hypertensive patients. The present study is the first to compare exercise and dobutamine echo exclusively in hypertensive patients with angina. The study included 197 middle-aged treated hypertensives (65 women) who were referred for coronary angiography. The result confirmed the poor specificity (56%) of exercise ECG in these patients.

Interestingly, as in other studies, the specificity and sensitivity of diagnostic methods were not influenced by the presence of echocardiographic LVH. Furthermore, the advantage of stress echo over ECG stress test was more obvious in women than in men especially in women with medium pre-test probability of CAD. Moreover, patients with coronary microangiopathy and LVH with diminished coronary flow reserve may have normal coronary angiogram. In these cases, stress echo should be recommended.

Impact of hypertension on the accuracy of exercise stress myocardial perfusion imaging for the diagnosis of coronary artery disease.

Elhendy A, van Domburg RT, Sozzi FB, Poldermans D, Bax JJ, Roelandt JR.
Heart 2001; **85**(6): 655–61.

BACKGROUND. Although the occurrence of myocardial perfusion abnormalities in hypertensive patients without epicardial CAD is well documented, the impact of this observation on the specificity and value of exercise stress myocardial perfusion scintigraphy for diagnosing CAD in a routine clinical setting is far from clear, and it is not known whether myocardial perfusion scintigraphy suffers particular limitations in hypertensive patients.

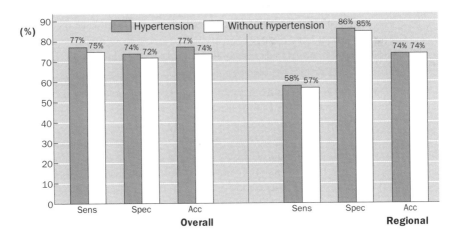

Fig. 10.1 Sensitivity (Sens), specificity (Spec), and accuracy (Acc) of exercise stress SPECT for the overall and regional diagnosis of CAD in patients with and without hypertension. Source: Elhendy *et al.* (2001).

INTERPRETATION. In the usual clinical setting, the value of exercise myocardial perfusion scintigraphy for diagnosing CAD is not degraded by the presence of hypertension.

Comment

This study set out to compare the accuracy of exercise stress myocardial perfusion single photon emission computed tomography imaging (SPECT with 99m technetium labelled agents) together with a symptom limited bicycle exercise stress test for the diagnosis of coronary artery disease in patients with and without hypertension. The test was performed in 332 patients (75 women and 137 hypertensives) without previous myocardial infarction (MI) who underwent coronary angiogram. The results showed that exercise SPECT has comparable diagnostic accuracy in both hyper- and normotensive patients. Quite rightly, the authors pointed out some potential limitations that may affect their study and these should not have changed the clinical value of exercise SPECT for diagnosing CAD in hypertensive patients in their study. However, it is worth pointing out that other diagnostic modalities should be used complementarily rather than mutually exclusively.

Left ventricular mass and function in hypertension

Introduction

Left ventricular hypertrophy and/or dilatation are common in hypertension. Indeed, increased echocardiographic-LVH is a stronger predictor for adverse cardiovascular (CV) events than any other risk factor (besides advanced age), in the general population, in those with hypertension, and in patients with CAD. Left ventricular (LV) geometric remodelling recently characterized by echocardiographic studies has found that patients with concentric LVH had the strongest mortality risk. Despite such potent risk of LVH or of increased LV mass, so far there have been no universally acceptable criteria for defining LV mass index (LVMI).

The patterns of echocardiographic LV geometry can be divided into either concentric or eccentric according to Ganau et al. |1|, and depend on the LVMI and relative wall thickness (RWT). Briefly, normal geometry is present when both LVMI and RWT are normal; increased RWT and normal LVMI identified concentric remodelling. Increased LVMI with normal RWT identified eccentric LVH; and increased both LVMI and RWT identified concentric LVH. Furthermore, the standardization for the assessment of LV systolic function in the presence of LVH also remains to be defined. The conventional chamber function measurements using LV endocardial fractional shortening or ejection fraction often report a normal or 'supranormal' systolic performance in hypertensive patients even in the absence of significant LVH. A newer method expressed as midwall fractional shortening (LV midwall mechanics) has been developed which takes into consideration the non-uniform wall thickness that contracts radially and longitudinally; the wall volume (myocardial mass) is assumed to be constant throughout the cardiac cycle. This model has been shown to substantially reduce the number of hypertensive patients with supranormal LV function and identified low LV myocardial performance in approximately one sixth of the patients, especially in those with an abnormal LV geometry. Such method eliminated the artefactual effect of the endocardial motion and is thus thought to be more representative of LV systolic function in hypertension-induced hypertrophy. Hence, this would allow a better assessment for improved myocardial performance and/or LV mass reduction with antihypertensive therapy. Indeed, decreased midwall fractional shortening has been identified as an independent predictor of CV morbidity and mortality and has been associated with diminished contractile reserve, abnormal diastolic function, LVH, and extracardiac target organ damage. Moreover, recent studies have also reported associations of low midwall fractional shortening with abnormal LV diastolic filling in selected hypertensive patients with normal LV fractional shortening.

Cardiovascular risk stratification in hypertensive patients: impact of echocardiography and carotid ultrasonography.

Cuspidi C, Lonati L, Macca G, *et al. J Hypertens* 2001; **19**(3): 375–80.

BACKGROUND. Decisions about the management of hypertensive patients should not be based on the level of BP alone, but also on the presence of other risk factors, target organ damage (TOD), and CV and renal disease.

INTERPRETATION. The detection of TOD by ultrasound techniques allowed a much more accurate identification of high-risk patients, who represented a very large fraction (45%) of the patient population seen in a hypertension clinic. In particular, a large proportion of patients classified as at moderate risk by routine investigations were instead found to be at high risk when ultrasound examinations were added. The results of this study suggest that CV risk stratification only based on simple routine work-up can often underestimate overall risk, thus leading to a potentially inadequate therapeutic management especially of low-medium risk patients.

Comment

The objective of this study was to evaluate the impact of echo and carotid ultrasonography in a more precise stratification of absolute CV risk stratified according to the criteria suggested by the 1999 World Health Organization/Isolated Systolic Hypertension (WHO/ISH) guidelines. LVH was defined as LVMI > 134 g/m^2 in men and > 110 g/m^2 in women; carotid plaque as focal thickening > 1.3 mm. Risk of TOD was initially evaluated by routine procedures only, and subsequently reassessed by using data on cardiac and vascular structure obtained by ultrasound examinations. According to the first classification 20% were low-risk patients, 50% medium-risk, 22% high-risk and 8% very-high-risk patients. A marked change in risk stratification was obtained when TOD was assessed by adding ultrasound examinations: low-risk patients 18%, medium-risk 28%, high-risk 45%, very-high-risk patients 9%. However, as demonstrated by the same author, the article below further showed us the wide variability in CV risk estimation by using different echocardiographic criteria. Nevertheless, a risk stratification chart for hypertension management is still a very useful simple tool for clinicians in order to identify those at higher CV risk or TOD though such a chart may not accurately identify patients in the lower risk range.

Influence of different echocardiographic criteria for detection of left ventricular hypertrophy on cardiovascular risk stratification in recently diagnosed essential hypertensives.

Cuspidi C, Macca G, Sampieri L, *et al. J Hum Hypertens* 2001; **15**(9): 619–25.

BACKGROUND. Hypertensive patients with LVH need a prompter and more intensive pharmacological treatment than subjects without evidence of cardiac involvement. So, the detection of LVH plays an important role for decision-making in hypertensives.

INTERPRETATION. The detection of LVH by echo allowed a much more accurate identification of high-risk patients. In particular the results suggest that: 1. CV risk stratification only based on a simple routine work-up can often underestimate overall risk; 2. a better standardisation in defining LVH is needed, considering that the impact of cardiac hypertrophy on risk stratification is markedly dependent on the echocardiographic criteria used to diagnose it.

Comment

The study evaluated the impact of six different echo criteria to define LVH in modifying the absolute CV risk of predominantly grade 1 and 2 essential hypertension. Risk was stratified according to the criteria suggested by the 1999 WHO/ISH guidelines. According to the first classification based on routine investigations, 46% were low risk and 54% were medium risk patients. However, LVH being assessed by echo, a significant percentage of patients, ranging from 9 to 25%, were found to having LVH according to different criteria and consequently moved from low and medium risk strata to high risk stratum. The wide variations in LVH prevalence observed in this and other studies stress the need of definite operative criteria in order to allow a more standardized stratification of CV risk in hypertensives.

Gender differences in systolic left ventricular function in hypertensive patients with electrocardiographic left ventricular hypertrophy (the LIFE study).

Gerdts E, Zabalgoitia M, Bjornstad H, Svendsen TL, Devereux RB. *Am J Cardiol* 2001; **87**(8): 980–3. A4.

BACKGROUND. Several studies have reported gender differences in LV adaptation to chronic pressure overload. The mechanisms by which gender influences cardiac adaptation to chronic pressure overload are, however, not fully understood.

INTERPRETATION. Female gender is an independent predictor of higher systolic LV function in hypertensive patients with ECG LVH.

Comment

This study is the first to demonstrate that female gender is associated with higher systolic LV function in older hypertensive patients with ECG LVH, independent of major confounders (CAD, serum creatinine and body mass index [BMI]), irrespective of whether LV systolic function is evaluated as ejection fraction, endocardial fractional shortening, midwall fractional shortening, or stress-corrected midwall fractional shortening. However, the findings of this cross-sectional study need to be confirmed in a cohort under longitudinal surveillance beginning at a point when hypertension and associated target organ damage were both milder.

Left ventricular midwall function improves with antihypertensive therapy and regression of left ventricular hypertrophy in patients with asymptomatic hypertension.

Schussheim AE, Diamond JA, Phillips RA. *Am J Cardiol* 2001; **87**(1): 61–5.

BACKGROUND. Recent evidence suggests that regression of LVH with antihypertensive therapy improves prognosis. The mechanism for this benefit is unknown but may be related to effects on myocardial performance. Midwall fractional shortening (mFS) is often depressed in patients with asymptomatic hypertension, is associated with LVH, and is a potent, independent predictor of outcome.

INTERPRETATION. Antihypertensive therapy and LV mass regression is associated with demonstrable improvements in cardiac performance when assessed using mFS. Determinations of mFS may have a promising role in identifying patients with early hypertensive heart disease, tracking responses to therapy, and in elucidating the potential beneficial effects associated with LV mass regression.

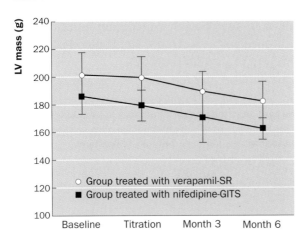

Fig. 10.2 LV mass (in grams) for both treatment groups at each of the 4 phases of the 6-month study. LV mass decreased significantly with treatment over time ($P < 0.05$). There were no significant differences between the two treatment groups. Source: Schussheim *et al.* (2001).

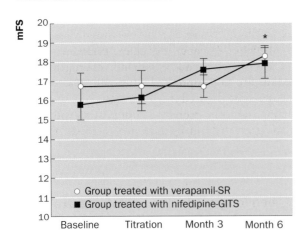

Fig. 10.3 Absolute mFS increased with treatment and was significantly increased compared with baseline after 6 months of therapy. There were no differences between therapies. *$P < 0.05$. Source: Schussheim *et al.* (2001).

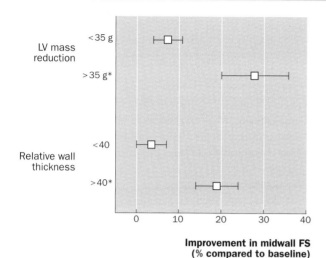

Fig. 10.4 Changes in mFS were more pronounced among patients who achieved a larger reduction in LV mass (> 35 g) and in those who had increased relative wall thickness (RWT > 0.40) at baseline. Symbols represent the percentage increase ± SEM in mFS for each group after 6 months of antihypertensive therapy. *$P < 0.05$. Source: Schussheim *et al.* (2001).

Comment

Again, this study tested whether antihypertensive therapy may improve midwall performance. mFS as well as conventional echocardiographic parameters were measured serially among 29 hypertensive persons during 6 months of drug therapy. Stress-adjusted and absolute midwall function improved by 10% and 11%, respectively, whereas no significant changes were detected in other measures of chamber function. Improvement in function was more pronounced in patients with concentrically remodelled ventricular geometry and in those who achieved greater reductions in LV mass.

Relationship between left ventricular diastolic relaxation and systolic function in hypertension: the Hypertension Genetic Epidemiology Network (HyperGEN) Study.

Bella JN, Palmieri V, Liu JE, *et al. Hypertension* 2001; **38**: 424–8.

BACKGROUND. The relation of impaired LV relaxation, as measured by prolonged isovolumic relaxation time (IVRT), to ventricular systolic function in hypertension remains uncertain in population-based samples.

INTERPRETATION. In hypertension, impaired LV relaxation parallels ventricular midwall dysfunction but not systolic chamber function. Whether combined diastolic and systolic dysfunction identifies hypertensive patients at especially high risk of CV events requires further study.

Comment

The study analysed 1457 echocardiograms of hypertensive participants in the Hypertension Genetic Epidemiology Network (HyperGEN) Study. The aim was to identify clinical and haemodynamic characteristics associated with impaired diastolic relaxation, as measured by prolonged IVRT, and to examine the relation of long IVRT to systolic LV function. Impaired IVRT was defined as IVRT > 100 ms. Patients with impaired LV relaxation were found to have lower LV myocardial function (as measured by stress-corrected MWS) and lower LV chamber contractility (as assessed by circumferential ejection systolic stress/end-systolic volume index) but LV mass and relative wall thickness were higher than for hypertensive patients with normal IVRT. The conclusion was that in hypertension, impaired LV relaxation, as measured by IVRT, parallels LV midwall dysfunction but not LV systolic chamber function. The parallelism between diastolic and systolic function may aid in the identification of hypertensive patients at high risk of future congestive heart failure.

Effect of electrocardiographic left ventricular hypertrophy on left ventricular systolic function in systemic hypertension (the Losartan Intervention For End-point (LIFE) Study).

Wachtell K, Rokkedal J, Bella JN, *et al. Am J Cardiol* 2001; **87**(1): 54–60.

BACKGROUND. LV ejection fraction is normal in most patients with uncomplicated hypertension, but the prevalence and correlates of decreased LV systolic chamber and myocardial function, as assessed by midwall mechanics, in hypertensive patients identified as being at high risk by the presence of LV hypertrophy on the electrocardiogram has not been established.

INTERPRETATION. In hypertensive patients with electrocardiographic LV hypertrophy, impaired LV performance occurs most often, and is associated with greater LV mass and relative wall thickness and may contribute to the high rate of CV events.

Comment

A notable finding of this study is that when midwall shortening was used rather than the conventional chamber function to assess LV systolic performance, a high prevalence (26%) of subnormal systolic performance was identified in hypertensive patients with ECG LVH. In addition, impaired LV function was independently associated with high relative wall thickness and LV mass within this population. However, a causal relationship could not be proved. Furthermore, the direct clinical significance of such LV impairment in the studied population is yet to be clarified though indirect evidence indicates poorer prognosis. It should also be noted that depressed endocardial shortening is most common in patients with eccentric LV hypertrophy, whereas impaired midwall shortening is most prevalent in patients with concentric remodelling or hypertrophy. Such geometric–dependent variations in LV performance assessments in these patients prompts the need for standardization of the methods though midwall shortening seems to be the better choice.

Relation of left ventricular geometry and function to systemic haemodynamics in hypertension: the LIFE Study.
Bella JN, Wachtell K, Palmieri V, *et al. J Hypertension* 2001; **19**: 127–34.

B ackground. LV geometry stratifies risk in hypertension, but the relationship between LV geometry and systemic haemodynamic patterns in moderately severe hypertension has not been fully elucidated. The objective was to clarify the relationship of systemic haemodynamic to LV geometric patterns in patients with moderate hypertension and target organ damage.

Interpretation. In patients with moderate hypertension and ECG-LVH, the levels of stroke volume (SV) and pulse pressure (PP)/SV, are associated with, and may be stimuli to different LV geometric phenotypes.

Comment

This study represents the first comprehensive evaluation in a large series of middle-aged and elderly patients with, on average, moderate hypertension and target organ damage, of the spectrum of LV geometric patterns in relation to the level of systemic volume load, haemodynamics and LV midwall function. Of LIFE patients who underwent echo, 47% had eccentric hypertrophy and 24% had concentric hypertrophy. When hypertensive patients were grouped by LV geometric phenotype, there was a stepwise increase in prevalent coronary disease from 7–8% in those with normal LV geometry or concentric remodelling to 14–17% in those with LV hypertrophy. In addition, cerebrovascular disease was nearly twice as common in patients with abnormal LV geometry than with normal geometry. Reduced or elevated SV appears to play a role in determining which hypertensive patients develop concentric LV remodelling or eccentric hypertrophy. Variations among hypertensive subgroups in estimated arterial stiffness, but not in mean arterial pressure or peripheral resistance, suggest that factors influencing arterial stiffness may also contribute to determining LV geometric phenotypes. The therapeutic interventions with losartan and atenolol in the LIFE study will make it possible to determine whether induced changes in SV (e.g. increase due to bradycardia or to beta-blockade) have the expected effects on LV geometry.

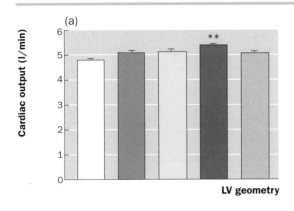

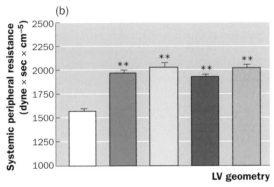

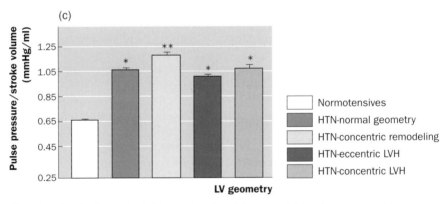

Fig. 10.5 (a) Cardiac output, (b) peripheral resistance and (c) pulse pressure/stroke volume in normotensive subjects and hypertensive patients with normal LV geometry, concentric remodelling, eccentric LVH and concentric LVH. Error bars indicate the mean and standard error of mean for each bar diagram. *$P < 0.05$ and **$P < 0.01$ *versus* the normotensive group. Source: Bella *et al.* (2001).

Ventricular and myocardial function following treatment of hypertension.

Aurigemma GP, Williams D, Gaasch WH, *et al. Am J Cardiol* 2001; **87**(6): 732–6.

BACKGROUND. Antihypertensive therapy has been associated with reductions in LV mass and changes in LV geometry. Most clinical studies of cardiac function before and after LV mass regression have used indexes of LV chamber function, none has performed an analysis of LV midwall mechanics.

INTERPRETATION. Reductions in LV mass associated with antihypertensive therapy are generally not accompanied by a decrement in LV chamber or myocardial function. Improvement in midwall shortening is more closely related to normalization of LV geometry than to reduction in LV mass.

Comment

The aim of this study was to investigate LV contractile function after treatment of hypertension, with an emphasis on midwall mechanics. LV mFS, in relation to stress, may be impaired in hypertensive patients with normal or supranormal LV ejection fraction (EF). The findings suggest that geometric remodelling preserves chamber indexes of function (endocardial shortening or EF) in the face of reduced myocardial shortening; the dissociation between chamber and myocardial indexes is directly related to RWT. Furthermore, improvement or deterioration in chamber or myocardial function was more closely related to changes in LV geometry than to changes in LV mass alone. In pressure overload hypertrophy or in subjects with high RWT, endocardial shortening may overestimate myocardial function. Moreover, previous studies have shown that depressed mFS predicts adverse outcome in hypertensive patients, especially in the subgroup with hypertrophy.

Effect of regression of left ventricular hypertrophy from systemic hypertension on systolic function assessed by midwall shortening (HOT echocardiographic study).

Zabalgoitia M, Rahman SN, Haley WE, *et al. Am J Cardiol* 2001; **88**(5): 521–5.

BACKGROUND. Depressed midwall shortening has been shown to be an independent predictor of CV morbid events in hypertensive patients with LVH despite normal endocardial fractional shortening. The effects of LV mass changes in hypertensive patients on midwall shortening are unclear.

INTERPRETATION. Midwall shortening is a more sensitive index of systolic function in subjects with pressure-overload hypertrophy, and it identifies high-risk patients who may benefit from a more aggressive antihypertensive programme. The disparity between midwall and endocardial shortening suggests reduced myofibril function in patients with hypertension-induced hypertrophy.

Comment

Hypercontractile LV systolic function measured at the endocardial level is frequently seen in patients with hypertensive LVH. Endocardial shortening merely reflects chamber dynamics whereas midwall shortening takes into consideration the non-uniform wall thickness (often seen in hypertensive LVH) and the wall volume (myocardial mass) i.e. LV geometry and hence may actually measuring the myocardial fibre shortening. This study assesses the impact of LVH regression on LV systolic function assessed at the endocardium and the midwall level in 508 patients with mild to moderate hypertension participating in the HOT study. Patients were prospectively studied by serial echo. From baseline to year 1, year 2, and end of the study, BMI was unchanged; however, diastolic BP (DBP) and systolic BP (SBP) as well as LVMI were significantly reduced. Over the same period of observation the endocardial fractional shortening did not change significantly; however, shortening at the midwall level showed improvement. The disparity observed confirms a reduced myocardial fibril shortening in hypertensive LVH and emphasizes the need to measure midwall shortening to unveil the beneficial mechanical impact of LVH regression.

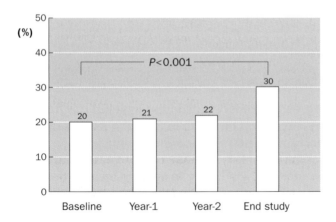

Fig. 10.6 Midwall fractional shortening improvement demonstrating a statistically significant improvement (*P* < 0.001) with time. Source: Zabalgoitia *et al.* (2001).

Relationship of the electrocardiographic strain pattern to left ventricular structure and function in hypertensive patients: the Losartan Intervention For End-point (LIFE) study.

Okin PM, Devereux RB, Nieminen MS, *et al.* J Am Coll Cardiol 2001; **38**(2): 514–20.

BACKGROUND. The classic ECG strain pattern, S-T segment depression and T-wave inversion, is a marker for LVH and adverse prognosis. However, the independence of the relation of strain to increased LV mass from its relation to coronary heart disease (CHD) has not been extensively examined.

INTERPRETATION. When clinical evidence of CHD is accounted for, ECG strain is likely to indicate the presence of anatomic LVH. Greater LV mass and higher prevalence of LVH in patients with strain offer insights into the known association of the strain pattern with adverse outcomes.

Comment

This study demonstrated that typical strain on the ECG in hypertensive patients identifies with greater LV mass, a higher prevalence of echocardiographic LVH that is more likely to be concentric, and lower myocardial contractility (as estimated by stress-corrected midwall shortening) and higher estimated myocardial oxygen demand, independent of the presence of clinically evident CHD and other demographic and clinical differences between patients with and without strain. The paper illustrated nicely the possible mechanisms of the abnormal repolarization of ECG strain. Future studies are needed to determine whether LVH regression is associated with reversal or reduction of the strain pattern, and whether serial evaluation of quantitative S-T segment and T-wave measurements will provide additional insight into this process.

However, the two conditions frequently co-exist. High pressure initially induces useful compensatory hypertrophy but later decompensation results in heart failure. Myocardial infarction may also play an important part in this decompensation.

Impact of coronary artery disease on left ventricular systolic function and geometry in hypertensive patients with left ventricular hypertrophy (the LIFE study).

Zabalgoitia M, Berning J, Koren MJ, *et al. Am J Cardiol* 2001; **88**(6): 646–50.

BACKGROUND. Hypertensive patients with LVH have a higher incidence of CV events than those without it. Coexistent clinical evidence of CAD and alterations in LV structure and function may contribute to their higher risk.

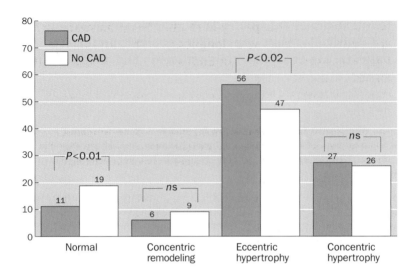

Fig. 10.7 Geometric distribution according to presence (dark grey bars) or absence (white bars) of CAD. The eccentric form of LV hypertrophy predominated over the other geometric forms. Moreover, the CAD group had a greater prevalence of eccentric hypertrophy than the non-CAD group, whereas the normal geometry pattern was seen more often in the non-CAD group. Source: Zabalgoitia *et al.* (2001).

INTERPRETATION. Clinical evidence of CAD in hypertensive patients with electrocardiographic evidence of LVH identifies subjects with structural and functional abnormalities at high risk for CV events. LV mass x circumferential end-systolic wall stress x ejection time, a non-invasive index that parallels myocardial oxygen demand per beat, is especially high in hypertensive patients with CAD.

Comment

The presence of LVH (especially concentric LVH) was associated with an attributable mortality risk greater than that of single and multivessel CAD or reduced LV ejection fraction. In the present study, eccentric LVH predominated in both groups but CAD group had a greater prevalence of eccentric LVH. Patients with CAD also had 80% higher LV mass and 20% higher LV wall stress, as a result, myocardial O_2 demand index was 1.2-fold higher than non-CAD group, and 2.15-fold greater than in normal adults. This may contribute to lower ischaemic threshold and thus increase frequency of morbid events. Follow-up of LIFE participants will provide important prognostic information.

Maximal exercise capacity is related to cardiovascular structure in patients with longstanding hypertension: a Losartan Intervention For End-point (LIFE) Reduction in Hypertension substudy.

Olsen MH, Wachtell K, Hermann KL, *et al. Am J Hypertens* 2001; **14**(12): 1205–10.

BACKGROUND. CV hypertrophy and remodelling in patients with never-treated hypertension has been associated with impaired exercise capacity, but whether this relationship remains in patients with longstanding hypertension and target organ damage is less elucidated.

INTERPRETATION. Patients with longstanding hypertension and target organ damage cannot achieve the predicted maximal workload. This impaired exercise capacity was associated with lower common carotid distensibility and lower oxygen reserve. The latter was independently related to LV hypertrophy, low systemic vascular compliance and peripheral vascular remodelling, suggesting that CV hypertrophy and remodelling might reduce exercise capacity by itself.

Comment

The study has demonstrated that patients with long-standing hypertension and electrocardiographic LV hypertrophy had impaired exercise capacity as they did not achieve the maximal workload predicted by age, gender and body composition. The impaired exercise capacity was related to lower common carotid distensibility. The strongest single correlate of impaired exercise capacity was low oxygen reserve, which was independently related to LV hypertrophy, low systemic vascular compliance and peripheral vascular remodelling. This suggests that CV hypertrophy and especially reduced vascular distensibility may by itself impair exercise capacity in patients with long-standing hypertension. It is well documented that antihypertensive treatment can improve exercise capacity, but it remains uncertain whether this improvement is due to either regression of CV remodelling, or merely due to the reduction in BP or both.

Blood pressure determinants of left ventricular wall thickness and mass index in hypertension: comparing office, ambulatory and exercise blood pressures.

Lim PO, Donnan PT, MacDonald TM. *J Hum Hypertens* 2001; **15**(9): 627–33.

BACKGROUND. LV mass relates positively and continuously to cardiac mortality and thus its regression is a rational therapeutic aim. Whilst the office BP relates poorly to

LV mass, it was unclear whether the 24-h ambulatory BP or the exercise SBP (ExSBP) was the stronger correlate of LV structural indices.

INTERPRETATION. Submaximal exercise BP measured at a workload comparable to physical activity encountered in daily life correlated more closely with the LV wall thickness and mass. The exercise BP should perhaps be normalized in hypertension management to optimize regression of LV hypertrophy.

Comment

The above findings are merely of scientific interest with little clinical relevance in the management of patients with hypertension because of its practicability. Furthermore, increased adrenosympathetic activations are a natural physiological response to exercise. It is unknown what BP level during exercise is considered abnormal and thus the need for treatment in order to optimize regression of LVH. Perhaps the associations of increased LV mass or hypertrophy with increased CV reactivity and isolated office ('white-coat') hypertension shown in other studies, and the ExSBP response seen in this study, are all related to a common pathogenesis pathway, secondary to chronic adrenosympathetic activations in these patients.

Ambulatory blood pressure monitoring

Introduction

Ambulatory blood pressure monitoring (ABPM) has become a widely used method of BP determination in clinical practice. Although the technique provides only intermittent readings throughout the 24-h period, average BPs obtained in this way are thought to be more representative of a patient's true BP (i.e. 'hypertensive load'). ABPM also reduces variability introduced by the observer such as digit preference, threshold avoidance and bias, and increases reproducibility. It has also been shown to correlate better with a variety of hypertensive end-organ damage indicators (parameters of LVH, microalbuminuria, retinal hypertensive changes), and is also a better prognostic marker for future CV events than office or clinic BP. Thus, a 24-h BP profile among hypertensive patients has allowed more detailed and accurate risk stratification as well as monitoring treatment.

Furthermore, ABPM has proved uniquely successful in distinguishing between true hypertension and 'white coat' hypertension. It has also established the important pathophysiological differences between normal nocturnal drop of BP (dippers) and those who exhibit a blunted fall in nocturnal BP (non-dippers). Notably, ABPM is increasingly used in newer drug therapy trials to evaluate the CV outcomes related to antihypertensive treatment. This has substantially reduced the risk of measuring a placebo effect, since patients without true persistent hypertension can be excluded during diagnostic procedures undertaken at study entry.

Indeed, the use of home (self-measured) BP, along with ABPM, has been recommended in the WHO/ISH guidelines as well as the Joint National Committee on

Table 10.1 The proposed limits of normal and elevated ambulatory BP

Parameter	Normotension	Hypertension
24-hour BP (mmHg)	< = 130/80	>135/85
Daytime BP (mmHg)	< = 135/85	>140/90
Night-time BP (mmHg)	< = 120/70	>125/75

BP=blood pressure

Source: Staessen *et al.* |**2**|.

Detection, Evaluation, and Treatment of High Blood Pressure (JNC) VI, as a complement to measurements in the clinic.

Although the use of ABPM is widespread, there has not been a consensus on the cut-off levels for diagnosing ambulatory hypertension that should be indicative for treatment. Many studies have been performed in selected tertiary centres and are therefore less representative of the general hypertensive population. In the past, large patient groups or convenient samples of normotensive and hypertensive patients were studied, and arbitrary cut-offs of the 90th or 95th percentile were chosen as the limit of normal BP. A summary of these data led to the suggestion of thresholds for defining ambulatory BP (Table 10.1). Ideally, such decisions should be based on outcome data or, at a minimum, on surrogate markers of hypertension damage.

Is resistant hypertension really resistant?

Brown MA, Buddle ML, Martin A. *Am J Hypertens* 2001; **14**(12): 1263–9.

BACKGROUND. Managing resistant hypertension is difficult and mostly involves expensive testing seeking an underlying secondary cause. This study was undertaken to determine 1. the extent of the white-coat phenomenon in patients with resistant hypertension, and 2. whether 24-h ABPM or having BP recorded by a nurse instead of the referring doctor could clarify how many apparently resistant hypertensives actually have controlled BP.

INTERPRETATION. The results show that approximately one in four patients with apparent resistant hypertension referred for ABPM have controlled BP and one-third of patients referred for initial evaluation of office or clinic hypertension have normal BP using ABPM, i.e. white-coat hypertension. Twenty-four-hour ABPM appears an appropriate initial step before further investigating or treating patients with apparently resistant hypertension.

Comment

Some 10% of hypertensive patients appear resistant to combinations of antihypertensive drugs, prompting referral for specialist care. Only about 10% of these patients are found to have a treatable secondary cause. Clearly defining patients with truly resistant hypertension, by excluding those with controlled BP in their usual environment, would reduce the considerable expense and inconvenience of investigations and adjustments to therapy for these patients.

This study confirms earlier studies that the prevalence of white coat hypertension is approximately 20% to 30% in patients with isolated office or clinic hypertension taking no antihypertensive drugs. For those taking antihypertensive medications, particularly those with apparent resistant hypertension (BP ≥140/ 90 mmHg despite taking at least three antihypertensive drugs in combination), 20% to 30% of patients referred for ABPM in fact have normal BP. On the assumption that this group has a better clinical outcome than those with true resistant hypertension, a hypothesis has yet to be tested formally. An important point in this small study was that increasing the number of antihypertensive drugs in those with apparent resistant hypertension did not influence the magnitude of the white coat effect. This highlights the clinical difficulties in treating such patients as their clinic or office BPs remain elevated despite increasing their antihypertensive drugs. On the other hand, this is a large study that reflects clinicians' patterns of use of 24-h ABPM to assess their patients with persistent or resistant hypertension. Considering the high cost of investigations and treatments for secondary causes of hypertension, ABPM would seem a sensible initial investigation in patients with apparent resistant hypertension.

The use of ambulatory blood pressure monitoring in managing hypertension according to different treatment guidelines.

Addison C, Varney S, Coats A. *J Hum Hypertens* 2001; **15**(8): 535–8.

BACKGROUND. Twenty-four-hour ABPM is thought to be more representative of a patient's true BP and is more reproducible than office BP measurements. It is also more closely related to the incidence of CV events and prevalence of end organ damage. Although ABPM has been in widespread use there has not been a consensus on the levels that should be used as guidelines for treatment.

INTERPRETATION. These results illustrate how patient management may differ markedly when treating in accordance either with the British Hypertension Society (BHS) guidelines for clinic readings or the suggested levels for ABP. More patients had abnormal BP levels according to ABPM, even though it is superior in detecting WCE and WCH. Clear guidelines for ABPM treatment levels need to be established.

Comment

This study investigated the use of ABPM in the management of hypertension in clinical practice and has illustrated the importance of introducing standardised ABPM treatment guidelines given the lack of consensus on the levels of normality of ABP and the disparities in recognising its prognostic value. The study clearly showed a disparity between the recommended guidelines for definite treatment between clinic and ABP, which is a difference of 20 mmHg SBP and 10 mmHg DBP. It also appears that if ABPM is performed it results in more patients being treated if O'Brien's (daytime ABP of ≥140 and/or 90 being probably abnormal and BP ≤135/85 probably normal) guidelines |3| are used (Table 10.3). As pointed out, we await with great interest the publication of the new guidelines from the BHS (how will they differ from the WHO/ISH guidelines?) and hope that ABPM thresholds are not ignored.

Table 10.2 Data split according to definitions

	Hypertension/ uncontrolled hypertension	Borderline between groups	Normal/well controlled BP
Clinical readings (BHS guidelines)	≥ 160 and/or ≥ 100 mmHg 722 (46%)	509 (33%)	≤ 139 and/or ≤ 89 mmHg 326 (21%)
Daytime ABPM lebels (O'Brien)	≥ 140 and/or ≥ 90 mmHg 1031 (67%)	190 (12%)	≤ 134 and/or ≤ 84 mmHg 336 (21%)

Source: Addison *et al.* (2001).

Table 10.3 Patients divided by treatment levels, according to their ABPM readings and clinic readings

ABP Clinic	Treatment or Increase in medication (≥ 140/90 mmHg)	Possible treatment (borderline)	No treatment/ no change in treatment (≤ 135/85 mmHg)	Total
Definite treatment or increase in medication (≥ 160/100 mmHg)	641	38	43	722
Possible treatment (borderline) (140–160/90–99 mmHg)	312	90	107	509
No treatment/no change in treatment (≤ 139/89 mmHg)	78	62	186	326
Total	1031	190	336	1557

Source: Addison *et al.* (2001).

Reproducibility of ambulatory blood pressure measurements in essential hypertension.

Zakopoulos NA, Nanas SN, Lekakis JP, *et al. Blood Press Monit* 2001; **6**(1): 41–5.

BACKGROUND. Data on the reproducibility of serial measurements of ambulatory BP in hypertensive patients are lacking. The purpose of this study was to examine 1. the reproducibility of four consecutive ambulatory BP measurements, and 2. the reproducibility of nocturnal falls in BP in hypertensive patients.

INTERPRETATION. Hourly SBP, DBP, heart rate, and nocturnal fall in BP were reproducible in four ambulatory BP monitorings recorded over 4 months. These findings suggest that ABPM is a reliable tool to monitor BP changes.

Comment

This study basically demonstrated the reliability of 24-h ABPM in clinical practice. In most studies the reproducibility of systolic and diastolic systemic BP was examined from two separate recordings. This study is unique in that it examined the reproducibility of hourly SBP and DBP, heart rate and of the nocturnal fall in BP by comparing four consecutive 24-h ABPMs recorded at 4-week intervals. A day/night difference in mean SBP and in mean DBP defined the nocturnal fall in BP. Twenty patients with mild to moderate essential hypertension were studied. The results were impressive: all measurements were highly reproducible during all periods of the recordings, whether over the entire 24 hours, during daytime, during night-times, even at one-hour intervals. Overall, the value of this method of determining BP resides in its ability to define accurately whole-day BP, including circadian fluctuations and differences between daytime and night-time BP values – important considerations when evaluating the efficacy of antihypertensive agents.

Home monitoring service improves mean arterial pressure in patients with essential hypertension: a randomized, controlled trial.

Rogers MA, Small D, Buchan DA, *et al. Ann Intern Med* 2001; **134**(11): 1024–32.

BACKGROUND. Technological advances in the distribution of information have opened new avenues for patient care. Few trials, however, have used telemedicine to improve BP in patients with essential hypertension.

INTERPRETATION. This telecommunication service was efficacious in reducing the mean arterial pressure of patients with established essential hypertension.

Comment

Home BP monitoring has become popular in clinical practice and several auto-mated devices for home BP measurements are now recommendable. Home BP is generally similar to daytime ambulatory BP but is lower than clinic or office BP as it eliminates the 'white coat' effect associated with office or clinic BP. The general trend in the literature suggests home BP monitoring may also improve compliance and BP control. This may well be a combined result of psychological factors, such as the feeling of being involved and reassurance by frequent measurements, thus paying closer attention to BP levels.

This is an interesting and innovative randomized controlled trial to determine the efficacy of a telecommunication service in reducing BP. The sample included 121 adults with essential hypertension under evaluation for a change in antihypertensive therapy either by usual care or home service consisting of automatic transmission of BP data over telephone lines, computerised conversion of the information into report forms, and weekly electronic transmission of the report forms to physicians and patients. Both groups had 24-h ABPM at baseline and exit. The results seem impressive: BP decreased in patients who used the service, while hypertension worsened in patients receiving usual care. The results were similar regardless of whether pressure was measured by a change in mean 24-h ABPM readings or by the percentage of BP readings above the target levels. Interestingly, it appears that African-American patients gained much better BP control from the service, mean arterial pressure (MAP) decreased by almost 10 mmHg in those receiving home service but increased by more than 5 mmHg in those receiving usual care.

Thus, the use of such technology in this population should be investigated further with a larger sample size, particularly since hypertension is considerably more prevalent in African-American patients. It is of note that the beneficial effect of home service was due in part to more frequent changes in type or dose of anti-hypertensive medications and possibly also due to better-motivated patients as well as physicians such that the 'service' rather than the 'technology' may account for the improvements. Unfortunately, the authors made no explanations on why patients who received usual care deteriorated from baseline BP levels, which is really surprising given the fact that most patients would at least improve simply by participating in a clinical study. Furthermore, the underlying reason(s) may invalidate the study's conclusion.

Association between albumin:creatinine ratio and 24-hour ambulatory blood pressure in essential hypertension.

Boulatov VA, Stenehjem A, Os I. *Am J Hypertens* 2001; **14**(4 Pt 1): 338–44.

BACKGROUND. Microalbuminuria is often found in essential hypertension (EH) and represents a sign of renal and CV damage. The present study aimed to look at the association between ambulatory BP and urinary albumin excretion (UAE).

INTERPRETATION. The threshold level of albumin:creatinine ratio (ACR) ≥ 3.0 mg/mmol currently used to define microalbuminuria may be not applicable to EH. Instead, a threshold level of ACR ≥ 1. 5 mg/mmol may be more appropriate.

Comment

Several studies have shown a positive correlation between UAE and office BP levels in hypertensive and normotensive individuals. However, a better relationship between the BP and UAE is observed when 24-h ABPM is used instead of office BP recordings. A positive correlation has been shown between 24-h, daytime, night-time SBP and DBP and UAE, as well as altered circadian BP profile in microalbuminuric patients. Despite an increased interest in the significance of microalbuminuria and EH, the methods used for the evaluation of UAE, and the threshold level of significant UAE remains debatable.

This study has shown that ACR measured in a single morning urine sample correlated with 24-h, daytime, and night-time SBP and DBP in hypertensive patients. All ABPM parameters were lower in subjects with normal albumin (ACR < 1.5 mg/mmol) excretion than in patients with borderline (1.5 ≤ ACR <3.0 mg/mmol) and overt microalbuminuria (ACR ≥3.0 mg/mmol). On the other hand, BP did not differ between the two microalbuminuric groups. The results obtained on the entire study population ($n = 140$) were further confirmed on selected patients with newly diagnosed untreated borderline to moderate hypertension. A close relationship between ABPM and ACR in the normoalbuminuric and borderline microalbuminuric range could mean that elevated UAE already exists in the early stages of essential hypertension, probably reflecting the functional alterations in renal haemodynamics.

Thus, it seems that that the threshold levels of ACR ≥ 3.0 mg/mmol currently used to define microalbuminuria may not be applicable to hypertension. More importantly, the mechanisms underlying the observed predictive role of ACR with regard to CV morbidity needs further clarification.

Relationships between 24-h blood pressure load and target organ damage in patients with mild-to-moderate essential hypertension.

Mule G, Nardi E, Andronico G, *et al. Blood Press Monit* 2001; **6**(3): 115–23.

BACKGROUND. To analyse the relationships between 24-h BP load (the percentage of SBP/DBPs exceeding 140/90 mmHg while awake and 120/80 mmHg during sleep) and some indices of hypertensive target organ involvement, independently of the mean level of 24-h BP.

INTERPRETATION. In mild-to-moderate arterial hypertension, a high 24-h SBP load may be associated, independently of the average level of 24-h systolic ambulatory BP, with an adverse CV risk profile.

Comment

In this study, 130 patients with mild-to-moderate hypertension underwent 24-h ABPM, ocular fundus examination, microalbuminuria assay and two-dimensional guided M-mode echocardiography. The study population was divided into subsets according to the systolic and diastolic 24-h BP load values predicted from the regression equation relating 24-h BP load to 24-h mean BP. The subjects with an observed load above this predicted value were included in the higher BP load groups, the remaining ones being included in the lower groups.

The study demonstrated that subjects with a higher SBP load had greater relative myocardial wall thickness and total peripheral resistance and lower mid-wall fractional shortening, end-systolic stress-corrected mid-wall fractional shortening and cardiac index. Moreover, the stroke index:pulse pressure ratio was reduced, and a greater prevalence of hypertensive retinopathy was observed in the higher systolic load group. On the contrary, no statistically significant difference was found for any of the cardiac, renal and funduscopic parameters examined when the two groups with a higher and lower 24-h DBP load were compared. Thus, 24-h SBP load related better to target organ damage than did 24-h DBP.

Left ventricular mass assessed by electrocardiography and albumin excretion rate as a continuum in untreated essential hypertension.
Bulatov VA, Stenehjem A, Os I. *J Hypertens* 2001; **19**(8): 1473–8.

BACKGROUND. To study an association between albumin excretion rate and left ventricular mass (LVM) determined by electrocardiogram-based criteria, and with respect to ambulatory BP, in patients with newly diagnosed and never-treated essential hypertension.

INTERPRETATION. The present findings show a continuous relationship between albumin excretion rate, LVM and ambulatory BP in newly diagnosed patients with essential hypertension, and suggest the occurrence of early effects on target organs (kidneys and heart). These associations were observed using easily applicable methods such as ECG monitoring and determination of the ACR in morning urine samples.

Comment

This is another study demonstrating the use of 24-h ABPM to assess the relationship between BP load and end-organ damage, in this case, albuminuria and increased LV mass.

The importance of 24-h blood pressure control.
Neutel JM. *Blood Press Monit* 2001; **6**: 9–16.

BACKGROUND. Two key areas are the development of antihypertensive therapies that enhance compliance through once-daily dosing and reduce BP consistently and smoothly throughout the dosing interval. In conjunction with these developments are changes in how drug therapy is assessed in clinical trials. The availability of ABPM provides a more detailed and accurate assessment of the effects of antihypertensive medications.

INTERPRETATION. Using the calculated trough:peak ratio, it has been found that agents with a ratio 0.50 are better able to control BP over the full 24 h while maintaining natural circadian patterns. ABPM studies assessing a recently introduced class of antihypertensive drugs, the angiotensin receptor blockers, have demonstrated 24-h efficacy with once-daily dosing, particularly with the newer agents.

Comment

Using ABPM, significant differences have been uncovered in how once-daily medications affect BP over the entire 24-h dosing interval. Additional insights into the CV risks associated with high BP loads and BP variability have also been provided. The introduction of the trough:peak ratio has allowed clinicians to evaluate the consistency and smoothness of the BP response to antihypertensive drug therapy.

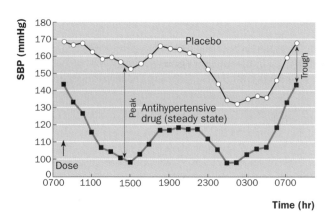

Time (hr)

Fig. 10.8 Fundamental approach to calculating the trough:peak ratio in an individual patient, showing how the time of the peak response is identified. The SBP measured following drug treatment (steady state) is subtracted from the SBP measured following placebo treatment in order to calculate the peak and trough responses. Source: Adapted with permission from Elliott HL. |**4**|

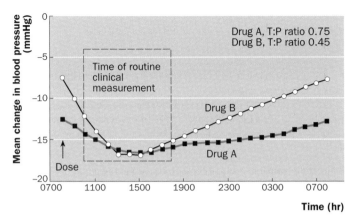

Fig. 10.9 Differences between drugs with different trough:peak ratios in providing 24-h BP control. Source: Adapted with permission from Elliott HL. |5|

This ratio describes the difference between a drug's effect at the end of the dosing interval (trough) and at the time of maximal effects (peak), usually seen a few hours after dosing. The ideal antihypertensive agent should provide drug effects that are smooth and consistent over 24 h to reduce BP variability. This is particularly important to ensure adequate reduction of total BP load and adequate coverage during the vulnerable early morning hours (typically the last 4–6 h of the dosing interval).

Microalbuminuria in hypertension

Introduction

Microalbuminuria is often found in essential hypertension and represents a sign of renal and CV complications and progression of disease i.e. a sign of end-organ damage. It is also a reliable marker of initial diabetic nephropathy, predicts the onset of overt proteinuria and the progression to chronic renal failure in both types of diabetes mellitus. Microalbuminuria has been shown to correlate with the presence of nephrosclerosis, while the presence of proteinuria generally indicates the existence of established renal parenchymatous damage. The prevalence of microalbuminuria varies greatly from one study to another ranging between 5% and 40%, dependent on the population characteristics, methods used and threshold levels.

Several studies have shown a positive correlation between various blood pressure components: 24-h, daytime, night-time SBP and DBP and UAE, as well as altered circadian blood pressure profile in microalbuminuric patients. Such

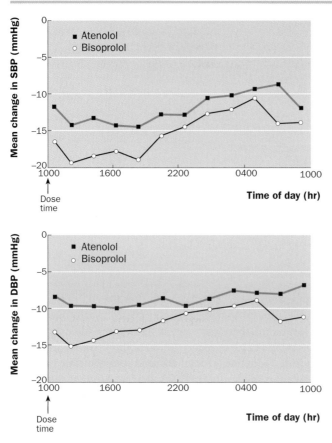

Fig. 10.10 Mean changes from baseline to end of treatment in 24-h ambulatory SBP and DBP in 96 patients treated with once-daily atenolol and 107 patients treated with once-daily bisoprolol. Although there was no difference in office BPs, bisoprolol produced significant reductions in SBP and DBP compared with atenolol during the day ($P < 0.05$ for 0600 h to 2200 h interval) and during the last 4 h of the dosing interval ($P < 0.05$ for 0600 h to 2200 h interval). Adapted from Neutel *et al.* |**6**|

relationship has been well documented with the advent of 24-h ambulatory BP monitoring. The relationship between increased urinary albumin excretion and major CV risk factors is also well recognised, even in those without clinical evidence of renal or CV disease. Indeed, non-diabetic hypertensive subjects with microalbuminuria are more likely to have dyslipidaemia, insulin resistance, be overweight, have increased serum uric acid levels and salt sensitivity. Microalbuminuria has been reported as an important and independent predictor for CV morbidity and mortality. Patients with raised UAE are more likely to demonstrate increased LVMI and LVH, thicker carotid plaque, pronounced atherosclerosis, and retinal vascular changes. Hence, there are important implications for the early identification and treatment of individuals at risk.

Table 10.4 Cardiovascular risk factors that cluster with microalbuminuria

Central obesity
Insulin resistance
Low HDL cholesterol levels
High triglyceride levels
Systolic hypertension
Absent nocturnal drop in blood pressure
Salt sensitivity
Male sex
Increased cardiovascular oxidative stress
Impaired endothelial function
Abnormal coagulation/fibrinolytic profiles

Source: Sowers *et al.* (2001).

Microalbuminuria in hypertensive patients with electrocardiographic left ventricular hypertrophy: the LIFE Study.
Wachtell K, Olsen MH, Dahlof B, *et al. J Hypertens* 2002; **20**(3): 405–12.

BACKGROUND. LV hypertrophy and albuminuria have both been shown to predict increased CV morbidity and mortality. However, the relationship between these markers of cardiac and renal glomerular damage has not been evaluated in a large hypertensive population with target organ damage. The present study was undertaken to determine whether albuminuria is associated with persistent ECG LVH, independent of established risk factors for cardiac hypertrophy, in a large hypertensive population with LVH who were free of overt renal failure.

INTERPRETATION. In patients with moderately severe hypertension, LVH on two consecutive ECGs is associated with increased prevalence of micro- and macroalbuminuria compared to patients without persistent ECG LVH. High albumin excretion was related to LVH independent of age, BP, diabetes, race, serum creatinine or smoking, suggesting parallel cardiac damage and albuminuria.

Comment

In this study, renal glomerular permeability was evaluated by urine albumin/creatinine (UACR, mg/mmol). Microalbuminuria was present if UACR > 3.5 mg/mmol and macroalbuminuria if UACR > 35 mg/mmol. The results showed that UACR was positively related to Sokolow–Lyon voltage criteria and Cornell voltage-duration product criteria. In multiple regression analysis, higher UACR was independently associated with older age, diabetes, higher BP, serum creatinine, smoking and LVH. ECG LVH was associated with a 1.6-fold increased prevalence of microalbuminuria and a 2.6-fold increased risk of macroalbuminuria compared to no LVH on the second ECG.

Microalbuminuria, central adiposity and hypertension in the non-diabetic urban population of the MONICA Augsburg survey 1994/95.

Liese AD, Hense HW, Doring A, Stieber J, Keil U. *J Hum Hypertens* 2001; **15**(11): 799–804.

BACKGROUND. **Microalbuminuria is a renal marker of general vascular endothelial damage and early atherosclerosis with adverse prognostic implications. Microalbuminuria is associated with diabetes, insulin resistance, central adiposity and hypertension.**

INTERPRETATION. Signs of early endothelial dysfunction manifested as microalbuminuria are strongly and independently associated with central adiposity and should be considered in the context of the metabolic or insulin resistance syndrome.

Comment

This study evaluated the degree of the association of components of the metabolic syndrome with microalbuminuria in a subsample of a non-diabetic study population. As part of the well-known MONICA population-based project with well-defined criteria, this study showed a graded, positive increase in prevalence of microalbuminuria across quintiles of waist-to-hip in both non-hypertensive and hypertensive men and women, but the microalbuminuria was uniformly higher among hypertensives. The study also revealed an independent association between microalbuminuria with central adiposity and hypertension.

The impact of antihypertensive drug groups on urinary albumin excretion in a non-diabetic population.

Monster TB, Janssen WM, de Jong PE, de Jong-van den Berg LT; PREVEND Study Group. *Br J Clin Pharmacol* 2002; **53**(1): 31–6.

BACKGROUND. **Microalbuminuria (30–300 mg in 24 h) is recognized to be independently associated with renal and CV risk. Antihypertensives may lower microalbuminuria. This study is to investigate whether the use of different antihypertensive drug classes in general practice influences microalbuminuria as related to BP in non-diabetic subjects.**

INTERPRETATION. This study suggests a disadvantageous effect of dihydropyridine calcium channel blockers on microalbuminuria compared with other antihypertensive drug groups. Thus, if microalbuminuria is causally related to an increased risk for CV morbidity and mortality, dihydropyridines do not seem to be agents of choice to lower BP. Furthermore, the combination of renin–angiotensin system inhibition and diuretics seems to act synergistically.

Comment

Microalbuminuria can be found in diabetic populations (prevalence: 10–30%), in hypertensive populations (5–25%), but also in non-diabetic, non-hypertensive populations (5–10%). It has been shown in various clinical trials that different antihypertensive drug classes vary in their proteinuria- and microalbuminuria-lowering effects. Indeed, various meta-analyses have also revealed that the angiotensin-converting enzyme inhibitors (ACEIs) are superior to other antihypertensives in lowering proteinuria and also microalbuminuria. More, recently, angiotensin II (Ang II) antagonists have been found to be equally effective in this regard as the ACE inhibitors.

Using the PREVEND IT (Prevention of REnal and Vascular Endstage Disease Intervention Trial) cohort data consisting of 8592 non-diabetic subjects, aged 28–75 years in the Netherlands, Monster *et al.* demonstrated that microalbuminuria was significantly associated with the use of dihydropyridine calcium channel blockers (odds ratio: 1.76 [1.22–2.54]), but not with other antihypertensive drug groups. In addition, the linear regression line of the relationship between BP and (log) urinary albumin excretion was also significantly steeper ($P = 0.0047$) for users of calcium channel blockers, but not for other antihypertensives, compared with subjects using no antihypertensive. Conversely, users of a combination of renin–angiotensin system inhibitors and diuretics had a less steep regression line ($P = 0.037$). This indicated that the use of dihydropyridine CCBs is associated with an elevated urinary albumin excretion which is in agreement with the recently published African American Study of Kidney Disease and Hypertension (AASK) which showed a staggering increase of almost 60% in protein excretion in patients treated with amlodipine whereas ramipril appeared to decrease proteinuria by 20%.

However, in the study by Monster *et al.*, the data did not show the expected superiority of ACEIs and Ang II antagonists in protecting against microalbuminuria, unless combined with a diuretic. As pointed out, there can be two reasons for this lack of effect. First, if it was already known that subjects had microalbuminuria there was a higher chance that they would be prescribed an ACEI or Ang II antagonist. Secondly, the lack of superiority could be due to the fact that in general practice the albuminuria lowering effect of ACEI therapy is not visible in the long term.

Microalbumin measurement alone or calculation of the albumin/creatinine ratio for the screening of hypertension patients?

Derhaschnig U, Kittler H, Woisetschlager C, Bur A, Herkner H, Hirschl MM.
Nephrol Dial Transplant 2002; **17**(1): 81–5.

BACKGROUND. Spot urine sampling seems to be a reliable screening method for the detection of microalbuminuria in hypertensive patients. It remains unclear whether microalbumin measurement alone or calculation of the ACR are more reliable for the detection of microalbuminuria in non-selected hypertensive patients.

INTERPRETATION. The ACR did not provide any advantage compared with microalbumin measurement alone, but requires an additional determination of creatinine and the use of gender-specific cut-off values. Therefore, measurement of microalbuminuria alone in the spot urine sample is more convenient in daily clinical practice and should be used as the screening method for hypertensive patients.

Comment

This study is interesting. Derhaschnig *et al.* compared the midstream spot urine sampling method for microalbuminuria with 24-h urinary collection method and examined the utility of the ACR in evaluating microalbuminuria in 264 hypertensive patients. Pathologic microalbuminuria was assumed when the microalbumin concentration exceeded 30 mg/l in the 24-h urine sample. They found no difference between the two methods in the measurement of microalbuminuria. The diagnostic performance expressed as area under the curve was 0.94 (95% confidence interval [CI] 0.90–0.98) for microalbumin measurement alone and 0.94 (95% CI 0.89–0.97) for ACR. The positive predictive value (PPV) and negative predictive value (NPV) were 44.2 and 97.9% for microalbumin measurement alone. ACR revealed a PPV of 29.3% and a NPV of 96.2% for males and 42.9 and 98% for females, if a cut-off value of 2.5 mg/mmol for males and of 4.0 mg/mmol for females was used.

References

1. Ganau A, Devereux RB, Roman MJ, de Simone G, Pickering TG, Saba PS, Vargiu P, Simongini I, Laragh JH. Patterns of left ventricular hypertrophy and geometric remodeling in essential hypertension. *J Am Coll Cardiol* 1992; **19**(7): 1550–8.

2. Staessen JA, O'Brien ET, Thijs L, *et al*. Modern approaches to BP measurement. *Occup Environ Med* 2000; **57**(8): 510–20.

3. O'Brien E, Owens P, Staessen JA, Imai Y, Kawasaki T, Kuwajima I. What are the normal levels for ambulatory blood pressure measurement? *Blood Press Monit* 1998; **3**(2): 131–2.

4. Elliott HL. Trough:peak ratio and 24-h blood pressure control. *J Hypertens* 1994; **12**(suppl 5): S29–S33.

5. Elliott HL. Benefits of 24-h blood pressure control. *J Hypertens* 1996; **14**(suppl 4): S15–S19.

6. Neutel JM, Smith DH, Ram CV, Kaplan NM, Papademetriou V, Fagan TC, Lefkowitz MP, Kazempour MK, Weber MA. Application of ambulatory blood pressure monitoring in differentiating between antihypertensive agents. *Am J Med* 1993; **94**(2): 181–7.

11

Other issues

Hypertension and cancer

Introduction

Antihypertensive treatment has been convincingly shown to reduce morbidity and mortality from cardiovascular (CV) and cerebrovascular events. However, some trials failed to demonstrate a reduction in all-cause mortality, thus raising the possibility that non-vascular mortality from other causes, such as malignancy, might potentially be higher in treated hypertensive patients.

Indeed, for several years now, antihypertensive treatment or even hypertension *per se* has been linked to an increased risk of malignancy. In recent years, several mainly retrospective studies and case reports have shown inconsistent results on the risk of cancer in hypertensive patients being treated with different antihypertensive drugs. At some point or another, nearly all antihypertensive drugs have been insinuated of increasing the risk of cancer. Some studies even found an association between hypertension and increased carcinogenesis. Certainly for calcium channel blockers (CCBs), beta-blockers and alpha-blockers, the available evidence seems to favour a neutral effect on cancer development and death rate. For angiotensin-converting enzyme inhibitors (ACEIs), the overall data suggest a similar neutral effect on cancer, and possibly, a small cancer protective effect. Perhaps the strongest evidence in favour of a link, although probably weak, between cancer and antihypertensive drugs is with the diuretics.

 Relation between drug treatment and cancer in hypertensives in the Swedish Trial in Old Patients with Hypertension 2: a 5-year, prospective, randomized, controlled trial.
Lindholm LH, Anderson H, Ekbom T, *et al. Lancet* 2001; **358**(9281): 539–44.

BACKGROUND. Is cancer related to hypertension and blood pressure (BP)? Do antihypertensive drugs promote cancer? Do antihypertensive drugs protect against cancer? We previously analysed the frequency of cardiovascular mortality and morbidity in elderly people who participated in the Swedish Trial in Old Patients with Hypertension 2 (STOP-Hypertension-2). We have also looked at the frequency of cancer in these patients.

INTERPRETATION. No difference in cancer risk was seen between patients randomly assigned to conventional drugs, calcium antagonists, or ACEIs. Thus, the general message to the practising physician is that more attention should be given to getting the BP down than to the risk of cancer.

Comment

The above retrospective study of cancer rates in the 5-year STOP-Hypertension-2 has shown no link between antihypertensive therapy and the risk of cancer. The STOP-Hypertension-2 cohort consists of 6614 elderly hypertensive men and women who were randomly assigned to 1 of 3 antihypertensive drug regimens: beta-blockers or diuretics; ACEIs; or calcium antagonists and followed for 5 years. The treated cohort developed 625 cases of cancer – very close to the incidence expected from the general Swedish population (standard incidence ratio [SIR] = 0.96). Analysis of the cancer rate by patient sex, by cancer type, and by time from randomization, did not reveal any significant deviation from the expected rate. The incidence of cancer was similar between treatment arms, and again did not differ from the general population (SIRs 0.92–0.99).

Antihypertensive therapy and cancer risk.
Felmeden DC, Lip GYH. *Drug Saf* 2001; **24**(10): 727–39.

BACKGROUND. The aim of this article is to provide an overview of the available data linking antihypertensive drug therapy to cancer risk. In recent years, a number of mainly retrospective studies have reached different conclusions on the risk of cancer in patients with hypertension being treated with different antihypertensive drugs. At some point or another, nearly all antihypertensive drugs have been suggested to increase the risk of cancer. Some studies have even found an association between hypertension itself and increased carcinogenesis. For calcium channel antagonists, beta-blockers and alpha-blockers, the available evidence seems to favour a neutral effect on cancer development and death rate. For ACEIs, the overall data suggest a similar neutral effect on cancer or, possibly, a small protective effect. Perhaps the strongest evidence in favour of a link, although probably weak, between cancer and antihypertensive drugs is with the diuretics.

INTERPRETATION. Until further solid data are available from prospective clinical trials, we suggest that the management of hypertension should continue according to current treatment guidelines with little fear of any substantial cancer risk.

Comment

The debate over the relationship between hypertension and cancer, and whether use of antihypertensive drugs affects a patient's risk of cancer has been going on for a long time. Several mainly retrospective studies and subgroup analyses have reported an increase in cancer risk associated with diuretics, beta-blockers, calcium antagonists, and even ACEIs. In contrast, one study from the Glasgow Blood Pressure clinic has suggested that ACEIs confer protection against malignancy.

Serum uric acid levels and cardiovascular risk

Introduction

The role of uric acid as an independent risk factor in the development of coronary heart disease (CHD) has been subject to considerable debate as serum urate is related to many of the established aetiological risk factors for CV disease that could confound the observed association. Previous studies of an association between uric acid and CV mortality have shown conflicting results. Data from the First National Health and Nutrition Examination Survey (NHANES I) follow-up study from 1971 to 1987 showed that baseline uric acid concentrations were an independent marker of ischaemic heart disease death but only in women. However, a recent analysis of Framingham Heart Study data found no association.

A number of epidemiological and clinical studies have shown a significant association between hyperuricaemia and hypertension. These findings in patients with essential hypertension may reflect early renal vascular involvement from hypertensive disease. But others have found elevated serum urate in the absence of significant clinical renal disease. More recent data suggested that raised serum urate may be an integral part of the cluster of risk factors associated with the insulin resistance syndrome.

Is serum uric acid a risk factor for coronary heart disease?
Wannamethee SG. *J Hum Hypertens* 1999; **13**(3): 153–6.

BACKGROUND. The role of uric acid as an independent risk factor in the development of CHD has been questioned as serum urate is related to many of the established aetiological risk factors for CV disease that could confound the observed association. This review assesses the role of elevated serum uric acid as an independent role for CHD.

INTERPRETATION. Raised serum urate is associated with many CV risk factors including hypertension, obesity, insulin resistance and hyperlipidaemia and established CHD. It also appears that raised serum urate may be an integral part of the cluster of risk factors associated with insulin resistance syndrome, particularly obesity and raised triglycerides. The evidence suggests that the influence of serum uric acid on CHD is probably explained by secondary associations of uric acid with other established etiological risk factors. The findings lend little support for an independent role of hyperuricaemia in the development of CHD.

Comment

This review provided an excellent summary of the controversial role of raised serum urate in the pathogenesis of CHD and its relationship with hypertension and hyperlipidaemia.

Serum uric acid and cardiovascular mortality: the National Health and Nutrition Examination Survey (NHANES) I epidemiologic follow-up study, 1971–1992.
Fang J, Alderman MH. *JAMA* 2000; **283**(18): 2404–10.

BACKGROUND. **Although many epidemiological studies have suggested that increased serum uric acid levels are a risk factor for CV mortality, this relationship remains uncertain.**

INTERPRETATION. The data suggest that increased serum uric acid levels are independently and significantly associated with risk of CV mortality.

Comment

Fang *et al.* report that raised levels of serum uric acid appear to be strongly associated with increased mortality, and this association holds for both men and women and blacks and whites. This analysis from an extension of the NHANES I follow-up from 1987 to 1992 found that serum uric acid levels bore a continuous, independent, specific, and significant positive relationship to CV mortality. This association was true for men and women as well as for blacks and whites. However, it was more robust among women and blacks than men and whites. In women, the association persisted through all levels of CV risk, regardless of diuretic use or menopausal status.

The differing results of this study and the Framingham analysis could be accounted for by differences in the populations studied. The homogeneous Framingham population was almost exclusively white, while NHANES was more heterogeneous, with 12.3% of the participants being black. Mortality rates were also much higher in the NHANES population, and CV mortality was twice as frequent as in the Framingham population.

Possible mechanisms that could underlie a causal association between uric acid and CV risk include accentuation of platelet aggregation and inflammation, and may also be implicated in the genesis of hypertension.

Hypertension and development

Introduction

There are two known important facts of hypertension development in humans: first, BPs rise with advancing age, and secondly, those individuals whose BP starts at a higher level tend to exhibit a faster age-related rise in pressure. This phenomenon of tracking is seen in all race and age groups, including infants. It implies that whatever the environmental factors influence BP, they exert their effect at a very early age. It is likely that an individual's susceptibility to environmental influences on higher BP development later in life is partly genetically determined. However, one interesting hypothesis has long been proposed to explain such early influence on human BP and later in life: the 'fetal origins hypothesis'. Put simply, the argument runs that poor nutrition *in utero* and in early life outside the womb programmes an infant to the risk, many years later, of CV problems. Indeed, a negative correlation between birth weight (excluding those with intrauterine growth retardation) and subsequent BP has been reported. The low birth weight may be related to poor socioeconomic and environmental conditions experienced by either infants or their mother during pregnancy. Accordingly, the hypothesis also follows that breast-feeding, which enhances the infant's natural nutritional supply may have a beneficial effect on childhood health and subsequent adult disease. The study reported by Atul Singhal *et al.* below showed that consumption of formula instead of human milk in infancy increases diastolic and mean arterial BP in later life.

Breast-feeding: primary prevention for hypertension?

Early nutrition in pre-term infants and later blood pressure: two cohorts after randomized trials.
Singhal A, Cole TJ, Lucas A. *Lancet* 2001; **357**: 413–19.

BACKGROUND. Despite data relating body size in early life to later CV outcomes, the hypothesis that nutrition affects such outcomes has not been established. Breast-feeding has been associated with lower BP in later life, but previous studies have not controlled for possible confounding factors by using a randomized design with prospective follow-up. This study designed to test the hypothesis that early diet programmes BP in later life in children randomly assigned different diets at birth.

INTERPRETATION. Breast milk consumption was associated with lower later BP in children born prematurely. The data provide experimental evidence of programming of a CV risk factor by early diet and further support the long-term beneficial effects of breast milk.

Comment

Two previous observational studies have shown a link between breast-feeding and lower BP in adulthood among those born at term. However, despite these data, a causal link between nutrition in early life and later outcomes could not be established by observational data alone. The present paper reported the first and would also probably be the last prospective randomized trial between human breast milk or breast-feeding and nutrient-enriched pre-term formula milk in premature born neonates. They tested the generic hypothesis that early nutrition influences later BP and the a *priori* specific hypothesis that consumption of human milk in infancy leads to lower BP in later life. The original cohort comprised 926 children. Of these, 216 (23%) were contacted between the ages of 13 and 16 years and BP measures taken. Mean arterial BP was significantly lower among the children assigned to receive banked breast milk (alone or in combination with mother's milk), than in the subjects assigned to pre-term formula. No significant difference was seen in the mean arterial pressure between those assigned to standard term formula and those receiving pre-term formula. Hence, it seems that just a month's worth of dietary manipulation has had an effect on a CV risk factor many years later. However, the results as they stand may not be generalizable to the full-term population, yet still provocative in light of the similar findings in full-term babies in the two observational studies.

Table 11.1 Mean arterial pressures at age 13–16 years among those assigned to two comparisons

End-point	Breast milk	Pre-term formula	P value	Term formula	Pre-term formula	P value
Mean arterial BP (mmHg)	81.9	86.1	0.001	85.5	84.5	0.51

Source: Singhal *et al.* (2001).

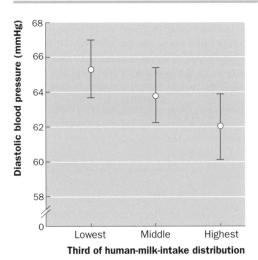

Fig. 11.1 Diastolic BP in thirds of proportional intake of human milk. Source: Singhal *et al.* (2001).

In addition to providing specific information relevant to the primary prevention of hypertension, this paper adds to the many publications reporting widespread effects of early nutritional state on later body composition, physiology and cognition. The difficulties lie in the impossibility of a randomized study and the frustration of having to wait 30 years plus for a truly prospective test.

Further reading

Part I Basic science

1. Joint National Committee on Detection, Evaluation and Treatment of High Blood Pressure. The Sixth Report of the Joint National Committee on Detection, Evaluation and Treatment of High Blood Pressure. *Arch Intern Med* 1997; **157**: 2413–46.

2. World Health Organization–International Society of Hypertension guidelines for the management of hypertension. *J Hypertens* 1999; **17**: 151–83.

3. Ramsay LE, Williams B, Johnston GD, MacGregor GA, Poston L, Potter JF, Poulter NR, Russell G. British Hypertension Society guidelines for hypertension management 1999: summary. *BMJ* 1999; **319**: 630–5.

4. Cushman WC. The clinical significance of systolic hypertension. *Am J Hypertens* 1998; **11**(pt 2): 182S–5S.

5. Silagy CA, McNeil JJ. Epidemiologic aspects of isolated systolic hypertension and implications for future research. *Am J Cardiol* 1992; **69**(3): 213–18.

6. Kaplan N. J-curve not burned off by Hypertension Optimal Treatment (HOT) study. *Lancet* 1998; **351**: 1748–9.

7. Hansson L, Lindholm LH, Ekbom T, Dahlöf B, Lanke J, Schersten B, Wester PO, Hedner T, de Faire U. Randomized trial of old and new antihypertensive drugs in elderly patients: cardiovascular morbidity and mortality; the Swedish Trial in Old Patients with Hypertension-2 Study. *Lancet* 1999; **354**: 1751–6.

8. Sever P. Abandoning diastole. *BMJ* 1999; **318**: 1773.

9. Domanski MJ, Davis BR, Pfeffer MA, Kastantin M, Mitchell GF. Isolated systolic hypertension: prognostic information provided by pulse pressure. *Hypertension* 1999; **34**: 375–80.

10. Stamler J, Stamler R, Neaton JD. Blood pressure, systolic and diastolic, and cardiovascular risks: US population data. *Arch Intern Med* 1993; **153**: 598–615.

11. Colhoun HM, Dong W, Poulter NR. Blood pressure screening, management and control in England: results from the health survey for England 1994. *J Hypertens* 1998; **16**: 747–52.

12. Hyman DJ, Paulik VN, Valbona C. Physician role in lack of awareness and control of hypertension. *J Clin Hypertens* 2000; **5**(2): 324–30.

13. Cushman WC. Alcohol consumption and hypertension. *J Clin Hypertens* 2001: **3**(3): 166–70.

14. Marmot MG, Elliott P, Shipley MJ, Dyer AR, Ueshima H, Beevers DG, Stamler R, Kesteloot H, Rose G, Stamler J. Alcohol and blood pressure: the INTERSALT study. *BMJ* 1994; **308**: 1263–7.

15. Weinberger MH. Salt sensitivity of blood pressure in humans. *Hypertension* 1996; **27** (pt 2): 481–90.

16. Bihorac A, Tezcan H, Ozener C, Oktay A, Akoglu E. Association between salt sensitivity and target organ damage in essential hypertension. *Am J Hypertens* 2000; **13**: 864–72.

Part II Hypertension and co-existing conditions

17. Kario K, Schwartz JE, Pickering TG. Ambulatory physical activity as a determinant of diurnal blood pressure variation. *Hypertension* 1999; **34**: 685–91.

18. Gifford RW, August PA, Cunningham G, *et al.* Report of the National High Blood Pressure Education Program Working Group on High Blood Pressure in Pregnancy. *Am J Obstet Gynecol* 2000; **183**: Sl–S22.

19. Lenfant C. Management of hypertension in pregnancy. *J Clin Hypertens* 2001: **3**(2): 71–2.

20. Seely EW. Hypertension in pregnancy: a potential window into long-term cardiovascular risk in women. *J Clin Endocrinol Metab* 1999; **84**: 1858–61.

21. Tight blood pressure control and risk of macrovascular and microvascular complications in type 2 diabetes: UK Prospective Diabetes Study Group (UKPDS) 38,. *BMJ* 1998; **317**: 703–13.

22. Effects of ramipril on cardiovascular and microvascular outcomes in people with diabetes mellitus: results of the HOPE study and MICRO-HOPE substudy. *Lancet* 2000; **355**: 253–59.

23. Ruggenenti P, Perna A, Gherardi G, Gaspari F, Benini R, Remuzzi G. Renoprotective properties of ACE-inhibition in non-diabetic nephropathies with non-nephrotic proteinuria. *Lancet* 1999; **354**: 359–64.

24. Haffner SM, Lehto S, Ronnemaa T, Pyorala K, Laakso M. Mortality from coronary heart disease in subjects with type 2 diabetes and in non-diabetic subjects with and without prior myocardial infarction. *N Engl J Med* 1998; **339**: 229–34.

25. Bakris GL, Williams M, Dworkin L, Elliott WJ, Epstein M, Toto R, Tuttle K, Douglas J, Hsueh W, Sowers J. Preserving renal function in adults with hypertension and diabetes: a consensus approach. National Kidney Foundation Hypertension and Diabetes Executive Committees Working Group. *Am J Kidney Dis* 2000; **36**(3): 646–61.

26. Giatras I, Lau J, Levey AS. Effect of angiotensin-converting enzyme inhibitors on the progression of non-diabetic renal disease: a meta-analysis of randomized trials. Angiotensin-Converting-Enzyme Inhibition and Progressive Renal Disease Study Group. *Ann Intern Med* 1997; **127**: 337–45.

27. Weber MA, Weir MR. Management of high-risk hypertensive patients with diabetes: potential role of angiotensin II receptor antagonists. *J Clin Hypertens* 2001; **3**: 225–35.

28. American Diabetes Association. Clinical practice recommendations 2000. *Diabetes Care* 2000; **23**(S1): S1–116.

Part III Therapy

29. Effect of antihypertensive drug treatment on cardiovascular outcomes in women and men. A meta-analysis of individual patient data from randomized, controlled trials. The INDANA Investigators. *Ann Intern Med* 1997; **126**: 761–7.

30. Mulrow C, Pignone M. What are the elements of good treatment for hypertension? in *Evidence-based hypertension*. London: BMJ Publishing Group 2001; 81–111.

31. Wright JM, Lee CH, Chambers GK. Systematic review of antihypertensive therapies. Does the evidence assist in choosing a first-line drug? *Can Med Assoc J* 1999; **161**: 25–32.

32. Davis BR, Cutler JA, Gordon DJ, Furberg CD, Wright JT, Cushman WC, Grimm RH, LaRosa J, Whelton PK, Perry HM, Alderman MH, Ford CE, Oparil S, Francis C,

Proschan M, Pressel S, Black HR, Hawkins M. Rationale and design for the Antihypertensive and Lipid Lowering Treatment to Prevent Heart Attack Trial (ALLHAT). *Am J Hypertens* 1996; **9**: 342–60.

33. MacMahon S, Neal B. Differences between blood-pressure-lowering drugs. *Lancet* 2000; **356**: 352–3.

34. Messerli FH, Grossman E. Beta-blockers and diuretics: to use or not to use. *Am J Hypertens* 1999; **12**(pt 1–2): 157S–163S.

35. Sica DA, Elliott WJ. Angiotensin-converting enzyme inhibitors and angiotensin receptor blockers in combination: theory and practice. *J Clin Hypertens* 2001; **3**(6): 383–7.

36. Elliott WJ. Therapeutic trials comparing angiotensin-converting enzyme inhibitors and angiotensin II receptor blockers. *Curr Hypertens Rep* 2000; **2**: 402–11.

37. Sica DA. Pharmacology and clinical efficacy of angiotensin-receptor blockers. *Am J Hypertens.* 2001; **14**: 242S–7S.

38. Ruggenenti P, Perna A, Gherardi G, Garini G, Zoccali C, Salvadori M, Scolari F, Schena FP, Remuzzi G. Renoprotective properties of ACE-inhibition in non-diabetic nephropathies with non-nephrotic proteinuria. *Lancet* 1999; **354**: 359–64.

39. Alderman MH, Cohen H, Roque R, Madhavan S. Effect of long-acting and short-acting calcium antagonists on cardiovascular outcomes in hypertensive patients. *Lancet* 1997; **349**: 594–8.

40. The Trials of Hypertension Prevention Collaborative Research Group. Effects of weight loss and sodium reduction intervention on blood pressure and hypertension incidence in overweight people with high-normal blood pressure. The Trials of Hypertension Prevention, Phase II. *Arch Intern Med* 1997; **157**: 657–67.

41. Serdula MK, Mokdad AH, Williamson DF, Galuska DA, Mendlein JM, Heath GW. Prevalence of attempting weight loss and strategies for controlling weight. *JAMA* 1999; **282**: 1353–8.

42. Appel LJ, Moore TJ, Obarzanek E, Vollmer WM, Svetkey LP, Sacks FM, Bray GA, Vogt TM, Cutler JA, Windhauser MM, Lin PH, Karanja N. A clinical trial of the effects of dietary patterns on blood pressure. DASH Collaborative Research Group. *N Engl J Med* 1997; **336**: 1117–24.

43. Maheswaran R, Beevers M, Beevers DG. Effectiveness of advice to reduce alcohol consumption in hypertensive patients. *Hypertension* 1992; **19**: 79–84.

44. Trials of Hypertension Prevention Collaborative Research Group. The effects of non-pharmacologic interventions on blood pressure of persons with high normal levels: results of the Trials of Hypertension Prevention, Phase I. *JAMA* 1992; **267**: 1213–20.

45. Trials of Hypertension Prevention Collaborative Research Group. Effects of weight loss, and sodium reduction intervention on blood pressure and hypertension incidence in overweight people with high-normal blood pressure: the Trials of Hypertension Prevention, Phase II. *Arch Intern Med* 1997; **157**: 657–67.

46. Whelton PK, Appel LJ, Espeland MA, Applegate WB, Ettinger WH Jr, Kostis JB, Kumanyika S, Lacy CR, Johnson KC, Folmar S, Cutler JA, for the TONE Collaborative Research Group. Sodium reduction and weight loss in the treatment of hypertension in older persons: a randomized controlled trial of non-pharmacologic interventions in the elderly (TONE). *JAMA* 1998; **279**: 839–46.

47. Ovik P. How smoking affects blood pressure. *Blood Pressure* 1996; **5**: 71–7.

Part IV Current practical issues

48. Laragh J. Laragh's lessons in pathophysiology and clinical pearls for treating hypertension. *Am J Hypertens* 2001; **14**: 84–9.

49. Benetos A, Rudnichi A, Safar M, Guize L. Pulse pressure and cardiovascular mortality in normotensive and hypertensive subjects. *Hypertension* 1998; **32**: 560–4.

50. Stergiopoulos N, Westerhof N. Determinants of pulse pressure. *Hypertension* 1998; **32**: 556–9.

51. Franklin SS, Khan SA, Wong ND, Larson MG, Levy D. Is pulse pressure useful in predicting risk for coronary heart disease? The Framingham heart study. *Circulation* 1999; **100**: 354–60.

52. Safar ME. Pulse pressure in essential hypertension: clinical and therapeutical implications. *J Hypertens* 1989; **7**: 769–76.

53. Franklin SS, Gustin W 4th, Wong ND, Larson MG, Weber MA, Kannel WB, Levy D. Hemodynamic patterns of age-related changes in blood pressure: the Framingham Heart Study. *Circulation* 1997; **96**: 308–15.

54. Blacher J, Asmar R, Djane S, London G, Safar M. Aortic pulse wave velocity as a marker of cardiovascular risk in hypertensive patients. *Hypertension* 1999; **33**: 1111–7.

55. Yudkin JS, Forrest RD, Jackson CA. Microalbuminuria as predictor of vascular disease in non-diabetic subjects. *Lancet* 1998; **2**: 530–3.

56. Luft FC, Agrawal B. Microalbuminuria as a predictive factor for cardiovascular events. *J Cardiovasc Pharmacol* 1999; **33**(S1): S11–S15.

57. Khattar RS, Swales JD, Banfield A, Dore C, Senior R, Lahiri A. Prediction of coronary and cerebrovascular morbidity and mortality by direct continuous ambulatory blood pressure monitoring in essential hypertension. *Circulation* 1999; **100**: 1071–6.

58. Verdecchia P. Prognostic value of ambulatory blood pressure: current evidence and clinical implications. *Hypertension* 2000; **35**: 844–51.

59. Staessen JA, Thijs L, Fagard R, O'Brien ET, Clement D, de Leeuw PW, Mancia G, Nachev C, Palatini P, Parati G, Tuomilehto J, Webster J. Predicting cardiovascular risk using conventional vs ambulatory blood pressure in older patients with systolic hypertension. *JAMA* 1999; **282**: 539–46.

60. Pickering TG, Kaplan NM, Krakoff L, Prisant LM, Sheps S, Weber MA, White WB, American Society of Hypertension Expert Panel. Conclusions and recommendations on the clinical use of home(self) and ambulatory blood pressure monitoring. *Am J Hypertens* 1996; **9**: 1–11.

61. Ward H. Uric acid as an independent risk factor in the treatment of hypertension. *Lancet* 1998; **352**: 670–1.

62. Culleton BF, Larson MG, Kannel WB, Levy D. Serum uric acid and risk for cardiovascular disease and death: the Framingham Heart Study. *Ann Intern Med* 1999; **131**: 7–13.

63. Pignone M, Mulrow CD. How do we best individualize treatment for patients based on their cardiovascular risk profile? in *Evidence-based hypertension*. London: BMJ Publishing Group 2001; 117-129.

List of abbreviations

11βHSD2	1β-hydroxysteroid dehydrogenase type 2	ARR	aldosterone–renin activity ratio
AASK	African-American Study of Kidney Disease	ASCOT	Anglo-Scandinavian Cardiac Outcomes Trial
AbnREL	abnormal relaxation	AT-1	angiotensin 1
ABP	ambulatory BP	AT1R	angiotensin 1 receptor
ABPM	ambulatory blood pressure monitoring	AT$_2$	angiotensin type 2
		ATP	adenosine triphosphate
ACE	angiotensin-converting enzyme	BHS	British Hypertension Society
		BLSA	Baltimore Longitudinal Study in Aging
ACEI	angiotensin-converting enzyme inhibitor	BMI	body mass index
ACR	albumin:creatinine ratio	BNP	brain natriuretic peptide
ACS	acute coronary syndrome	BP	blood pressure
ADA	American Diabetes Association	BPH	benign prostatic hyperplasia
		BPLT	Blood Pressure Lowering Treatment
ADVANCE	Action in Diabetes and Vascular disease – PreterAx and DiamicroN MR Controlled Evaluation	BRS	baroreceptor reflex sensitivity
		C	compliance
		CA	cardiac arrhythmia
AGE	advanced glycosylation end-product	CAD	coronary artery disease
		CAI	carotid amplification index
AGT	angiotensinogen	CALM	candesartan and lisinopril microalbuminuria
AHA	American Heart Association		
AIR	acetylcholine-induced relaxation	CANDLE	Candesartan versus Losartan Efficacy Comparison
ALLHAT	Antihypertensive and Lipid-Lowering treatment to prevent Heart Attack Trial	CAPPP	Captopril Prevention Project
		CB	centre-based
		CCB	calcium channel blocker
AMI	acute myocardial infarction	CHD	coronary heart disease
Ang	angiotensin	CHF	congestive heart failure
ANOVA	analysis of variance	CI	confidence interval
ANP	atrial natriuretic peptide	COER	controlled-onset extended release
APA	aldosterone-producing adenoma		
		CONVINCE	Controlled ONset Verapamil INvestigation of Cardiovascular End-points
ARA	ACEI and AT1R antagonists		
ARB	angiotensin receptor blocker		
ARIC	Atherosclerosis Risk in Communities Study	CrCl	creatinine clearance
		CRI	chronic renal insufficiency

CRP	C-reactive protein
CSDH	combined SDH
CT	computed tomography
CTA	computed tomography angiography
CV	cardiovascular
CVD	cardiovascular disease
DAE	due to adverse events
Dahl S	Dahl salt-sensitive hypertensive rat
DASH	Dietary Approaches to Stop Hypertension
DBP	diastolic blood pressure
DC	distensibility coefficient
DM	diabetes mellitus
ECG	electrocardiography
echo	echocardiography
ECTIM	Etude Cas-Témoin de l'Infarctus Myocarde
ED	erectile dysfunction
EF	ejection fraction
EH	essential hypertension
ELSA	European Lacidipine Study on Atherosclerosis
ER	extended release
ERA	Estrogen Replacement and Atherosclerosis
ERK	extracellular signal-related protein kinase
ESRD	end-stage renal disease
EST	exercise stress testing
ET	endothelin
ET-1	endothelin −1
ETT	exercise tolerance test
ExSBP	exercise systolic blood pressure
FA	Framingham Algorithm
FBF	forearm blood flow
FBPP	Family Blood Pressure Program
FCHL	familial combined hyperlipidaemia
FDH	familial dyslipidaemic hypertension
FFA	free fatty acids
FH	family history of hypertension
FRS	Framingham risk score

GENOA	Genetic Epidemiology Network of Atherosclerosis
GFR	glomerular filtration rate
GITS	gastrointestinal treatment system
GR	glucocorticoid receptors
HARVEST	Hypertension and Ambulatory REcording Venetia Study
HB	home-based
HCTZ	hydrochlorothiazide
HDL	high-density lipoprotein
HDL-C	high-density lipoprotein cholesterol
HERS	Heart and Estrogen-progestin Replacement Study
HF	heart failure
HHD	hypertensive heart disease
HHP	Honolulu Heart Program
HOMA	homeostasis model assessment
HOPE	Heart Outcomes Prevention Evaluation
HOT	Hypertension Optimal Treatment
HPS	Heart Protection Study
HR	heart rate
HRres	heart rate reserve
HRT	hormone replacement therapy
HTN	hypertension
HyperGEN	Hypertension Genetic Epidemiology Network
HYVET	Hypertension in the Very Elderly Trial
I	insertion
IDNT	Irbesartan Diabetic Nephropathy Trial
IHA	idiopathic hyperaldosteronism
IHH	isolated home hypertension
iLVH	inappropriate left ventricular hypertrophy
IM	intima media
IMPRESS	Inhibition of metalloprotease by BMS-186716 in a randomized exercise and symptoms study
IMT	intima-media thickness
INDANA	Individual Data Analysis of Antihypertension Intervention Trials

INSIGHT	Intervention as a Goal in Hypertension Treatment	MRC	Medical Research Council
INVEST	International Verapamil SR/Trandolapril	MRI	magnetic resonance imaging
IO	isolated office	MSNA	multiunit discharges
IOH	in-office hypertension	MWS	midwall shortening
IR	insulin resistance	n	number
IRMA	IRbesartan MicroAlbuminuria	NCEP	National Cholesterol Education Programs
ISH	isolated systolic hypertension	NE	norepinephrine
IVRT	isovolumic relaxation time	NEP	neutral endopeptidase
JNC VI	Sixth Joint National Committee on Prevention, Detection, Evaluation and Treatment of High Blood Pressure	NF-κB	nuclear factor-κB
		NHANES	National Health and Nutrition Examination Survey
		NHLBI	National Heart, Lung and Blood Institute
KIHD	Kuopio Ischaemic Heart Disease	NIDDM	non-insulin dependent diabetes mellitus
LBBB	left bundle branch block	NIH	National Institutes of Health
LDL	low-density lipoprotein	NKCC2	Na,K,2Cl-cotransporter
LIFE	Losartan Intervention For End-point Reduction in Hypertension	NN	normotensive non-pregnant
		NNT	number needed to treat
		NO	nitric oxide
L-NMMA	N(G)- monomethyl-L-arginine	NORDIL	Nordic Diltiazem
		NP	normal pregnancy
LV	left ventricular	NPV	negative predictive value
LVET	left ventricular rejection time	NT	normotensive
LVH	left ventricular hypertrophy	NX-NaC1	nephrectomy and high NaCl loading
LVM	left ventricular mass	NYHA	New York Heart Association
LVMI	left ventricular mass index	OBP	office BP
MAP	mean arterial pressure	OD/od	odds ratio
MARVAL	Microalbuminuria Reduction with Valsartan	OHyp	offspring of hypertensive parents
MBP	mean BP	ONorm	offspring of normal parents
mFS	midwall fractional shortening	OR	odds ratio
mg	milligrams	P	probability
MI	myocardial infarction	PA	primary aldersteronism
MIRACL	Myocardial Ischaemia Reduction with Aggressive Cholesterol Lowering	PAC	plasma aldersterone concentration
		PAD	peripheral arterial disease
MMSE	Mini Mental State Examination	PAF	population-attributable fraction
MONICA	Monitoring Trends and Determinants in Cardiovascular Diseases	PAI-1	plasminogen activator inhibitor 1
		PAMELA	Pressione Arteriose Monitorate E Loro Associazioni
MPA	medroxyprogesterone acetate		
MR	mineralocorticoid receptor		
MRA	magnetic resonance angiography	PAT	population-attributable fraction

PATS	Post-stroke Antihypertensive Treatment Study	SAPPHIRe	Stanford Asian Pacific Program in Hypertension and Insulin Resistance
PE	pre-eclampsia		
Per/Ind	Perindopril/Indapamide	SBP	systolic blood pressure
PHYLLIS	Plaque Hpertension Lipid Lowering Italian Study	SCI	silent cerebral infarcts
		SCOPE	Study on COgnitive and Prognosis in the Elderly
PIH	pregnancy-induced hypertension	SD	standard deviation
PP	pulse pressure	SDH	systolic diastolic hypertension
PPP	Primary Prevention Project	SECURE	Study to evaluate carotid ultrasound changes in patients treated with ramipril and vitamin E
PPV	positive predictive value		
PRA	plasma renin activity		
PRESERVE	Prospective Randomized Enalapril Study Evaluation Regresssion of Ventricular Enlargement		
		SEM	standard error of the mean
		SH	systemic hypertension
		Sham	sham-operation on a normal diet
PREVENT	Prospective Randomized Evaluation of the Vascular Effects of Norvasc Trial	SHARE-AP	Study of Health Assessment and Risk Evaluation in Aboriginal Peoples
PRIMe	PRogram for Irbestan Mortality and Morbidity Evaluations	SHEAF	Self-measurement of blood pressure at Home in the Elderly: Assessment and Follow-up
PROBE	Prospective Randomized Open Blinded End-Points		
PROGRESS	Perindopril pROtection aGainst REcurrent Stroke Study	SHEP	Systolic Hypertension in the Elderly
		SHR	spontaneously hypertensive rat
PVR	peripheral vascular resistance	SHRSP	spontaneously hypertensive rat – stroke prone
PWV	pulse wave velocity	SHS	Strong Heart Study
RAS	renin–angiotensin system	SIR	standard incidence ratio
RENAAL	Reduction of Endpoints in NIDDM with the Angiotensin II Antagonist Losartan	SL	Sokolow–Lyon voltage
		SPECT	single photon emission computed tomography imaging
RIA	radioimmunoassay		
RMANOVA	Repeated Measures Analysis of Variance	SR-SH	salt-resistant spontaneous hypertension
ROC	receiver-operating characteristic	SR-V	slow release - verapamil
		SSH	salt-sensitive hypertension
ROS	reactive oxygen period	SS-SH	salt-sensitive spontaneous hypertension
RR	relative risk		
RRR	relative risk reduction	STOP	Swedish Trial in Old Patients
RWT	relative wall thickness	SV	stroke volume
SAMPLE	Study on Ambulatory Monitoring of Blood Pressure and Lisinopril Evaluation	SWEAT	Sedentary Women Exercise Adherence Trial
		Syst-Eur	Systolic Hypertension in Europe

TC	total serum cholesterol	VALUE	Valsartam Antihypertensive Long-term Use Evaluation
TEMI	transient episodes of myocardial ischaemia	VEGF	vascular endothelial growth factor
TIA	transient ischaemic attack	VHAS	Verapamil in Hypertension
TOD	target organ damage		and Atherosclerosis Study
TOHP	Trials for the Hypertension Prevention Research Group	VPI	vasopeptidase inhibitor
TOMHS	Treatment of Mild Hypertension Study	vWf	von Willebrand factor
		WCH	white-coat hypertension
TONE	Trial Of Non-pharmacologic interventions in the Elderly	WCSH	white-coat syndrome hypertensive
TRF	terminal restriction fragments	WCSN	white-coat syndrome normotensive
UACR	urine albumin/creatinine		
UAE	urinary albumin excretion	WHO	World Health Organization
UAER	urinary albumin excretion rate	WHO/ISH	World Health Organization/International Society of Hypertension
UKPDS	United Kingdom Prospective Diabetes Study		
UP/Cr	urine protein–creatinine ratio	WKY	Wistar-Kyoto rat

Index of Papers Reviewed

older individuals. Results from the trial of non-pharmacologic interventions in the elderly (TONE). *Arch Intern Med* 2001; **161**: 685–93. **243**

Asmar RG, London GM, O'Rourke ME, Safar ME. Improvement in blood pressure, arterial stiffness and wave reflections with a very-low-dose Perindopril/Indapamide combination in hypertensive patient: a comparison with atenolol. REASON Project Coordinators and Investigators. *Hypertension* 2001; 38(4): 922–6. **288**

Asmar R, Rudnichi A, Blacher J, London GM, Safar ME. Pulse pressure and aortic pulse wave are markers of CV risk in hypertensive populations. *Am J Hypertens* 2001; 14(2): 91–7. **281**

Asmar R, Topouchian J, Pannier B, Benetos A, Safar M. Pulse wave velocity as endpoint in large-scale intervention trial. The Complior Study. Scientific, quality control, coordination and investigation committees of the Complior Study. *J Hypertens* 2001; 19(4): 813–8. **295**

Asmar R, Safar M, Queneau P. Evaluation of the placebo effect and reproducibility of blood pressure measurement in hypertension. *Am J Hypertens* 200; 14(6 Pt 1): 546–52. **48**

Asmar R, Vol S, Brisac AM, Tichet J, Topouchian J. Reference values for clinic pulse pressure in a non-selected population. *Am J Hypertens* 2001; 14(5 Pt 1): 415–8. **274**

Aurigemma GP, Williams D, Gaasch WH, Reda DJ, Materson BJ, Gottdiener JS. Ventricular and myocardial function following treatment of hypertension. *Am J Cardiol* 2001; 87(6): 732–6. **311**

Aviv A. Pulse pressure and human longevity. *Hypertension*. 2001; 37: 1060–6. **280**

Ayala DE, Hermida RC. Influence of parity and age on ambulatory monitored blood pressure during pregnancy. *Hypertension* 2001; 38(3 Pt 2): 753–8. **122**

Bakris G. A practical approach to achieving recommended blood pressure goals in diabetic patients. *Arch Intern Med*. 2001; 161: 2661–7. **132**

Bakris G, Gradman A, Reif M, Wofford M, Munger M, Harris S, Vendetti J, Michelson EL, Wang R. Antihypertensive efficacy of candesartan in comparison to losartan: the CLAIM study. *J Clin Hypertens* (Greenwich) 2001; 3(1): 16–21. **173**

Bella JN, Devereux RB, Roman MJ, Palmieri V, Liu JE, Paranicas M, Welty TK, Lee ET, Fabsitz RR, Howard BV. Separate and joint effects of systemic hypertension and diabetes mellitus on left ventricular structure and function in American Indians (the Strong Heart Study). *Am J Cardiol* 2001; 87(11): 1260–5. **136**

Bella JN, Palmieri V, Liu JE, Kitzman DW, Oberman A, Hunt SC, Hopkins PN, Rao DC, Arnett DK, Devereux RB. Relationship between left ventricular diastolic relaxation and systolic function in hypertension: The Hypertension Genetic Epidemiology Network (HyperGEN) Study. *Hypertension* 2001; 38: 424–8. **307**

Bella JN, Wachtell K, Palmieri V, Liebson PR, Gerdts E, Ylitalo A, Koren MJ, Pedersen OL, Rokkedal J, Dahlof B, Roman MJ, Devereux RB. Relation of left ventricular geometry and function to systemic haemodynamic in hypertension: The LIFE Study. *J Hypertension* 2001; 19: 127–134. **309**

Benetos A, Thomas F, Bean K, Gautier S, Smulyan H, Guize L. Prognostic value of systolic and diastolic blood pressure in treated hypertensive men. *Arch Intern Med*. 2002; 162(5): 577–81. **12**

Benetos A, Okuda K, Lajemi M, Kimura M, Thomas F, Skurnick J, Labat C, Bean K, Aviv A. Telomere length as an indicator of biological aging. The gender effect and relation with pulse pressure and pulse wave velocity. *Hypertension* 2001; 37: 381–5. **280**

Tuomilehto J. Hypertension in the Very Elderly Trial (HYVET): protocol for the main trial. *Drugs & Aging* 2001; 18(3): 151–64. **26**

Burchardt M, Burchardt T, Anastasiadis AG, Kiss AJ, Baer L, Pawar RV, de la Taille A, Shabsigh A, Ghafar MA, Shabsigh R. Sexual dysfunction is common and overlooked in female patients with hypertension. *J Sex Marital Ther* 2002; 28(1): 17–26. **256**

Burchardt M, Burchardt T, Anastasiadis AG, Kiss AJ, Shabsigh A, de La Taille A, Pawar RV, Baer L, Shabsigh R. Erectile dysfunction is a marker for cardiovascular complications and psychological functioning in men with hypertension. *Int J Impot Res* 2001; 13(5): 276–81. **259**

Campese VM, Lasseter KC, Ferrario CM, Smith WB, Ruddy MC, Grim CE, Smith RD, Vargas R, Habashy MF, Vesterqvist O, Delaney CL, Liao WC. Omapatrilat *versus* lisinopril: efficacy and neurohormonal profile in salt-sensitive hypertensive patients. *Hypertension* 2001; 38(6): 1342–8. **208**

Canzanello VJ, Jensen PL, Hunder I. Rapid adjustment of antihypertensive drugs produces a durable improvement in blood pressure. *Am J Hypertens* 2001; 14: 345–50. **38**

Cheng JWM, Schwartz AM. Patient-reported adherence to guidelines of the Sixth Joint National Committee on Prevention, Detection, Evaluation, and Treatment of High Blood Pressure. *Pharmacotherapy* 2001; 21(7): 828–41. **41**

Churchill D, Beevers DG. Differences between office and 24-hour ambulatory blood pressure measurement during pregnancy. *Obstet Gynecol* 1996; 88(3): 455–61. **123**

Collaborative Group of the Primary Prevention Project. Low-dose aspirin and vitamin E in people at cardiovascular risk: a randomized trial in general practice. *Lancet* 2001; 357(9250): 89–95. **224**

Cooper AR, Moore LA, McKenna J, Riddoch CJ. What is the magnitude of blood pressure response to a programme of moderate intensity exercise? Randomized controlled trial among sedentary adults with unmedicated hypertension. *Br J Gen Pract* 2000; 50(461): 958–62. **230**

Cox K, Burkea V, Morton AR, Gillam HF, Beilin LJ, Puddey IB. Long-term effects of exercise on blood pressure and lipids in healthy women aged 40–65 years: the Sedentary Women Exercise Adherence Trial (SWEAT). *J Hypertens* 2001; 19: 1733–43. **230**

Cushman WC, Materson BJ, Williams DW, Reda DJ. Pulse pressure changes with six classes of antihypertensive agents in a randomized, controlled trial. *Hypertension* 2001, 38: 953–7. **289**

Cuspidi C, Lonati L, Macca G, Sampieri L, Fusi V, Severgnini B, Salerno M, Michev I, Rocanova JI, Leonetti G, Zanchetti A. Cardiovascular risk stratification in hypertensive patients: impact of echocardiography and carotid ultrasonography. *J Hypertens* 2001; 19(3): 375–80. **303**

Cuspidi C, Macca G, Sampieri L, Fusi V, Severgnini B, Michev I, Salerno M, Magrini F, Zanchetti A. Target organ damage and non-dipping pattern defined by two sessions of ambulatory blood pressure monitoring in recently diagnosed essential hypertensive patients. *J Hypertens* 2001; 19(9): 1539–45. **99**

Cuspidi C, Macca G, Sampieri L, Michev I, Fusi V, Salerno M, Severgnini B, Corti C, Magrini F, Zanchetti A. Influence of different echocardiographic criteria for detection of left ventricular hypertrophy on cardiovascular risk stratification in recently diagnosed essential hypertensives. *J Hum Hypertens* 2001; 15(9): 619–25. **304**

Heart Attack Trial (ALLHAT) and other studies of hypertension. *Ann Intern Med* 2001; **135**: 1074–8. **198**

Gasowski J, Fagard RH, Staessen JA, Grodzicki T, Pocock S, Boutitie F, Gueyffier F, Boissel JP; INDANA Project Collaborators. Pulsatile BP component as predictor of mortality in hypertension: a meta-analysis of clinical trial control groups. a meta-analysis of clinical trial control groups. *J Hypertens* 2002; **20**(1): 145–51. **297**

Gerdts E, Papademetriou V, Palmieri V, Boman K, Bjornstad H, Wachtell K, Giles TD, Dahlof B, Devereux RB. Correlates of pulse pressure reduction during antihypertensive treatment (losartan or atenolol) in hypertensive patients with electrocardiographic left ventricular hypertrophy (the LIFE study). *Am J Cardiol* 2002; **89**(4): 399–402. **273**

Gerdts E, Zabalgoitia M, Bjornstad H, Svendsen TL, Devereux RB. Gender differences in systolic left ventricular function in hypertensive patients with electrocardiographic left ventricular hypertrophy (the LIFE study). *Am J Cardiol* 2001; **87**(8): 980–3. A4 **305**

Giles TD, Sander GE. Beyond the usual strategies for blood pressure reduction: therapeutic considerations and combination therapies. *J Clin Hypertens* 2001; **3**(6): 346–53. **174**

Glanz M, Garber AJ, Mancia G, Levenstein M. Meta-analysis of studies using selective alpha1-blockers in patients with hypertension and type 2 diabetes. *Int J Clin Pract* 2001; **55**(10): 694–701. **206**

Glen SK, Elliott HL, Curzio JL, Lees KR, Reid JL. White-coat hypertension as a cause of cardiovascular dysfunction. *Lancet* 1996; **348**(9028): 65–7. **264**

Glynn RJ, L'Italien GJ, Sesso HD, Jackson EA, Buring JE. Development of predictive models for long-term cardiovascular risk associated with systolic and diastolic

blood pressure. *Hypertension* 2002; **39**:105–10. **27**

Gradman AH, Lewin A, Bowling BT, Tonkon M, Deedwania PC, Kezer AE, Hardison JD, Cushing DJ, Michelson EL. Comparative effects of candesartan cilexetil and losartan in patients with systemic hypertension. Candesartan *versus* Losartan Efficacy Comparison (CANDLE) Study Group. *Heart Dis* 1999; **1**(2): 52–7. **172**

Grandi AM, Broggi R, Colombo S, Santillo R, Imperiale D, Bertolini A, Guasti L, Venco A. Left ventricular changes in isolated office hypertension: a blood pressure-matched comparison with normotension and sustained hypertension. *Arch Intern Med.* 2001; **161**(22): 267–81. **264**

Greenwood JP, Scott EM, Stoker JB, Walker JJ, Mary DA. Sympathetic neural mechanisms in normal and hypertensive pregnancy in humans. *Circulation* 2001; **104**(18): 2200–4. **120**

Gress TW, Nieto FJ, Shahar E, Wofford MR, Brancati FL. Hypertension and antihypertensive therapy as risk factors for type 2 diabetes mellitus. Atherosclerosis Risk in Communities Study. *N Engl J Med* 2000; **342**(13): 905–12. **202**

Grimm RH Jr, Margolis KL, Papademetriou V, Cushman WC, Ford CE, Bettencourt J, Alderman MH, Basile JN, Black HR, DeQuattro V V, Eckfeldt J, Hawkins CM, Perry HM Jr, Proschan M. Baseline characteristics of participants in the Antihypertensive and Lipid lowering Treatment to prevent Heart Attack Trial (ALLHAT). *Hypertension* 2001; **37**: 19–27. **200**

Grossman E, Messerli FH, Goldbourt U. High blood pressure and diabetes mellitus: are all antihypertensive drugs created equal? *Arch Intern Med* 2000; **160**(16): 2447–52. **221**

Hansson L, Lithell H, Skoog I, Baro F, Banki CM, Breteler M, Castaigne A,

Correia M, Degaute JP, Elmfeldt D, Engedal K, Farsang C, Ferro J, Hachinski V, Hofman A, James OF, Krisin E, Leeman M, de Leeuw PW, Leys D, Lobo A, Nordby G, Olofsson B, Opolski G, Prince M, Reischies FM. Study on Cognitive and Prognosis in the Elderly (SCOPE): Baseline Characteristics. *Blood Press* 2000; 9: 146–151. **69**

Hansson L, Zanchetti A, Carruthers SG, Dahlof B, Elmfeldt D, Julius S, Menard J, Rahn KH, Wedel H, Westerling S. Effects of intensive blood-pressure lowering and low-dose aspirin in patients with hypertension: principal results of the Hypertension Optimal Treatment (HOT) randomized trial. HOT Study Group. *Lancet* 1998; 351(9118): 1755–62. **224**

Harrington F, Saxby BK, McKeith IG, Wesnes K, Ford GA. Cognitive performance in hypertensive and normotensive older subjects. *Hypertension* 2000; 36(6): 1079–82. **67**

Herrington DM, Reboussin DM, Brosnihan KB, Sharp PC, Shumaker SA, Synder TE, Furberg CD, Kowalchuk GJ, Stuckey TD, Rogers WJ, Givens DH, Waters D. Effects of estrogen replacement on the progression of coronary-artery atherosclerosis. *N Engl J Med* 2000; 343(8): 522–9. **74**

Haenni A, Reneland R, Lind L, Lithell H. Serum aldosterone changes during hyperinsulinemia are correlated to body mass index and insulin sensitivity in patients with essential hypertension. *J Hypertens* 2001; 19: 107–12. **89**

Hermida RC, Ayala DE. Evaluation of the blood pressure load in the diagnosis of hypertension in pregnancy. *Hypertension* 2001; 38: 723–9. **122**

Higashi Y, Sasaki S, Nakagawa K, Matsuura H, Chayama K, Oshima T. Effect of obesity on endothelium-dependent, nitric oxide-mediated vasodilation in normotensive individuals and patients with essential hypertension. *Am J Hypertens* 2001; 14(10): 1038–45. **87**

Hsu CY. Does treatment of non-malignant hypertension reduce the incidence of renal dysfunction? A meta-analysis of ten randomized, controlled trials. *J Hum Hypertens* 2001; 15(2): 99–106. **154**

Hsu CY, Bates DW, Kuperman GJ, Curhan GC. Blood pressure and angiotensin converting enzyme inhibitor use in hypertensive patients with chronic renal insufficiency. *Am J Hypertens* 2001; 14(12): 1219–25. **151**

Hulley S, Grady D, Bush T, Furberg C, Herrington D, Riggs B, Vittinghoff E. Randomized trial of estrogen plus progestin for secondary prevention of coronary heart disease in postmenopausal women. *JAMA* 1998; 280(7): 605–13. **73**

Hyman DJ, Pavlik VN. Characteristics of patients with uncontrolled hypertension in the United States. *N Engl J Med* 2001; 345(7): 479–86. **35**

Izzo JL Jr, Manning TS, Shykoff BE. Office blood pressures, arterial compliance characteristics, and estimated cardiac load. *Hypertension* 2001; 38: 1467–70. **286**

Jafar TH, Schmid CH, Landa M, Giatras I, Toto R, Remuzzi G, Maschio G, Brenner BM, Kamper A, Zucchelli P, Becker G, Himmelmann A, Bannister K, Landais P, Shahinfar S, de Jong PE, de Zeeuw D, Lau J, Levey AS. Angiotensin-converting enzyme inhibitors and progression of non-diabetic renal disease. A meta-analysis of patient-level data. *Ann Intern Med* 2001; 135(2): 73–87. **162**

James PT, Leach R, Kalamara E, Shayeghi M. The worldwide obesity epidemic. *Obes Res* 2001; 9(suppl 4): 228S–33S. **77**

Kannel WB. Elevated systolic blood pressure as a cardiovascular risk factor. *Am J Cardiol* 2000; 85(2): 251–5. **18**

PHASTE study. Conventional antihypertensive drug therapy does not prevent the increase of pulse pressure with age. *Hypertension.* 2001; 38: 958–61. **290**

Mukamal KJ, Maclure M, Muller JE, Sherwood JB, Mittleman MA. Prior alcohol consumption and mortality following acute myocardial infarction. *JAMA* 2001; 285(15): 1965–70. **58**

Mule G, Nardi E, Andronico G, Cottone S, Raspanti F, Piazza G, Volpe V, Ferrara D, Cerasola G. Relationships between 24-h blood pressure load and target organ damage in patients with mild-to-moderate essential hypertension. *Blood Press Monit* 2001; 6(3): 115–23. **322**

Neldam S. Forsen B. Multicentre Study Group. Antihypertensive treatment in elderly patients aged 75 years or over: a 24-week study of the tolerability of candesartan cilexetil in relation to hydrochlorothiazide. *Drugs & Aging* 2001; 18(3): 225–32. **180**

Nelson M, Reid C, Krum H, McNeil J. A systematic review of predictors of maintenance of normotension after withdrawal of antihypertensive drugs. *Am J Hypertens* 2001; 14(2): 98–105. **37**

Neutel JM. The importance of 24-h blood pressure control. *Blood Press Monit* 2001; 6: 9–16. **324**

Niskanen L, Hedner T, Hansson L, Lanke J, Niklason A. Reduced cardiovascular morbidity and mortality in hypertensive diabetic patients on first-line therapy with an ACE inhibitor compared with a diuretic/ß-blocker-based treatment regimen. A subanalysis of the Captopril Prevention Project. *Diabetes Care* 2001; 24: 2091–6. **140**

Nussberger J, Wuerzner G, Jensen C, Brunner HR. Angiotensin II suppression in humans by the orally active renin inhibitor Aliskiren (SPP100): comparison with enalapril. *Hypertension* 2002; 39(1): E1–8. **210**

Obarzanek E, Sacks FM, Vollmer WM, Bray GA, Miller ER 3rd, Lin PH, Karanja NM, Most-Windhauser MM, Moore TJ, Swain JF, Bales CW, Proschan MA. Effects on blood lipids of a blood pressure-lowering diet: the Dietary Approaches to Stop Hypertension (DASH) Trial. *Am J Clin Nutr* 2001; 74(1): 80–9. **240**

Okin PM, Devereux RB, Nieminen MS, Jern S, Oikarinen L, Viitasalo M, Toivonen L, Kjeldsen SE, Julius S, Dahlof B. Relationship of the electrocardiographic strain pattern to left ventricular structure and function in hypertensive patients: the LIFE study. Losartan Intervention For End-point. *J Am Coll Cardiol* 2001; 38(2): 514–20. **313**

Oliveria SA, Lapuerta P, McCarthy BD, L'Italien GJ, Berlowitz DR, Asch SM. Physician-related barriers to the effective management of uncontrolled hypertension. *Arch Intern Med* 2002; 162: 413–20. **39**

Olsen MH, Wachtell K, Hermann KL, Bella JN, Andersen UB, Dige-Petersen H, Rokkedal J, Ibsen H. Maximal exercise capacity is related to cardiovascular structure in patients with longstanding hypertension. A LIFE substudy. Losartan Intervention For Endpoint-Reduction in Hypertension. *Am J Hypertens* 2001; 14(12): 1205–10. **315**

Onder G, Gambassi G, Landi F, Pedone C, Cesari M, Carbonin PU, Bernabei R Investigators of the GIFA Study (SIGG-ONLUS). Trends in antihypertensive drugs in the elderly: the decline of thiazides. *J Hum Hypertens* 2001; 15(5): 291–7. **185**

Orchard TJ, Forrest KY, Kuller LH, Becker DJ. Lipid and blood pressure treatment goals for type 1 diabetes. Ten-year incidence data from the Pittsburgh Epidemiology of Diabetes Complications Study. *Diabetes Care* 2001; 24: 1053–9. **138**

Pahor M, Psaty BM, Alderman MH, Applegate WB, Williamson JD,

Cavazzini C, Furberg CD. Health outcomes associated with calcium antagonists compared with other first-line antihypertensive therapies: a meta-analysis of randomized controlled trials. *Lancet* 2000; 356: 1949–54. **192**

Palmieri V, Bella JN, Arnett DK, Liu JE, Oberman A, Schuck MY, Kitzman DW, Hopkins PN, Morgan D, Rao DC, Devereux RB. Effect of type 2 diabetes mellitus on left ventricular geometry and systolic function in hypertensive subjects. *Circulation* 2001; 103: 102–7. **135**

Papademetriou V, Devereux RB, Narayan P, Wachtell K, Bella JN, Gerdts E, Chrysant SG, Dahlof B. Similar effects of isolated systolic and combined hypertension on left ventricular geometry and function: the LIFE Study. *Am J Hypertens* 2001; 14(8 Pt 1): 768–74. **20**

Parving HH, Lehnert H, Brochner-Mortensen J, Gomis R, Andersen S, Arner P. The effect of irbesartan on the development of diabetic nephropathy in patients with type 2 diabetes. IRbesartan MicroAlbuminuria type 2 diabetes mellitus in hypertensive patients (IRMA II). *N Engl J Med* 2001; 345(12): 870–8. **146 169**

Pasierski T, Szwed H, Malczewska B, Firek B, Kosmicki M, Rewicki M, Kowalik I, Sadowski Z. Advantages of exercise echocardiography in comparison to dobutamine echocardiography in the diagnosis of coronary artery disease in hypertensive subjects. *J Hum Hypertens* 2001; 15(11): 805–9. **300**

Pedersen-Bjergaard U, Agerholm-Larsen B, Pramming S, Hougaard P, Thorsteinsson B. Activity of angiotensin-converting enzyme and risk of severe hypoglycaemia in type 1 diabetes mellitus. *Lancet* 2001; 357(9264): 1248–53. **165**

Perry HM Jr, Davis BR, Price TR, Applegate WB, Fields WS, Guralnik JM, Kuller L, Pressel S, Stamler J, Probstfield JL. Effect of treating isolated systolic hypertension on the risk of developing various types and subtypes of stroke: the Systolic Hypertension in the Elderly Program (SHEP). *JAMA* 2000; 284(4): 465–71. **183**

Phillips RA, Sheinart KF, Godbold JH, Mahboob R, Tuhrim S. The association of blunted nocturnal blood pressure dip and stroke in a multiethnic population. *Am J Hypertens* 2000; 13(12): 1250–5. **102**

Picano E, Palinkas A, Amyot R. Diagnosis of myocardial ischaemia in hypertensive patients. *J Hypertens* 2001; 19(7): 1177–83. **299**

Pickering TG. Obesity and hypertension: a growing problem. *J Clin Hypertens* 2001; 3(4): 252–4. **77**

Pini R, Cavallini MC, Bencini F, Stagliano L, Tonon E, Innocenti F, Baldereschi G, Marchionni N, Di Bari M, Devereux RB, Masotti G, Roman MJ. Cardiac and vascular remodelling in older adults with borderline isolated systolic hypertension: The ICARe Dicomano Study. *Hypertension* 2001; 38: 1372–6. **21**

Pitt B, Byington RP, Furberg CD, Hunninghake DB, Mancini GB, Miller ME, Riley W. Effect of amlodipine on the progression of atherosclerosis and the occurrence of clinical events. PREVENT Investigators. *Circulation* 2000; 102(13):1503–10. **188**

Pocock SJ, McCormack V, Gueyffier F, Boutitie F, Fagard RH, Boissel JP. A score for predicting risk of death from CV disease in adults with raised BP, based on individual patient data from randomized controlled trials. *BMJ* 2001; 323(7304): 75–81. **29**

Port S, Demer L, Jennrich R, Walter D, Garfinkel A. Systolic blood pressure and mortality. *Lancet* 2000; 355(9199): 175–80. **18**

Primatesta P, Brookes M, Poulter NR. Improved hypertension management and control: results from the health survey for

Hypertension (DASH) diet. DASH-Sodium Collaborative Research Group.*N Engl J Med* 2001; **344**(1): 3–10. **237**

Sanmuganathan PS, Ghahramani P, Jackson PR, Wallis EJ, Ramsay LE. Aspirin for primary prevention of coronary heart disease: safety and absolute benefit related to coronary risk derived from meta-analysis of randomized trials. *Heart* 2001; **85**(3): 265–71. **225**

Sawicki PT, Siebenhofer A. Betablocker treatment in diabetes mellitus. *J Intern Med* 2001; **250**(1): 11–7. **203**

Schussheim AE, Diamond JA, Phillips RA. Left ventricular midwall function improves with antihypertensive therapy and regression of left ventricular hypertrophy in patients with asymptomatic hypertension. *Am J Cardiol* 2001; **87**(1): 61–5. **305**

Schwartz GG, Olsson AG, Ezekowitz MD, Ganz P, Oliver MF, Waters D, Zeiher A, Chaitman BR, Leslie S, Stern T. Effects of atorvastatin on early recurrent ischemic events in acute coronary syndromes. The MIRACL Study: a randomized controlled trial. *JAMA*. 2001; **285**: 1711–18. **91**

Scuteri A, Bos AJ, Brant LJ, Talbot L, Lakatta EG, Fleg JL. Hormone replacement therapy and longitudinal changes in blood pressure in postmenopausal women. *Ann Intern Med* 2001; **135**(4): 229–38. **71**

Sega R, Trocino G, Lanzarotti A, Carugo S, Cesana G, Schiavina R, Valagussa F, Bombelli M, Giannattasio C, Zanchetti A, Mancia G. Alterations of cardiac structure in patients with isolated office, ambulatory, or home hypertension. Data from the general population (Pressione Arteriose Monitorate E Loro Associazioni [PAMELA] Study). *Circulation*. 2001; **104**: 1385–92. **265**

Seshadri S, Wolf PA, Beiser A, Vasan RS, Wilson PW, Kase CS, Kelly-Hayes M, Kannel WB, D'Agostino RB. National Heart, Lung, and Blood Institute's Framingham Study, Framingham, MA, USA. Elevated midlife blood pressure increases stroke risk in elderly persons. The Framingham Study. *Arch Intern Med* 2001; **161**: 2343–50. **28**

Sharma AM, Pischon T, Engeli S, Scholze J. Choice of drug treatment for obesity-related hypertension: where is the evidence? *J Hypertens* 2001; **19**(4): 667–74. **80**

SHEP Cooperative Research Group. Prevention of stroke by antihypertensive drug treatment in older persons with isolated systolic hypertension. Final results of the Systolic Hypertension in the Elderly Program (SHEP). *JAMA* 1991; **265**(24): 3255–64. **183**

Sica DA. The Heart Outcomes Prevention Evaluation (HOPE) Study: Limitations and strengths. *J Clin Hypertens* 2000; **2**(6): 406–9. **220**

Simon JA, Hsia J, Cauley JA, Richards C, Harris F, Fong J, Barrett-Connor E, Hulley SB. Postmenopausal hormone therapy and risk of stroke: The Heart and Estrogen-progestin Replacement Study (HERS). *Circulation* 2001; **103**(5): 638–42. **72**

Singhal A, Cole TJ, Lucas A. Early nutrition in pre-term infants and later blood pressure: two cohorts after randomized trials. *Lancet* 2001; **357**: 413–19. **335**

Sleight P, Yusuf S, Pogue J, Tsuyuki R, Diaz R, Probstfield J. Blood-pressure reduction and cardiovascular risk in HOPE study. *Lancet* 2001; **358**: 2130–31. **218**

Solomon CG, Hu FB, Stampfer MJ, Colditz GA, Speizer FE, Rimm EB, Willet WC, manson JE. Moderate alcohol consumption and risk of coronary heart disease among women with type 2 diabetes mellitus. *Circulation* 2000; **102**(5): 494–9. **53**

Solomon CG, Seely EW. Brief review: hypertension in pregnancy: a manifestation of the insulin resistance syndrome? *Hypertension* 2001; **37**: 232–9. **119**

Vasan RS, Larson MG, Leip EP, Evans JC, O'Donnell CJ, Kannel WB, Levy D. Impact of high-normal blood pressure on the risk of cardiovascular disease. *N Engl J Med* 2001; 345(18): 1291–7. **5**

Vasan RS, Larson MG, Leip EP, Kannel WB, Levy D. Assessment of frequency of progression to hypertension in non-hypertensive participants in the Framingham Heart Study: a cohort study. *Lancet* 2001; 358: 1682–6. **4**

Verdecchia P, Porcellati C, Reboldi G, Gattobigio R, Borgioni C, Pearson TA, Ambrosio G. Left ventricular hypertrophy as an independent predictor of acute cerebrovascular events in essential hypertension. *Circulation* 2001; 104: 2039–44. **105**

Vokó Z, Bots ML, Hofman A, Koudstaal PJ, Witteman JC, Breteler MM. J-shaped relation between blood pressure and stroke in treated hypertensives. *Hypertension* 1999; 34: 1181–85. **22**

Vollmer WM, Sacks FM, Ard J, Appel LJ, Bray GA, Simons-Morton DG, Conlin PR, Svetkey LP, Erlinger TP, Moore TJ, Karanja N. Effects of diet and sodium intake on blood pressure: subgroup analysis of the DASH-Sodium Trial. *Ann Intern Med* 2001; 135(12): 1019–28. **240**

Wachtell K, Olsen MH, Dahlof B, Devereux RB, Kjeldsen SE, Nieminen MS, Okin PM, Papademetriou V, Mogensen CE, Borch-Johnsen K, Ibsen H. Microalbuminuria in hypertensive patients with electrocardiographic left ventricular hypertrophy: the LIFE study. *J Hypertens* 2002; 20(3): 405–12. 327

Wachtell K, Rokkedal J, Bella JN, Aalto T, Dahlof B, Smith G, Roman MJ, Ibsen H, Aurigemma GP, Devereux RB. Effect of electrocardiographic left ventricular hypertrophy on left ventricular systolic function in systemic hypertension (The LIFE Study). Losartan Intervention For Endpoint. *Am J Cardiol* 2001; 87(1): 54–60. **308**

Wang JG, Staessen JA. Antihypertensive drug therapy in older patients. *Curr Opin Nephrol Hypertens* 2001; 10(2): 263–9. **17 279**

Wannamethee SG. Is serum uric acid a risk factor for coronary heart disease? *J Hum Hypertens* 1999; 13(3):153–6. 333

Weber MA, Neutel JM, Smith DH. Contrasting clinical properties and exercise responses in obese and lean hypertensive patients. *J Am Coll Cardiol* 2001; 37(1): 169–74. **82**

Weinberger MH, Fineberg NS, Fineberg SE, Weinberger M. Salt sensitivity, pulse pressure, and death in normal and hypertensive humans. *Hypertension* 2001; 37 (2 suppl): 429–32. **294**

White WB. Ambulatory blood pressure monitoring: dippers compared with non-dippers. *Blood Press Monit* 2000; 5(Suppl 1):S17–23. **104**

White WB, Johnson MF, Black HR, Elliott WJ, Sica DA. Gender and age effects on the ambulatory blood pressure and heart rate responses to antihypertensive therapy. *Am J Hypertens* 2001; 14(12): 1239–47. **47**

Wofford MR, Anderson DC Jr, Brown CA, Jones DW, Miller ME, Hall JE. Antihypertensive effect of alpha- and beta-adrenergic blockade in obese and lean hypertensive subjects. *Am J Hypertens* 2001; 14(7 Pt 1): 694–8. **81**

Xin X, He J, Frontini MG, Ogden LG, Motsamai OI, Whelton PK. Effects of alcohol reduction on blood pressure: a meta-analysis of randomized controlled trials. *Hypertension* 2001; 38(5): 1112–7. **251**

Yusuf S, Sleight P, Pogue J, Bosch J, Davies R, Dagenais G. Effects of an angiotensin-converting-enzyme inhibitor, ramipril, on cardiovascular events in high-risk patients. The Heart Outcomes Prevention Evaluation Study Investigators. *N Engl J Med* 2000; 342(3): 145–53. **212**

Zabalgoitia M, Berning J, Koren MJ, Stoylen A, Nieminen MS, Dahlof B, Devereux RB. Impact of coronary artery disease on left ventricular systolic function and geometry in hypertensive patients with left ventricular hypertrophy (the LIFE study). *Am J Cardiol* 2001; 88(6): 646–50. **313**

Zabalgoitia M, Rahman SN, Haley WE, Yarows S, Krause L, Anderson LC, Oraby MA, Amarena J. Effect of regression of left ventricular hypertrophy from systemic hypertension on systolic function assessed by midwall shortening (HOT echocardiographic study). *Am J Cardiol* 2001; 88(5): 521–5. **311**

Zakopoulos NA, Lekakis JP, Papamichael CM, Toumanidis ST, Kanakakis JE, Kostandonis D, Vogiazoglou TJ, Rombopoulos CG, Stamatelopoulos SF, Moulopoulos SD. Pulse pressure in normotensives: a marker of cardiovascular disease. *Am J Hypertens* 2001; 14(3): 195–9. **273**

Zakopoulos NA, Nanas SN, Lekakis JP, Vemmos KN, Kotsis VT, Pitiriga VC, Stamatelopoulos SF, Moulopoulos SD. Reproducibility of ambulatory blood pressure measurements in essential hypertension. *Blood Press Monit* 2001; 6(1): 41–5. **320**

Zanchetti A, Crepaldi G, Bond MG, Gallus GV, Veglia F, Ventura A, Mancia G, Baggio G, Sampieri L, Rubba P, Collatina S, Serrotti E. Systolic and pulse blood pressures (but not diastolic blood pressure and serum cholesterol) are associated with alterations in carotid intima–media thickness in the moderately hypercholesterolaemic hypertensive patients of the Plaque Hypertension Lipid Lowering Italian Study. *J Hypertens* 2001; 19(1): 7–8. **293**

Zanella MT, Kohlmann O Jr, Ribeiro AB. Treatment of obesity hypertension and diabetes syndrome. *Hypertension* 2001; 38(3 Pt 2): 705–8. **79**

Index

KEEPING UP TO DATE IN ONE VOLUME

The Year in Hypertension

The Year in Hypertension
appears on a regular basis

To receive more information about the next issue,
or to reserve a copy on publication,
please contact the address below:

Clinical Publishing Services Ltd
Oxford Centre for Innovation
Mill Street
Oxford OX2 0JX, UK

T: +44 1865 811116
F: +44 1865 251550
E: info@clinicalpublishing.co.uk
W: www.clinicalpublishing.co.uk

KEEPING UP TO DATE IN ONE SERIES

"The Year in ..."

EXISTING AND FUTURE VOLUMES

The Year in Hypertension 2000   ISBN 0 9537339 0 4

The Year in Rheumatic Disorders 2001   ISBN 0 9537339 1 2

The Year in Neurology 2001   ISBN 0 9537339 5 5

The Year in Gynaecology 2001   ISBN 0 9537339 2 0

The Year in Hypertension 2001   ISBN 0 9537339 4 7

The Year in Diabetes 2001   ISBN 0 9527339 6 3

The Year in Dyslipidaemia 2002   ISBN 0 9537339 3 9

The Year in Interventional Cardiology 2002   ISBN 0 9537339 7 1

The Year in Rheumatic Disorders 2002   ISBN 0 9537339 9 8

The Year in Gynaecology 2002   ISBN 1 904392 01 6

To receive more information about these books and future volumes,
or to order copies, please contact the address below:

Clinical Publishing Services Ltd

Oxford Centre for Innovation

Mill Street

Oxford OX2 0JX, UK

T: +44 1865 811116

F: +44 1865 251550

E: info@compuserve.com

W: www.clinicalpublishing.co.uk

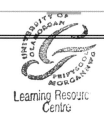